Cognitive and Behavioral Rehabilitation

THE SCIENCE AND PRACTICE OF NEUROPSYCHOLOGY
A Guilford Series

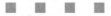

Robert A. Bornstein, *Series Editor*

Cognitive and Behavioral Rehabilitation:
From Neurobiology to Clinical Practice
Jennie Ponsford, Editor

Aphasia and Language: Theory to Practice
Stephen E. Nadeau, Bruce A. Crosson,
and Leslie J. Gonzalez Rothi, Editors

Pediatric Neuropsychology: Research, Theory, and Practice
Keith Owen Yeates, M. Douglas Ris, and H. Gerry Taylor, Editors

The Human Frontal Lobes: Functions and Disorders
Bruce L. Miller and Jeffrey L. Cummings, Editors

Cognitive and Behavioral Rehabilitation

■ ■ ■ ■

From Neurobiology to Clinical Practice

Edited by Jennie Ponsford

Series Editor's Note by Robert A. Bornstein

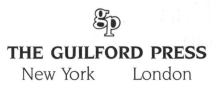

THE GUILFORD PRESS
New York   London

Library of Congress Cataloging-in-Publication Data

Cognitive and behavioral rehabilitation : from neurobiology to clinical practice /
edited by Jennie Ponsford.
    p. cm. — (Science and practice of neuropsychology)
  Includes bibliographical references and index.
  ISBN 1-57230-990-3 (Hardcover: alk. paper)
  1. Cognition disorders—Rehabilitation.   2. Behavior therapy.   I. Ponsford,
Jennie.   II. Series.
  RC553.C64C625 2004
  616.8′043—dc22

                                  2003025017

To my great mentor, Kevin Walsh,
whose insights continue to inspire me.

—J. P.

About the Editor

Jennie Ponsford is Associate Professor in the Department of Psychology at Monash University and Director of the Monash–Epworth Rehabilitation Research Centre at Epworth Hospital, both in Melbourne, Australia. She completed a master's degree in clinical neuropsychology at the University of Melbourne and a PhD, on the assessment and rehabilitation of attentional deficits following head injury, at LaTrobe University in Melbourne. Dr. Ponsford has spent the past 23 years engaged in clinical work and research focusing on the assessment and rehabilitation of individuals with brain injury. She has published over 50 journal articles and book chapters on this subject, as well as a book—*Traumatic Brain Injury: Rehabilitation for Everyday Adaptive Living*— on the management of traumatic brain injury.

Dr. Ponsford directs a doctoral program in clinical neuropsychology at Monash University and is regularly invited to speak at international conferences. She has served on the Governing Board of the International Neuropsychological Society and as president of both the International Association for the Study of Traumatic Brain Injury and the Australian Society for the Study of Brain Impairment, of which she is an Honorary Fellow. Currently she is a Governor of the International Brain Injury Association. She is also an Associate Editor of the *Journal of the International Neuropsychological Society* and *Brain Injury*, and serves on the Editorial Board of the journals *Brain Impairment*, *Neuropsychological Rehabilitation*, and *NeuroRehabilitation*.

Contributors

Anne Aimola Davies, PGDipClinPsych, PhD, Department of Psychology, Australian National University, Canberra, Australia; Macquarie Centre for Cognitive Sciences, Macquarie University, Sydney, Australia

Nick Alderman, MAppSci, PhD, CPsychol, FBPsS, Kemsley Division, St. Andrew's Hospital, Northampton, United Kingdom

Jan Cioe, PhD, Department of Psychology, Okanagan University College, Kelowna, British Columbia, Canada

Elizabeth L. Glisky, PhD, Department of Psychology, University of Arizona, Tucson, Arizona

Bryan Kolb, PhD, Canadian Centre for Behavioural Neuroscience, University of Lethbridge, Lethbridge, Alberta, Canada

Brian Levine, PhD, Rotman Research Institute and Departments of Psychology and Medicine (Neurology), University of Toronto, Toronto, Ontario, Canada

Stephen E. Nadeau, MD, Department of Neurology, University of Florida College of Medicine; Geriatric Research, Education and Clinical Center; Brain Rehabilitation Research Center; and Rehabilitation Outcomes Research Center, Malcom Randall Department of Veterans Affairs Medical Center, Gainesville, Florida

Jennie Ponsford, MA(Clin Neuropsych), PhD, MAPsS, Department of
Psychology, Monash University, and Monash–Epworth Rehabilitation
Research Centre, Epworth Hospital, Melbourne, Australia

Leslie J. Gonzalez Rothi, PhD, Brain Rehabilitation Research Center,
Malcom Randall Department of Veterans Affairs Medical Center, Gainesville,
Florida

Gary R. Turner, MA, Rotman Research Institute and Department of
Psychology, University of Toronto, Toronto, Ontario, Canada

Catherine Willmott, MSc(Clin Neuropsych), MAPsS, Department of
Psychology, Epworth Hospital, and Department of Psychology, Monash
University, Melbourne, Australia

Series Editor's Note

Cognitive and Behavioral Rehabilitation: From Neurobiology to Clinical Practice, edited by Jennie Ponsford, is the fourth volume in the Guilford series The Science and Practice of Neuropsychology. The scientific foundations and evidence of efficacy for rehabilitation of cognitive and behavioral disorders arising from brain injury and illness have matured rapidly over the last decade. Rigorous scientific inquiry is expanding and, in some cases, substantially altering our previously held views. The promise of innovative rehabilitation strategies, combined with new pharmacological interventions and other biological interventions such as trophic factors, stem cells, and fetal transplant that can limit or prevent permanent neurological loss, will radically transform the landscape of the rehabilitation potential for patients suffering from brain illness or injury. The future vistas of nanotechnology will provide opportunities that today can barely be conceptualized. It is timely, therefore, that as we look toward this new frontier we pause to take stock of where we have been, and to take a critical look at what we think we know at this stage in the evolution of our knowledge.

In this series, neuropsychology is defined broadly as the study of brain–behavior relationships, incorporating the perspectives of the full range of related disciplines. Although some volumes in the series will undoubtedly be of greater interest to specific subsets of readers, it is intended that the series be of interest to scientists and practitioners in all of the disciplines that address questions of brain and behavior in research and/or applied contexts. A wide range of topics will be covered, including reviews of emerging technologies and their potential impact on the science and clinical understanding of neuropsychology.

This volume on the rehabilitation of cognitive and behavioral disorders reflects the progress that has been made over the past decades. In their infancy, techniques were developed and applied in the absence of rigorous scientific data to support their efficacy. That situation has dramatically changed over the past two decades, as reflected by the stellar group of investigators and practitioners who have contributed to the present volume. This volume includes a synthesis of the discoveries in the neurosciences that provide the foundation for current models of rehabilitation. In addition, it demonstrates the integration of these scientific foundations in the treatment of deficits in several key cognitive and behavioral domains, and provides us with a glimpse into the future. The dynamic nature of the field of cognitive and behavioral rehabilitation provides one of the clearest and most exciting opportunities to translate the discoveries from the laboratory to the arena of patient care.

ROBERT A. BORNSTEIN, PHD

Acknowledgments

I am deeply indebted to Bryan Kolb and Jan Cioe, Catherine Willmott, Elizabeth Glisky, Stephen Nadeau and Leslie Gonzalez Rothi, Anne Aimola Davies, Gary Turner and Brian Levine, and Nick Alderman for their significant contributions to this volume. Some of them had to be extremely patient while other chapters were being completed, and I am very grateful for this. All of us have been challenged to bridge the gap between neurobiology and clinical practice. This resulted in the exchange of dozens of e-mails with Bryan Kolb, whose willingness to communicate his research in a clinically meaningful way and to exchange ideas enabled this book to achieve its goal.

The original concept for the book was put to me by Bob Bornstein who, as Series Editor, has offered much encouragement along the way. Rochelle Serwator of The Guilford Press has been a most patient, enthusiastic, and supportive editor. I am also deeply indebted to Deborah Goff, Monique Roper, and Meagan Carty for their editorial assistance and moral support. My colleague Greg Savage also offered helpful advice. The ultimate inspiration for this book came from the many brain-injured individuals with whom I have had the privilege of working over the past 23 years.

My husband, Lew, daughters, Isabelle and Alice, and my parents and friends have been sorely neglected at times, and I thank them for their continuing love and support.

Contents

Cognitive
and Behavioral
Rehabilitation

Introduction

Jennie Ponsford

The field of neurological rehabilitation has shown rapid growth over the past few decades, but it has a long history. As pointed out in a historical review by Prigatano (1999), interest in the impact of neuronal injury and recovery was expressed as early as 1888 by John Hughlings-Jackson, who speculated on mechanisms of recovery from hemiplegia and wrote:

> Why do patients recover from hemiplegia when the loss of nerve tissue is permanent? . . . I should put down paralysis at the onset to the destruction effected, and attribute degrees of recovery to degrees of compensation; nervous arrangements near to those destroyed, having closely similar duties, come to serve, not as well, but, according to the degree of gravity of the lesion, next and next as well as those destroyed. (cited in Prigatano, 1999, pp. 6–7)

In 1938, Karl Lashley (cited in Prigatano, 1999, p. 11) acknowledged the multifactorial processes of recovery, stating that

> functional loss may be due to destruction of essential structures, to temporary pathological changes in the cells, to shock or diaschisis, to metabolic disturbances, or to lowered tonic activity. In each case, the mechanism of recovery will be different, and we rarely know, in any instance, to what extent these various factors have contributed to the symptoms.

Until the 1980s, most neuropsychological rehabilitation programs focused on language disorders. In the mid-1800s Paul Broca administered language rehabilitation programs. This was followed by the influential work of Shepherd Franz. In 1905, Franz reportedly speculated that "new brain paths are opened in the reeducation process" and that "it is probable that the right side of the cerebrum takes part" in this process (cited in Boake, 2003, p. 13). Franz also used forelimb restraint as a means of improving motor performance in hemiparetic monkeys (Ogden & Franz, cited in Boake, 2003, p. 13), an approach advocated to this day.

During and after World War I, Kurt Goldstein established the first brain injury rehabilitation programs for brain-injured soldiers in Germany, which had facilities for psychological assessment and workshops for vocational retraining, using compensatory methods, and emphasizing the importance of observing functional performance. Goldstein (1942) was also the first to describe impairment of "abstract attitude" as a basis for inappropriate social behavior.

During World War II Alexander Romanovich Luria developed an approach to the study of higher cerebral functions, their recovery, and rehabilitation, based on his work with victims of missile wounds. This approach formed the foundation on which much of modern neuropsychology and neuropsychological rehabilitation has been built. In his texts *The Working Brain* and *Restoration of Function after Brain Injury*, Luria (1963, 1973) acknowledged the presence of functional systems mediating cognitive functions, components of which might be located in different brain regions. The manifestations of cerebral dysfunction would therefore differ according to which part of the functional system was disrupted by injury. Luria emphasized the importance of a detailed neuropsychological examination of the brain-injured person as a means of establishing the precise nature of the cognitive impairment. This, in turn, formed the basis of an individualized rehabilitation program. He advocated extensive practice as a means of retraining the impaired function in order to rebuild new habits. He also acknowledged the influence of a number of factors on the extent of recovery, including the nature of the lesion, most particularly its size and the presence of complications in the recovery process, the state of the brain before the injury, including the age of the brain, and the person's premorbid personality and coping style.

Despite these cogent insights, which remain relevant to today's practice of neurological rehabilitation, this field was slow to develop after World War II and remained more focused on the alleviation of physical disability. During the 1970s, however, there was a growing awareness of the needs of individuals with traumatic brain injury. Improved medical management following the example of pioneers such as Bryan Jennett and Graeme Teasdale from Glasgow, led to a growth in the number of survivors of traumatic brain injury, who were predominantly young adults. It became apparent that rehabilitation models developed for people with primarily physical disabilities did not meet the needs of individuals with brain injury. While physical disabilities were present for some, the more prominent and common impairments were psychological in nature: impairments of attention, memory, reasoning, and other cognitive abilities; communication difficulties; changes in behavior and personality. There was frequently a perplexing lack of self-awareness of these changes, which, in turn, created severe stress among family members. The youth of this group meant they would be living with these difficulties for many years and faced failure to attain important developmental milestones such as completing study, establishing a vocation, and forming long-term personal and social relationships.

In an attempt to address the unique impairments of the survivor of brain injury, neuropsychologists began to apply their techniques to impairments other than aphasia and thus developed the field, which became known as cognitive rehabilitation. Cognitive impairments were identified via traditional neuropsychological assessment methods and broken down into their underlying components. Repeated practice was given on tasks exercising different components of the deficit, with the aim of restoring the impaired function.

The development of this new field of cognitive rehabilitation was led by pioneers such as Leonard Diller and Yehuda Ben-Yishay from New York University and Rusk Institute of Rehabilitation Medicine. One of Diller's major contributions was the scientific evaluation of the impact of various remedial strategies for visuospatial disorders in stroke patients, most notably retraining of scanning abilities in patients with unilateral spatial neglect (Diller et al., 1974). This was one of the first well-designed controlled evaluations of a cognitive intervention and it had a significant influence on the field.

Yehuda Ben-Yishay worked with victims of head trauma. In the early 1970s he had developed a treatment program in Israel for victims of missile wounds, and he developed this concept further at New York University (Ben-Yishay et al., 1978). In addition to cognitive retraining exercises, clients received psychotherapy and participated in a therapeutic community, designed to enhance self-awareness and self-esteem and acceptance of change, in addition to cognitive function. The group of clients and staff spent many hours interacting as a group, discussing and learning to accept the changes in themselves, while also rebuilding their self-confidence. Realizing the importance of motivation in the rehabilitation process, Ben-Yishay was the first to address one of the greatest challenges which still faces clinicians to this day. This approach has been further developed by George Prigatano at the Barrow Neurological Institute in Phoenix and others (Prigatano et al., 1986; Prigatano, 1999).

During the late 1970s and early 1980s there was a surge in the availability of computer software designed for the retraining of various cognitive abilities by neuropsychologists such as William Lynch, Odey Bracy, and Rosamund Gianutsos. This software began to be used routinely in rehabilitation units. Controlled research studies evaluating the impact of such interventions was scant, however. Toward the end of the 1980s a number of studies were conducted evaluating the impact of such interventions, the majority focusing on attention. These studies which are reviewed in other chapters of this book have had mixed findings. Overall, there is evidence of improvement on tasks being trained and other tasks which are similar, but limited evidence of generalization to everyday life.

These early cognitive interventions were generally evaluated using neuropsychological measures, which were similar to the tasks used for training. During the 1980s there was realization of the need to evaluate outcome from a broader perspective. Since that time many measures have been developed and applied, although there has been little agreement and uniformity in the use of criteria or measures. Initially emphasis was placed on the measurement of disability using a range of activities of daily living scales. More recently, there has been a greater emphasis on evaluating the performance of different social roles, such as the ability to live independently; to pursue work, study, and/or recreational pursuits; and to form personal and social relationships, using measures such as the Craig Handicap Assessment and Reporting Technique (CHART), developed by Whiteneck, Charlifue, Gerhart, Overholser, and Richardson (1992), and the Community Integration Questionnaire (CIQ), developed by Willer, Ottenbacher, and Coade (1994). Outcome has been measured not only from the perspective of the therapist but also from that of the injured person and close others. There has been greater emphasis on investigating not just how well individuals are functioning but also how they and their close others are feeling, and how they perceive their quality of life. With these developments in outcome measurement, follow-up studies have identified a significant number of individuals who continue to experience many difficulties in their daily lives over many years after they leave the rehabilitation setting.

As a consequence, there has been a trend toward the development of community-based models of rehabilitation. Transitional living centers were established to provide *in vivo* training in living skills. More recently such programs are being conducted within the context of the home or workplace, with retraining or support services being supplied as needed to maximize independence. All these developments have been constrained by decreasing funding support, particularly in the United States. Hospital stays and entitlements to rehabilitation services have been significantly reduced in the last decade. They have also been influenced by the growing application of evidence-based medicine and what is perceived as a lack of scientific evidence regarding the efficacy of rehabilitative interventions. This has been largely due to methodological weaknesses in much of the research which has been conducted to date (Chesnut et al., 1999; Cicerone et al., 2000; Carney, Chestnut, Maynard, Mann, & Hefland, 1999).

Paralleling all this has been an enormous body of basic neurosciences research focusing on mechanisms of neuronal injury associated with traumatic brain injury, stroke, and a range of degenerative diseases and processes occurring following injury, largely through animal studies. There have been trials of a number of pharmacological interventions. Mechanisms of neuronal regrowth, sprouting, and dendritic reorganization and factors that facilitate and hinder these processes have also been studied. Major developments include the isolation of trophic factors, which appear to enhance regrowth and reorganization, fetal transplants, and work with stem cells as potential mediators of neuronal regeneration. The influence of different environmental situations or inputs and their interaction with recovery mechanisms has also been vigorously explored. Cognitive neurosciences research has developed our understanding of the brain mechanisms that underpin a range of cognitive functions, an understanding that has developed significantly with the advent of functional neuroimaging techniques.

Unfortunately, however, these bodies of work in human rehabilitation, animal studies of mechanisms of injury and repair, and the development of the cognitive neurosciences have been conducted in parallel, with minimal communication between them. Relatively little rehabilitation research has been based on neurosciences research or even solid theoretical underpinnings. Indeed many rehabilitation therapists are not cognizant of research in these other areas, which has profound implications for their work. Although there are a number of texts that focus on either theories of neurological recovery of function or approaches to rehabilitation, relatively few books have successfully integrated the scientific evidence relating to impairment and recovery of specific cognitive and behavioral disorders with the clinical application of rehabilitative interventions in adults.

This book aims to bridge this gap. In the first chapter Bryan Kolb and Jan Cioe outline basic principles of neuronal organization that underpin relationships between the brain and behavior, the physiological events associated with brain damage, and the factors that affect neuronal change after injury. In the second chapter, Bryan Kolb explores mechanisms of recovery from neuronal injury, the potential for plasticity in the normal and injured brain, and factors that affect recovery, exploring the potential for interventions which might enhance recovery.

With this as background, Chapters 3–7 cover five core cognitive domains—nonspatial attention, memory, language, visuospatial attention, executive function and self-awareness. Chapter 8 focuses on disorders of behavior. Each is written by a specialist in that field, who has worked at both a theoretical or experimental and a clinical level with individuals with disorders in that domain. In these chapters an attempt has been made to discuss, within a theoretical framework, anatomical, biochemical, and/or physiological aspects of the function and the pathophysiological basis of impairments resulting form different forms of brain injury and to suggest or review remedial interventions in light of this framework. The final chapter discusses the application of information from each of these chapters to the rehabilitation of cognitive and behavioral disorders associated with the two most common causes of acquired neurological disability—traumatic brain injury and stroke. The book thus attempts to bridge the gap between basic neuroscience and clinical practice and will, ideally, be read by practitioners at both ends of the spectrum.

REFERENCES

Ben-Yishay, Y., Ben-Nachum, Z., Cohen, A., Gross, Y., Hofien, A., Rattok, Y., et al. (1978). Digest of a two-year comprehensive clinical rehabilitation research program for out-patient head injured Israeli veterans (Oct. 1975–Oct. 1977). In *Working approaches to remediation of cognitive deficits in brain damaged persons* (Rehabilitation Monograph No. 59, pp. 1–61). New York: Institute of Rehabilitation Medicine, New York University Medical Center.

Boake, C. (2003). Stages in the history of neuropsychological rehabilitation. In B. A. Wilson (Ed.), *Neuropsychological rehabilitation: Theory and practice.* Lisse: Swets & Zeitlinger.

Carney, N., Chestnut, R. M., Maynard, H., Mann, N. C., & Hefland, M. (1999). Effect of cognitive rehabilitation on outcomes for persons with traumatic brain injury: A systematic review. *Journal of Head Trauma Rehabilitation, 14,* 277–307.

Chesnut, R. M., Carney, N., Maynard, H., Mann, N. C., Patterson, P., & Helfand, M. (1999). Summary report: Evidence for the effectiveness of rehabilitation for persons with traumatic brain injury. *Journal of Head Trauma Rehabilitation, 14,* 176–188.

Cicerone, K. D., Dahlberg, C., Kalmar, K., Langenbahn, D. M., Malec, J. F., Bergquist, T., et al. (2000). Evidence-based cognitive rehabilitation: Recommendations for clinical practice. *Archives of Physical Medicine and Rehabilitation, 81,* 1596–1615.

Diller, L., Ben-Yishay, Y., Gerstman, L. J., Goodkin, R., Gordon, W., & Weinberg, J. (1974). *Studies in cognition and rehabilitation in hemiplegia* (Rehabilitation Monograph No. 50). New York: Institute of Rehabilitation Medicine, New York University Medical Center.

Goldstein, K. (1942). *Aftereffects of brain injuries in war: Their evaluation and treatment; the application of psychologic methods in the clinic.* New York: Grune & Stratton.

Luria, A. R. (1963). *Restoration of function after brain injury* (B. Haigh, Trans.). New York: Macmillan. (Original work published 1948)

Luria, A. R. (1973). *The working brain.* London: Penguin Press.

Prigatano, G. P. (1999). *Principles of neuropsychological rehabilitation.* New York: Oxford University Press.

Prigatano, G. P., Fordyce, D. J., Zeiner, H. K., Roueche, J. R., Pepping, M., & Wood, B. C. (1986). *Neuropsychological rehabilitation after brain injury.* Baltimore: Johns Hopkins University Press.

Whiteneck, G. G., Charlifue, S. W., Gerhart, K. A., Overholser, D., & Richardson, G. N. (1992). Quantifying handicap: A new measure of long-term rehabilitation outcomes. *Archives of Physical Medicine and Rehabilitation, 73,* 519–526.

Willer, B., Ottenbacher, K., & Coade, M. (1994). The Community Integration Questionnaire: A comparative examination. *American Journal of Physical Medicine and Rehabilitation, 73,* 103–111.

1

■ ■ ■ ■

Neuronal Organization and Change after Neuronal Injury

Bryan Kolb
Jan Cioe

One basic challenge we face in designing rehabilitative strategies after brain injury is to identify some regularities in the brain's organization and to establish a set of principles that can help us to understand how the nervous system works. Having done this, we can then examine what happens when the brain is injured and its function is disrupted. But not all brains are the same; thus we must also identify those factors that influence the functioning of the normal brain and the dysfunctioning of the abnormal brain.

CONCEPTS OF BRAIN AND BEHAVIOR

It would be presumptuous to believe that the organization and functioning of the human brain could be described in a few pages (see Kolb & Whishaw, 2003, for an extensive discussion). But it is possible, however, to identify a few basic concepts that underlie brain organization and function.

1. *The brain has evolved as an organ that creates a representation of the external world and produces behavior in response to the world.* Perhaps the simplest statement of the brain's functions is that it produces behavior. There is

7

more to this statement than is immediately apparent, however. For the brain to produce behavior it must have information about the world, such as information about the objects around us—their size, shape, movement, and so forth. Thus, behaviors are made in response to the external world. But what is this external world? Although we like to think that it is just as we experience it, much like a photograph of a scene, the external world is created by the nervous system, and the perception of what the external world is like depends on the complexity and organization of the nervous system. Consider the visual world that most people see in a rich blanket of colors. Although we take color for granted, not all species, and certainly not even all people, perceive color the way most humans do. Behaviors that depend on the ability to distinguish different hues therefore depend on a neural machinery that can detect the difference between, for example, red and pink.

This idea may be abstract, but it is central to understanding how the brain functions. Consider the task of answering a telephone. The brain directs the body to pick up the receiver when the nervous system responds to vibrating molecules of air by creating the subjective experience of a ring. We perceive this sound, and react to it, as if it actually existed, when in fact the sound is merely a fabrication of the brain. That fabrication is produced by a chain reaction that occurs when vibrating air molecules hit the eardrum. In the absence of the nervous system, especially the brain, there is no such thing as sound. Rather, there is only the movement of air molecules.

But there is more to understanding the brain's fundamental functions. For a link between sensory processing and behavior to be made, the brain must also have a system for accumulating, integrating, and using knowledge. Hearing a telephone ring is only useful if we have knowledge of what a telephone is. Whenever the brain collects sensory information it is essentially creating knowledge about the world, knowledge that can be used to produce more effective behaviors. The knowledge currently being created in one sensory domain can be compared with both past knowledge and knowledge gathered in other domains.

We can now identify the brain's three primary functions: (1) to produce behavior, (2) to create a sensory reality, and (3) to create knowledge that integrates information from different times and sensory domains, using that knowledge to guide behavior.

Each of the brain's three functions requires specific machinery. There must be systems in the brain to create the sensory world, systems to produce behavior, and systems to integrate the two.

A fundamental difference between the human brain and that of other animals is that it is larger relative to body size. The increase in brain size is related, in part, to an expansion of our perceptual abilities. Stated differently, as our brain grew larger in evolution, its representation of the external world became more complex. But, as the brain grew larger in evolution, the amount of information processed and generated as knowledge grew so large that there needed to be mechanisms for organizing all this information. One solution to the problem of categorizing information is to create some form of coding system, of which language is the extreme example. We can see then that the loss of language will not only interfere with communication with others but could also disrupt the organization of our understanding of the perceptual world.

    2. *The brain is composed of neurons and glia.* The brain has two main types of cells: neurons and glia (Figure 1.1). There are about 80 billion neurons and 100 billion glia in a human brain. Neurons are the cells that carry out the brain's major behavioral functions, as described later. Glia were once thought to be little more than a type of glue that held the nervous system together, but we now know that glia play an active, and neural complementary, role in brain functioning.

    There are two major categories of glial cells: the macroglia and microglia. The macroglia include astrocytes and oligodendrocytes, the latter being the cells that form myelin. Astrocytes actively produce factors (such as neurotrophic factors) that influence neuronal activity and function. They also have receptors for various chemicals, including some neurotransmitters (e.g., noradrenaline), and thus their activity can be influenced by neurons. Although neurons and astrocytes have quite different functions in the brain, they are closely related developmentally, and there is now some suspicion that it is possible for astrocytes to turn into neurons under the right circumstances in the mature nervous system. Furthermore, it is clear that astrocytes play an important role in neuronal repair, and thus their activities are central to understanding recovery from brain injury.

    In contrast to neurons and macroglia, microglia derive from a different cell population in the body, namely, blood cells. Microglia are scavenger cells and increase in number dramatically after injury.

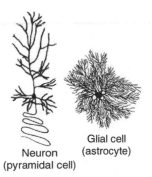

Neuron
(pyramidal cell)

Glial cell
(astrocyte)

FIGURE 1.1. Neurons and glia are the two principal cell types in the brain.

3. *The neuron is the basic unit of anatomy, physiology, and cognition.* Nerve cells, no matter where they are found in the nervous systems of different animals are remarkably similar. Most neurons have some type of mechanism both for receiving information (a dendritic field) and for sending information (an axon). But simply acting as a way station for information serves little purpose: Neurons also act to alter the incoming information before passing it on. The inputs to a neuron at any given moment are "summed up," and the neuron sends out signals to other neurons that reflect this summation. The summation is more than just a matter of adding up equally weighted inputs. Some inputs have a greater influence than others on the receiving neuron, and the simultaneous occurrence of certain inputs may have effects that far exceed their simple sum. The summation of information, then, allows that information to be transformed in some way before being passed on to other neurons. This makes the summation process partly one of creating new information.

A fundamental tenet of the neuron doctrine developed by Ramón y Cajál and others early in the 20th century was that this creation of information by neurons makes individual neurons the basic unit of information processing, plasticity, and even cognition. We now know, for example, that drugs act at the level of individual neurons; experience changes individual neurons; neurons communicate with one another to generate sensory experience and to produce behavior; and differences between brains represent differences in neuron distribution, organization, and connectivity. We hasten to note, however, that although neurons are individuals, each with a role in behavior, as brains have grown larger through evolution, the number of neurons performing similar functions has expanded exponentially.

Simple nervous systems, such as in the 302-neuron-large nervous system of the worm *C. elegans*, are designed such that each neuron has a specific job. If one neuron should die or dysfunction, the entire system is affected. As brains have grown larger, however, the creation of a brain to an exact blueprint becomes much more difficult, and nature's solution has been to create extra neurons with the strategy of being able to shed unused or unneeded neurons. This solution has the advantage of not only allowing much more flexibility in adapting to specific environmental conditions but also in freeing the nervous system from depending on the survival and functioning of each individual neuron. Stated differently, although the neurons in our brain are the basic units of the brain's operation, the death of a neuron in our brain does not lead to the death of some mental or behavioral process.

4. *The synapse is the key site of neuronal communication and learning.* Although the neuron is the fundamental unit of the nervous system, it is the connections between neurons (i.e., the synapses) that provide a mechanism for information processing and storage. Indeed, the importance of the synapse in

perceptual processing led Hebb (1949) to make the synapse the central feature of his now classic theory of brain and behavior.

Synapses are most often between axon terminals of one cell and the dendrite, cell body, or axon of another cell, and the primary mode of communication across most synapses is chemical. The action of the chemical is either to alter cellular channels on the receiving cell or to initiate changes in the cell membrane that will, in turn, initiate biochemical events (so-called second messengers) in the receiving cell. There are several ways in which synaptic activity can be influenced. Because most synapses are chemical, the simplest way to change synaptic activity is to affect either the release of a chemical (by increasing or decreasing it) or the action of the chemical on its receptor (by attenuating or potentiating the effect on the postsynaptic membrane). This is, of course, the direct route of action of most drugs. But, there are less direct routes too.

One effect of repeated exposure to drugs is to alter either the characteristics of the postsynaptic membrane (such as the number of receptor sites) or the number of synapses. The number of synapses can be increased by adding synapses to the existing cell or by increasing the synaptic space by adding more dendritic material. Changes in receptor or synaptic number are required for processes that are likely involved in events such as learning and drug addiction. Indeed, synaptic change is required for virtually any behavioral change, whether it be related to learning, development, and aging or recovery from injury. Because synaptic change is the key to behavioral change, it follows that factors that increase (or decrease) synaptic change, such as drugs, hormones, or experiences, will stimulate (or retard) behavioral changes. Therefore, new treatments for behavioral change necessarily must be designed to maximize synaptic change.

5. *The central nervous system has multiple levels of function.* As we mentioned earlier, as the brain expanded in evolution, it increased its capacity for sensory processing and knowledge production. But these additions did not simply reflect the expansion of existing brain regions but, rather, were added according to the following rule: "descent with modification." Practically speaking, this meant that as the brain evolved, new areas were added but old ones were also retained. At the turn of the last century, John Hughlings-Jackson suggested that the addition of new brain structures during evolution could be viewed as adding new levels of nervous system control. The lowest level is the spinal cord, the next level is the brainstem, and the highest level is the forebrain. These levels are not autonomous, however. To move the arms, the brainstem must use circuits in the spinal cord. Similarly, to make independent movements of the arms and fingers, as in tying a shoelace, the cortex must use circuits in both the brainstem and the spinal cord. Each new level offers a refinement and elaboration of the motor control provided by one or more lower levels.

We can observe the operation of functional levels in the behavior of people with brain injuries. Someone whose spinal cord is disconnected from the brain cannot voluntarily move a limb because the brain has no way to control the movement. But the limb can still move automatically to withdraw from a noxious stimulus because the circuits for moving the muscles are still intact in the spinal cord. Similarly, if the forebrain is not functioning but the brainstem is still connected to the spinal cord, a person can still move, but the movements are relatively simple: There is limited limb use and no digit control.

The principle of multiple levels of function can also be applied to the cortex in mammals, which evolved by adding new areas, mostly sensory processing ones. The newer areas essentially added new levels of control that provide more and more abstract analysis of inputs. Consider the recognition of an object, such as a car. The simplest level of analysis represents the features of this object such as its size, shape, and color. A higher level of analysis recognizes this object as a car. And an even higher level of analysis recognizes this as Jennie's car, which has a dent in the fender. Probably the highest levels are cortical regions that substitute one or more words for the object (Ford Escort, for instance) and can think about the car in its absence.

When we consider the brain as a structure composed of multiple levels of function, it is clear that these levels must be extensively interconnected to integrate their processing and create unitary perceptions or movements.

6. *Functions in the brain are both localized and distributed.* We have seen that sensory information, knowledge, and the control of movement are all represented at multiple levels in the nervous system, beginning at the spinal cord and ending in multiple cortical areas. Implicit in this idea of multiple levels of representation is the idea that functions can be localized to specific locations in the brain. Although the concept of localization makes intuitive sense, it turns out to be controversial. One of the great debates in the history of brain research has been over what aspects of different functions are actually localized in specific brain regions. Perhaps the fundamental problem is that of defining a function. Consider language. Language includes comprehension of spoken words, written words, signed words (as in American Sign Language), and even touched words (as in Braille). Language also includes processes of producing words, both orally and in writing, as well as constructing whole linguistic compositions, such as stories, poems, songs, and essays. Because there are many aspects of the function we call language, it is not surprising that these functions reside in widely separated areas of the brain. We see evidence of this widespread distribution in language-related brain injuries. People with injuries in different locations may selectively lose the abilities to produce words, understand words, read words, write words, and so forth. Specific language-related abilities, therefore, are found in specific locations, but language, per se, is distributed over a wide region of the brain.

Language is hardly unique. Virtually every other psychological function, such as memory, perception, emotion, attention, and motivation, is similarly distributed. Although we tend to think of these hypothetical processes as things, the brain organizes functions in terms of the underlying processes necessary for different aspects of the functions. Thus, to return to language, the brain localizes functions such as the perception of speech sounds, the production of movements, and so on. It is these functions that are localized. Perhaps the extreme example is the lateralization of language. Although it is tempting to conclude that language is lateralized, it is more accurate to conclude that processes that are needed to produce language are lateralized. Viewed in this way, it is easier to appreciate why other functions, such as certain aspects of spatial analysis, also are lateralized: They rely on a particular set of neural processes that are located together in one hemisphere. (For a more extensive discussion of this principle, see Kolb & Whishaw, 2003.)

Because many functions are both localized and distributed in the brain, damage to a small brain region produces only focal symptoms. It requires massive brain damage to completely remove some function. For instance, a relatively small injury could impair some aspect of language functioning, but it would take a widespread injury to completely remove all language abilities. In fact, one of the characteristics of dementing diseases, such as Alzheimer's, is that people can have widespread deterioration of the cortex yet maintain remarkably normal language functions until late stages of the disease.

7. *The nervous system works through excitation and inhibition.* Not all symptoms of brain injury or disease result from a loss of a specific function or group of functions. Symptoms may also result more indirectly through a loss of inhibition or excitation. Neurons can pass on information to other neurons either by being active or by being silent. That is, they can be "on" or "off." Some neurons in the brain function primarily to excite other neurons, whereas others function to inhibit neurons. These excitatory and inhibitory effects are produced by various neurotransmitters, hormones, or other chemicals that turn the neurons on or off.

Just as individual neurons can act to excite or inhibit other neurons, brain nuclei (or cortical layers) can do the same to other nuclei (or layers). These actions are especially obvious in the motor systems. A loss of inhibition of small movements can produce hand tremor or continuous tongue movements, symptoms known as dyskinesias. But a loss of inhibition can be seen more grossly too, such as in people with frontal lobe injury. Such people are often unable to inhibit behaviors, such as talking at inappropriate times or using certain words (e.g., swear words). In contrast, people with injury to the speech zones of the left hemisphere may be unable to talk at all because the injury is in an area that normally initiates the behavior of speech. These contrasting symptoms lead to an important conclusion: Brain injury can produce either a loss of behavior or a release of behavior. Behavior is lost when the damage prevents excitatory instructions; behavior is released when the damage prevents inhibitory instructions.

8. *Patterns of neural organization are plastic.* The brain is plastic in two fundamental ways. First, although we tend to think of regions of the brain as having fixed functions, a conclusion that follows directly from the idea of localization of function, the brain has a capacity to adapt to different experiences by changing the relative representation of functions. Second, the brain is also plastic in the sense that the connections among neurons in a given functional system are constantly changing in response to experience. This type of plastic change is reflected in our capacity for learning, and subsequently for recalling, learned material. There are clearly limits to plasticity, however. Reorganization of sensory representations is limited by the boundaries of the inputs. For example, the extent of the somatosensory representation is limited by the inputs from the somatosensory thalamus. Adjacent regions, which receive input from the motor or visual thalamic nuclei, cannot assume somatosensory functions because they are connected with the different receptors. The brain assumes that input going to the visual areas is visual in nature. Similarly, although neurons can grow new dendrites in response to experience, there are limits to how much a given neuron can change and how many connections can be placed on a neuron. Not only are there biophysical limits with respect to the effects of new connections on membrane potentials, but there are metabolic limitations. They are not designed to have cell bodies a centimeter in diameter! The nature of brain plasticity and its role in functional recovery is the topic of the next chapter.

PHYSIOLOGICAL EVENTS ASSOCIATED WITH BRAIN DAMAGE

Although we may be able to point to a specific proximal cause of a brain injury, such as a stroke, the end result of brain injury is not the result of a single causative event. Rather, there is an initial event followed by a cascade of cellular events that can seriously compromise the injured brain as well as brain regions that were not directly injured. Consider what happens after a stroke in which there is an interruption of the blood supply to one of the cerebral arteries.

The first stage of a stroke is a lack of blood (ischemia), which results in a cascade of events that progress even if the blood flow is restored. As illustrated in Figure 1.2, over the first seconds to minutes there are changes in the ionic balance of the affected regions, including changes in pH and properties of the cell membrane. These ionic changes result in a variety of pathological events including the release to massive amounts of glutamate and the prolonged open-

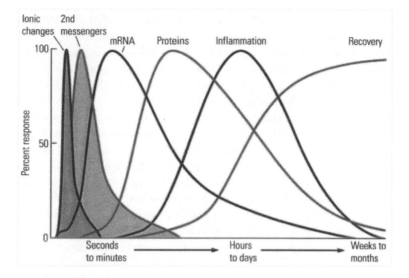

FIGURE 1.2. The cascade of poststroke events. There are immediate changes in the brain followed by changes that may last hours or days and finally changes that may take months to evolve.

ing of calcium channels. The open calcium channels allow toxic levels of calcium to enter the cell and not only to produce direct toxic effects but to instigate various second messenger pathways that can also prove to be harmful to the neurons. Over the ensuing minutes to hours there is a stimulation of mRNA, which in turn alters the production of proteins in the neurons, which again may prove toxic to the cells.

About 24 hours postinjury there is considerable edema (swelling). Edema probably results from both extracellular fluid accumulation, especially in the white matter, and astrocytic swelling (Nieto-Sampedro & Cotman, 1985). Edema is particularly problematic in the brain because swelling means that there is an increase in volume of the brain but the skull is not accommodating. Thus, the swelling acts to put pressure on the brain, which can cause neuronal dysfunction and injury. Luckily, many of the effects of edema are transient and functions return as the swelling reduces. A good example is seen in the postsurgical recovery of IQ in patients with temporal or frontal lobectomies for the treatment of epilepsy. Milner (1975) reported that IQ had dropped about 15 points when measured 2 weeks after surgery, but by 1 year it had returned to preoperative levels. Although the IQ drop may result from factors in addition to edema, treatment with anti-inflammatories such as cortisone decreases the IQ drop and speeds up recovery.

Along with the development of edema, there may also be changes in the metabolism and/or glucose utilization of an injured hemisphere that may persist for days. These metabolic changes can have severe effects on brain functioning in otherwise normal tissue. It has been shown, for example, that after a cortical stroke there is a drop of about 60% in glucose metabolism throughout the rest of the damaged hemisphere and, surprisingly, a drop of about 25% in the undamaged hemisphere (e.g., Pappius, 1981).

Although neuronal death resulting from an injury will occur rather quickly, there is also a significant loss of neurons not directly affected by the injury (Figure 1.3). Thus, about 48 hours after the lesion, more distal neurons begin to die as result of the changes in blood flow, metabolism, pH, edema, and so on. The secondary cell death can be quite extensive and may even be larger than the cell death resulting directly from the injury itself.

Both microglia and macroglia are present in the region of injury within 48 hours. The microglia act as phagocytes, clearing away degenerative debris, a process that may take months to complete. Astrocytes adjacent to the lesion area enlarge and extend fibrous processes that isolate the surfaces of the injury from the surrounding tissue. At about the same time fibroblasts from nearby connective tissue invade the injury site and produce a scar that prevents axons from reentering the injured region (Figure 1.3).

In addition to symptoms resulting from cell death, most brain injuries produce a form of neural shock that von Monakow called diaschisis. von Monakow noted that after the brain is injured, not only is localized neural tissue and its function lost but areas related to the damaged area suffer a sudden withdrawal of excitation or inhibition. Such sudden changes in input can lead to a temporary loss of function both in areas adjacent to an injury and in regions that may be quite distal.

Treatments for cerebral injury can be directed at different targets in the postinjury cascade. For example, drugs can be used to block calcium channels or prevent ionic imbalance. Such drugs are called neuroprotectants because it is hoped that they will protect neurons from the cascade of toxic events that follow an ischemic episode. Other drugs can be used to reduce swelling or to enhance metabolic activity. The effect of neuroprotectants and anti-inflammatories is obviously quite different than the effect of treatments that are hoped to stimulate plasticity and functional compensation. The latter treatments would not be protecting compromised brain, but rather they would be designed to stimulate plastic changes in the remaining brain, changes that could potentially underlie functional compensation.

One important consideration in the immediate postinjury period is what types of activities might actually make cell death worse. In the course of studies designed to promote functional recovery after injury, Schallert and his colleagues (e.g., Kozlowski, James, & Schallert, 1996) accidentally found that initiating intense therapy after a stroke may actually make the stroke damage worse. In these studies rats were fitted with a restraint harness that prevented

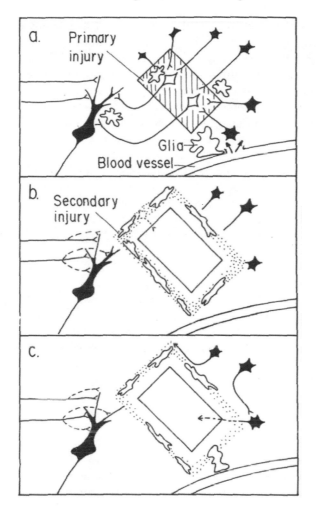

FIGURE 1.3. Major cellular events after a brain injury. (a) Cells in the area of primary injury die immediately while cells in adjacent regions are alive but disrupted. (b) Cells in the disrupted region (secondary injury) die at a later time. Glia proliferate (dotted area) and form a boundary between normal and abnormal brain tissue. Reactive sprouts begin to innervate deafferented cells (lower left). (c) Regenerating axonal sprouts (upper right) are unable to penetrate the glial boundary and either die or form inappropriate connections. From Nieto-Sampredro and Cotman (1985). Copyright 1985 by The Guilford Press. Reprinted by permission.

the animals from using the forelimb ipsilateral to a sensorimotor cortex injury. The idea was to force animals to use the impaired limb and, it was hoped, stimulate recovery. The problem was that the animals wore the harness 24 hours a day, and the continual forced use of the affected limb significantly enlarged the lesion cavity and subsequent functional outcome. Importantly, this effect is not simply due to stress or some nonspecific effect because a similar treatment did not increase the size of injury to animals with visual cortex injuries (De Bow, Kolb, McKenna, & Colbourne, 2003). Although few human stroke treatments would be so intense, the Schallert studies emphasize the question as to when therapy should be commenced and how intense it should be, which remains to be determined.

COMPENSATORY PROCESSES FOLLOWING BRAIN INJURY

Once the cascade of neurobiological events triggered by an injury abates, the nervous system begins reparative processes, many of which enhance synaptic formation (Figure 1.4). Although none of these reparative processes will completely replace the lost tissue, there is often an associated behavioral improvement. It thus seems reasonable to look for therapies that can enhance these reparative processes and in so doing afford greater functional improvement after injury. We briefly consider five of the most important reparative processes, including (1) regeneration, (2) sprouting, (3) denervation supersensitivity, (4) reactive synaptogenesis, and (5) neural and glial genesis.

Regeneration

Regeneration is the process by which neurons damaged by trauma regrow connections to the area they previously innervated. Although regeneration is well known in the peripheral nervous system, it is not common in the central nervous system. One of the main problems is the scarring we noted earlier. One solution is to build artificial tubes or bridges across the area of scarring (e.g., Aguayo, 1985). These bridges can be either glial tubes or relatively undifferentiated embryonic tissue, both of which can provide a medium through which regenerating fibers can grow. There are also ways to promote fiber growth. One is the use of factors that promote fiber outgrowth, an example of which are neurotrophic factors, such as nerve growth factor, a high-molecular-weight protein that is either produced or taken up from glia by nerve terminals and then transported to the cell body to play some role in maintaining normal cell growth or health. Another approach is based on the idea that there are molecules in the developed nervous system that inhibit new axonal growth after the brain is mature. After brain damage, if these molecules themselves could be inhibited temporarily, then regrowth could occur. One example can be seen in

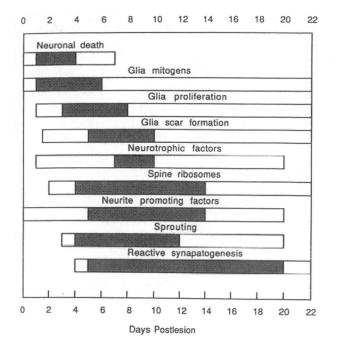

FIGURE 1.4. Time course of events following central nervous system injury. The beginning of the bars indicates the time postlesion when the event is initiated. The intensity of the shading parallels the intensity of the phenomenon indicated by the bar. Adapted from Nieto-Sampedro and Cotman (1985). Copyright 1985 by The Guilford Press. Adapted by permission.

work of Martin Schwab and his colleagues. In the course of trying to stimulate the bisected spinal cord of rats to regenerate lost connections, Schwab discovered that there was a protein that prevented regenerating fibers from passing, a protein aptly called "no go." The solution to no go's actions was to infuse a neutralizing antibody to no go. Indeed, when the antibody was infused there was not only an enhanced regeneration of the spinal cord axons but an associated behavioral improvement as well (e.g., Merkler, et al., 2001).

Sprouting

Sprouting is the growth of nerve fibers to innervate new targets, particularly if they have been vacated by other terminals. Sprouting can be seen by the growth of axon terminals as well as by the expansion of postsynaptic dendritic fields, the latter providing more space for the incoming axon terminals and their synapses. The hippocampus of the rat provides a nice model of this type of phenomenon. If the entorhinal cortex of rats is removed unilaterally, there is a loss of more than 85% of the synapses from the distal regions of the hippocampal granule cells in the same hemisphere. This massive denervation of the cells leads to a reorganization of the connections of the dentate gyrus (for a review, see Steward, 1991). During the first few days there is a retraction of the denervated dendrites, followed by a regrowth as new axon terminals from connections originating in the contralateral entorhinal cortex invade the previously denervated area (Figure 1.4). The sprouting of new connections is correlated with a partial return of performance on neuropsychological learning tasks (e.g., Loesche & Steward, 1977).

Like regeneration, sprouting can be enhanced by the use of factors that fiber outgrowth. One example is inosine. For example, Chen, Goldberg, Kolb, Lanser, and Benowitz (2002) have shown not only that infusing inosine after middle cerebral artery occlusion in rats can stimulate the sprouting of axonal projections from the normal to the injured hemisphere but that these projections can support functional compensation. Such studies are promising for rehabilitative efforts and lead to the question whether functional improvement might be enhanced if animals are given behavioral therapies at the same time they receive the chemical treatments.

Reactive Synaptogenesis

Restoration of damaged circuitry requires that regenerating fibers reach their targets and functional synapses are formed (e.g., Nieto-Sampedro & Cotman, 1985). The new synapses do not replace the original ones but result in the formation of a different neural circuit. The generation of the new synapses has two components. There is the presynaptic side where axon terminals must form synaptic boutons and make the appropriate presynaptic apparatus, such as making synaptic vesicles, and there is the postsynaptic side in which the dendrite must make the postsynaptic receptor surface and, for most excitatory synapses, also a spine structure. It is not yet known what factors influence these two processes.

Neural and Glial Genesis

A stem cell is a cell with an extensive capacity for self-renewal. It divides and produces two stem cells, one of which dies while the other goes on to divide again. This process is repeated over and over throughout a person's lifetime. In an adult, the neural stem cells line the ventricles and form the ventricular zone. It is reasonable to presume that the stem cells lining the ventricles have some function, although it is not clear exactly what that function might be. It is known, however, that stem cells can give rise to so-called progenitor (or precursor) cells. These progenitor cells can also divide, and they eventually produce nondividing cells, known as neuroblasts and glioblasts. Neuroblasts and glioblasts, in turn, become neurons and glia when they mature. Neural stem cells, then, are the cells that give rise to all the many specialized cells of the brain and spinal cord. Stem cells remain capable of producing neurons and glia not just into early adulthood but even in an aging brain, at least in the olfactory bulb and hippocampus. The fact that neurogenesis can continue into adulthood and even into senescence is important because it means that neurons that die in an adult could be replaceable.

Altman (see Altman & Bayer, 1993) was the first to show that stem cells could be mobilized after cerebral injury. He made small lesions in the posterior cortex of rats and using a radioactive label, tritiated thymidine, he was able to show that a small number of new neurons were generated and migrated to the region of the lesion. The problem for rehabilitation therapy is to stimulate the brain to generate a much larger number of cells than Altman's rats generated.

One way to stimulate neuronal generation is to infuse growth factors such as epidermal growth factor (EGF) and basic fibroblast growth factor (bFGF) into the ventricle after a cerebral injury. EGF and bFGF act to stimulate stem cell division *in vitro*, and thus it is reasonable to suppose that they could have a similar function *in vivo*. Indeed, they do. It has been shown that infusions of EGF and bFGF mobilize thousands, and perhaps millions of cells that migrate from the subventricular zone and occupy the space of injured cells (see Schallert, Leasure, & Kolb, 2000, Figure 1.4). The difficulty is that these cells do not differentiate properly into neurons and glia and subsequently die. What is required is some type of factor that can stimulate the cells to differentiate. One candidate is erithropoetin. Recently, Weiss and Kolb have shown in unpublished studies that erithropoetin can stimulate differentiation of both neuronal and glial phenotypes after cerebral stroke and that these cells migrate to the area of lesion. Such studies are still a long way from the clinic, but they do suggest that it might be possible to regenerate at least some of the lost neurons and glia, which in turn could facilitate functional improvement after injury (see also Kolb, Gibb, Gorny, & Whishaw, 1998).

FACTORS AFFECTING NEURONAL CHANGES AFTER BRAIN INJURY

We have seen that there is a cascade of neuronal and glial changes that unfolds after a cerebral injury. In addition, we have considered some types of reparative processes that can be triggered after an injury and potentially help facilitate the outcome of behavioral therapies after brain injury. We now consider several factors that can influence both the cascade of changes and the reparative processes that may underlie functional improvement. Although there have been extensive studies looking at factors affecting cell death in the first hours after injury (so-called neuroprotectants), these studies have had controversial results and for the most part they have had little impact on rehabilitation strategies. Our focus, therefore, will be on those factors that are likely to have longer-term impacts on reparative processes in the brain. Our discussion is not exhaustive but provides general examples of how functional outcome can vary so widely after cerebral injury.

Age

At the time an egg is fertilized by a sperm, a human embryo consists of just a single cell. But this cell soon begins to divide, and by the 14th day the embryo resembles a fried egg. It is made of several sheets of cells with a raised area in the middle. The raised area is the primitive body. By 3 weeks after conception there is a primitive brain, which is essentially a sheet of cells at one end of the embryo. This sheet of cells rolls up to form the neural tube, much as a flat sheet of paper can be curled to make a cylinder.

The body and the nervous system change rapidly over the next 3 weeks of development. By 7 weeks of age (or 49 days) the embryo begins to resemble a miniature person and the brain looks distinctly human by about 100 days after conception, but it does not begin to form gyri and sulci until about 7 months. By the end of the ninth month, the brain has the gross appearance of the adult human brain, even though its cellular structure is different.

As we more carefully investigate the development of the child's brain, we can identify a series of changes that occur in a relatively fixed sequence. These include (1) the generation of cells, (2) the migration of cells, (3) the formation and growth of axons, (4) the formation of dendrites, (5) the formation of synaptic connections, (6) the pruning of cells and synapses, and (7) myelination. This program of development has two extraordinary features. First, subcomponents of the nervous system are formed from cells whose destination and function are largely predetermined before they migrate from the wall of the ventricles. Second, development is marked by an initial abundance of cells, branches, and connections, with an important part of subsequent maturation consisting of cell death or pruning back of the initial surfeit.

Because of deficits in the genetic program, intrauterine trauma, the influence of toxic agents, or other factors, peculiarities or errors in development can occur that may contribute to obvious and severe deformities, such as those listed in Table 1.1. Less pronounced deficits may become manifest in such problems as learning disabilities or may appear only as subtle changes in behavior.

As we shall see in the next chapter, brain injury has different effects depending on the precise time of injury. The most thorough studies of timing effects have been conducted in rodents, and primarily in rats (e.g., Kolb, 1995). As a general rule of thumb, we can conclude that recovery from cerebral injury

TABLE 1.1. Types of Abnormal Development

Type	Symptom
Anencephaly	Absence of cerebral hemispheres, diencephalon, and midbrain
Holoprosencephaly	Cortex forms as a single undifferentiated hemisphere
Lissencephaly	Brain fails to form sulci and gyri and corresponds to a 12-week embryo
Micropolygyria	Gyri are more numerous, smaller, and more poorly developed than normal
Macrogyria	Gyri are broader and less numerous than normal
Microencephaly	Development of the brain is rudimentary and the person has low-grade intelligence
Porencephaly	Symmetrical cavities in the cortex, where cortex and white matter should be
Heterotopia	Displaced islands of gray matter appear in the ventricular walls or white matter, caused by aborted cell migration
Agenesis of the corpus callosum	Complete or partial absence of the corpus callosum
Cerebellar agenesis	Portions of the cerebellum, basal ganglia, or spinal cord are absent or malformed

is poor during the period of neural migration and relatively good during the periods of mitosis and synaptogenesis. The latter period is particularly labile insofar as at that age there is evidence of considerable regeneration, sprouting, and cell genesis.

In the human, mitosis is largely complete around the beginning of the third trimester, which in turn is characterized by extensive migration. Migration is largely complete around birth and synaptogensis peaks during the first year of life. The straightforward prediction from the studies of laboratory animals is that the worst time for cerebral injury is in the third trimester and the best time is probably around 8–12 months of age.

The Nature of the Injury

The adult brain can be injured in numerous ways, including stroke, head trauma, and neurosurgical excision for disease. The literature on functional recovery and rehabilitation quite reasonably has assumed that after the initial postinjury period, patients with different types of brain injuries are likely to benefit similarly from treatments. This presumption rests on the assumption, however, that the reparative processes that spontaneously begin after injury are similar for different types of injuries. A recent study by Gonzalez and Kolb (2003) leads us to question this assumption.

These authors gave rats equivalent lesions of the sensorimotor cortex but produced the damage either by aterial occlusion, vascular stripping, or surgical suction. The behavioral outcomes were similar in three groups, with severe chronic motor symptoms in the contralateral limbs. Similarly, the infarct volumes were essentially identical across the groups. What was surprising, however, was that when the authors examined the morphology of neurons in the striatum and perilesional area, they found that each group was different. For instance, the brains with suction lesions showed atrophy of dendritic fields, much like the middle panel in Figure 1.5, whereas the brains with vascular stripping showed reconfigured fields, much like those in the bottom panel of Figure 1.5. The important feature of this study is not only that different types of injuries

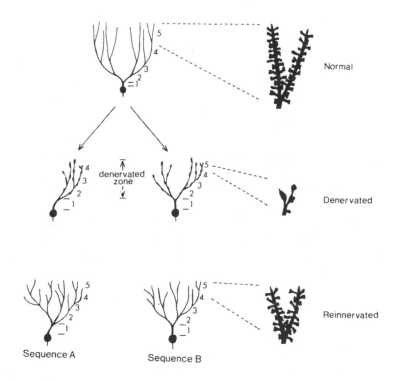

FIGURE 1.5. Changes in dendritic morphology of the hippocampal granule cells after denervation. The dendrites initially retract and then regrow. The regrowth is not the same as the original growth, and the dendrites remain somewhat stunted. Adapted from Steward (1991). Copyright 1991 by Plenum Press. Adapted by permission.

have different morphological sequelae but also that the capacity for further sprouting and regeneration is not equivalent (see also Szele, Alexander, & Chesselet, 1995). That is, because there are limitations to the amount of reparative change that may be possible after injury, it seems likely that cells with no spontaneous change may have the potential for greater change than those that have significantly remodeled without intervention. This conclusion has obvious implications for rehabilitation of human patients, although we unaware of any direct studies on this issue.

Hormones

The levels of circulating hormones play a role not only in determining the structure of the developing brain but also in controlling the morphology of neurons in the adult brain both with and without injury. The complexity of the effects of circulating hormones on neuronal morphology in the adult is clearly illustrated in a comparison of two cerebral regions. For example, Gould, Tanapat, Rydel, and Hastings (2000) have shown that estrogen levels are correlated with synapse density in the hippocampus: Ovariectomy produces a dramatic drop in spine density that is reversed by estrogen replacement. Curiously, the opposite is true in the neocortex: Ovariectomy produces a significant increase in spine density that is reversed by estrogen (e.g., Stewart & Kolb, 1994).

These estrogen-related changes have important implications for post-injury reparative processes. The presence of estrogen ought to stimulate synaptogenesis in the hippocampus but inhibit synaptogenesis in the cortex, which presents an obvious conundrum for brain-injured postmenopausal women on hormone replacement therapy. Presumably a decision must be made about the extent of injury and potential for reparative processes in the hippocampus versus neocortex. We note, too, that circulating hormones may have a different effect on neuronal survival after injury than they do on subsequent reparative processes. For example, although it is frequently argued that estrogen may be neuroprotective after cortical injury, Forgie and Kolb (1998, 2003) have found estrogen to disrupt recovery from cortical injury. This is clearly an emerging issue in women's health that requires systematic investigation. Indeed, recent studies have suggested that hormone replacement therapy with estrogen and progestin may hasten cognitive decline in older women, a result that was unexpected and potentially important (Rapp et al., 2003; Shumaker et al., 2003).

Genetic Factors

Like all cells, neurons have the machinery to produce a wide variety of proteins, which for neurons can be used for manufacturing synaptic structures, axons, neurochemicals, and so on. The production of proteins is ultimately controlled by messenger RNA (ribonucleic acid) so anything that influences the genetic code has the potential to influence reparative processes in the brain. One mechanism for influencing genetic expression is through the production of immediate early genes. Two such genes, *c-fos* and *c-jun*, have been studied extensively (e.g., Dragunow, Currie, Faull, Robertson, & Jansen, 1989). These genes are virtually unexpressed in quiet conditions but can be activated by a wide range of sensory stimuli and behaviors. Thus, within an hour or so of some particular experience there can be genetic changes that can influence protein production in neurons. Hence, it appears that experience can modify behavior through changes in gene expression. This is potentially important for designing therapies for brain-injured patients because we could predict that the optimal conditions for therapeutic effectiveness will be under conditions that favor genetic changes. The development of new genetic screening procedures, known as gene-chip arrays, have allowed investigators to look at something on the order of 30,000 genes at once. To date, there have been no studies demonstrating how different therapies can influence the expression of genes in such studies, but this is clearly the grist for studies in the future.

Unmasking and Latent Pathways

Wall and Egger (1971) used microelectrode recordings to map the somatosensory thalamus of rats, finding that tactile stimulation of the hindlimb and forelimb activated distinctly different regions of the thalamus. They then cut the pathway from the spinal cord carrying information from the hindleg and once again they stimulated the forelimb or hindlimb. As expected, there was no response in the hindlimb regions, but the forelimb region was normal. After 3 days, however, there was a remarkable change. About two-thirds of the region that had previously exhibited evoked potentials upon stimulation of the hindleg now responded to stimulation of the forelimb.

In later experiments, Merill and Wall (1978) used cooling to block the same projections from the hindlimb to the thalamus and again looked for aberrant responses in the thalamus. Once again tactile stimulation of the hindlimb had no effect, but now they could find some cells in the hindlimb region that responded to forelimb stimulation. When the spinal cord was rewarmed these cells no longer responded to forelimb stimulation. The virtually immediate reorganization (and reversal) of the tactile thalamus led Wall and Egger (1971) to conclude that there could not have been generation of new connections or synapses. Rather, it seemed more likely that fibers from the forelimb were always connected to the hindlimb area but were kept under some form of inhibition and thus were not functional. The lesions and cooling acted to "unmask" the normally latent pathways.

Few studies have directly demonstrated that unmasking can support functional compensation after cerebral injury. There are hints that this may be possible, however. For example, Cowey and Stoerig (1989) examined the visual thalamocortical projections of monkeys with long-standing visual cortex ablations. Normally the cells in the thalamus degenerate after their cortical targets are removed, but Cowey and Stoerig (1989) were able to show that some cells remained in the lateral geniculate nucleus. These cells survived because they still had projections to regions outside the visual cortex. The authors suggested that the spared neurons participated in the residual vision that the monkeys displayed in spite of their visual cortex lesions.

Redundancy and Multiple Representations

We began the chapter by outlining principles of cerebral organization, which included the idea that functions are represented at multiple levels and in a localized and distributed manner. One implication of this organization is that there is some built-in redundancy in the brain. That is, functions can be performed using more than one brain network, albeit not as efficiently. Consider, for example, that people with surgical excision of Broca's area often have significant recovery of language functions and in some cases may have only subtle impairments (e.g., Zangwill, 1975). This is not to suggest that Broca's area is not necessary for normal language functioning; it obviously is. What we are suggesting is that the brain has a significant capacity for reorganizing neural networks representing both the external world and knowledge. This reorganization has the capacity to allow the brain to compensate for brain injury. It is the nature of this compensation that is the topic of the next chapter.

REFERENCES

Aguayo, A. J. (1985). Axonal regeneration from injured neurons in the adult mammalian central nervous system. In C. W. Cotman (Ed.), *Synaptic plasticity* (pp. 457–484). New York: Guilford Press.

Altman, J., & Bayer, S. (1993). Are new neurons formed in the brains of adult mammals?: A progress report, 1962–1992. In A. C. Cuello (Ed.), *Neuronal cell death and repair* (pp. 203–225). New York: Elsevier.

Chen, P., Goldberg, D., Kolb, B., Lanser, M., & Benowitz, L. (2002). Axonal rewiring and improved function induced by inosine after stroke. *Proceedings of the National Academy of Sciences* (USA), 99, 9031–9036.

Cowey, A., & Stoerig, P. (1989). Projection patterns of surviving neurons in the dorsal lateral geniculate nucleus following discrete lesions of striate cortex: Implications for residual vision. *Experimental Brain Research, 75,* 631–638.

De Bow, S., Kolb, B., McKenna, J., & Colbourne, F. (2003). *Sensorimotor overstimulation induces cell death after injury to sensorimotor but not visual cortex.* Manuscript submitted for publication.

Dragunow, M., Currie, R. W., Faull, R. L., Robertson, H. A., & Jansen K. (1989).

Immediate-early genes, kindling and long-term potentiation. *Neuroscience and Biobehavioral Reviews, 13,* 301–313.

Forgie, M. L., & Kolb, B. (1998) Manipulation of gonadal hormones in neonatal rats alters the morphological response to cortical neurons to brain injury in adulthood. *Behavioral Neuroscience, 117,* 257–262.

Forgie, M. L., & Kolb, B. (2003). *Estrogen disrupts recovery from cortical injury in rats.* Manuscript submitted for publication.

Gould, E., Tanapat, P., Rydel, T., & Hastings, N. (2000). Regulation of hippocampal neurogenesis in adulthood. *Biological Psychiatry, 48,* 715–720.

Gonzalez, C., & Kolb, B. (2003). A comparison the behavioral and anatomical sequelae of different models of stroke in rats. *European Journal of Neuroscience, 18,* 1950–1962.

Hebb, D. O. (1949). *Organization of behavior.* New York: McGraw-Hill.

Kolb, B. (1995). *Brain plasticity and behavior.* Mahwah, NJ: Erlbaum.

Kolb, B., Gibb, R., Gorny, G., & Whishaw, I. Q. (1998). Possible brain regrowth after cortical lesions in rats. *Behavioral Brain Research, 91,* 127–141.

Kolb, B., & Whishaw, I. Q. (2003). *Fundamentals of human neuropsychology* (5th ed.). New York: Worth/Freeman.

Kozlowski, D. A., James, D. C., & Schallert, T. (1996). Use-dependent exaggeration of neuronal injury after unilateral sensorimotor cortex lesions. *Journal of Neuroscience, 16*(15), 4776–4786.

Loesche, J., & Steward, O. (1977). Behavioral correlates of denervation and reinnervation of the hippocampal formation of the rat: Recovery of alternation performance following unilateral cortex lesions. *Brain Research Bulletin, 2,* 31–39.

Merill, E. G., & Wall, P. D. (1978). Plasticity of connection in the adult nervous system. In C. W. Cotman (Ed.), *Neuronal plasticity* (pp. 97–111). New York: Raven Press.

Merkler, D., Metz, G. A., Raineteau, O., Dietz, V., Schwab, M. E., & Fouad, K. (2001). Locomotor recovery in spinal cord-injured rats treated with an antibody neutralizing the myelin-associated neurite growth inhibitor Nogo-A. *Journal of Neuroscience, 21*(10), 3665–3673.

Milner, B. (1975). Psychological aspects of focal epilepsy and its neurosurgical management. *Advances in Neurology, 8,* 299–321.

Nieto-Sampedro, M., & Cotman, C. W. (1985). Growth factor induction and temporal order in central nervous system repair. In C. W. Cotman (Ed.), *Synaptic plasticity* (pp. 407–456). New York: Guilford Press.

Pappius, H. M. (1981). Local cerebral glucose utilization in thermally traumatized rat brain. *Annals of Neurology, 9,* 484–491.

Rapp, S. R., Espeland, M. A., Shumaker, S. A., Henderson, V. W., Brunner, R. L., Manson, J. E., et al. (2003). Effect of estrogen plus progestin on global cognitive function in postmenopausal women: The Women's Health Initiative Memory Study: A randomized controlled trial. *Journal of the American Medical Association, 289,* 2663–2672.

Schallert, T., Leasure, J. L., & Kolb, B. (2000). Experience-associated structural events, subependymal cellular proliferative activity, and functional recovery after injury to the central nervous system. *Journal of Blood Flow and Metabolism, 11,* 1513–1528.

Shumaker, S. A., Legault, C., Thal, L., Wallace, R. B., Ockene, J. K., Hendrix, S. L., et al. (2003). Estrogen plus progestin and the incidence of dementia and mild cognitive impairment in postmenopausal women: The Women's Health Initiative Memory Study: A randomized controlled trial. *Journal of the American Medical Association, 289,* 2651–2662.

Steward, O. (1991). Synapse replacement on cortical neurons following denervation. In A. Peters & P. G. Jones (Eds.), *Cerebral cortex* (Vol. 9, pp. 81–132). New York: Plenum Press.

Stewart, J., & Kolb, B. (1994). Dendritic branching in cortical pyramidal cells in response to ovariectomy in adult female rats: suppression by neonatal exposure to testosterone. *Brain Research, 654,* 149–154.

Szele, F. G., Alexander, C., & Chesselet, M. F. (1995). Expression of molecules associated with neuronal plasticity in the striatum after aspiration and thermocoagulatory lesions of the cerebral cortex in adult rats. *Journal of Neuroscience, 15,* 4429–4448.

Wall, P. D., & Egger, M. D. (1971). Formation of new connections in adult rat brains after partial deafferentation. *Nature, 232,* 542–545.

Zangwill, O. (1975). Excision of Broca's area without persistent aphasia. In K. J. Zulch., O. Creutzfeldt., & G. C. Galbraith (Eds.), *Cerebral localization* (pp. 179–196). Berlin: Springer-Verlag.

2

■ ■ ■ ■

Mechanisms of Cortical Plasticity after Neuronal Injury

Bryan Kolb

Perhaps the most significant and perplexing question facing rehabilitation researchers and practitioners is the issue of how to repair the injured nervous system in order to restore lost functions. Until recently it was generally presumed that when the nervous system was damaged, little could be done to initiate repair within the brain itself. Although it was recognized that the brain showed acute inflammatory and related responses to injury, the organization of the brain was seen as a relatively static organ after injury. Thus, rehabilitative strategies were largely aimed at developing behavioral therapies. This view, of course, ignored the fact that behavioral therapies have the potential to alter brain organization and function. It is now clear that environmental and other events can alter the organization of the normal and the injured brain, a property of the brain usually referred to as *plasticity*. It follows that if neural circuits can be modified after injury, one might anticipate some type of functional change as well. Furthermore, if neural circuits are plastic after injury, rehabilitation efforts should be designed to facilitate the plastic changes. Indeed, it is not unreasonable to suppose that some types of rehabilitation programs could actually act in a manner that interferes with plasticity, which is not an ideal situation.

In principle, there are two ways the brain could show plastic changes that might support recovery. First, recovery could result from the reorganization of remaining circuits. The general idea is that the nervous system could reorganize in some way to do "more with less." It seems unlikely, however, that a complexly integrated structure such as the cerebral cortex could undergo a wholesale reorganization of cortical connectivity, at least in the adult. Rather, recovery from cortical injury would most likely result from a change in the intrinsic organization of local cortical circuits in regions directly or indirectly disrupted by the injury. The change in the intrinsic circuitry would likely involve an increase in the number of neuronal connections, an increase that could actually be quite substantial. Second, cerebral reorganization could be stimulated by the exogenous application of different treatments that would facilitate synaptic formation. The treatments could take the form of some sort of behavioral therapy, or it might involve the application of some sort of pharmacological agent that would influence reparative processes in the remaining brain. Once again, it would seem most likely that the induced neuronal changes would be in the intrinsic organization of the cortex. One might predict that the changes are likely to be more extensive than in the case of endogenous change, in part because the treatment could act upon the whole brain. This is a double-edged sword, however, because plastic changes across the entire nervous system may not necessarily be beneficial.

The remainder of this chapter summarizes findings from studies that provide evidence that plastic changes in the brain are correlated with behavioral restitution. We begin by considering the assumptions and ideas that underlie the idea that synaptic change is related to behavioral change. We then consider the ways in which plasticity can be measured in the normal and injured brain and finally consider some of the factors that influence recovery.

ASSUMPTIONS UNDERLYING RECOVERY FROM INJURY

As we consider the properties of the brain that make it plastic, we need to consider five underlying assumptions.

1. *Structural changes in the brain underlie behavioral change*. Historically, behavioral scientists have seen the structure of the brain as incidental to the study of its function, but this is not the view of behavioral neuroscientists. Rather, the basic assumption is that not only do plastic changes in the brain underlie behavioral changes but also it is possible to identify and potentially influence those changes. It follows then that if we can understand which morphological changes are associated with functional recovery, we can direct our attentions to designing treatments that will stimulate such plastic changes. An important corollary of this assumption is that if such plastic

changes do not occur after an injury, there will be an absence of functional recovery.

2. *Plasticity is a property of the synapse.* There are both behavioral and anatomical grounds for believing that the neuron is the functional unit of the nervous system. The idea that individual neurons are the units of the nervous system is the basis of the neuron doctrine popularized by Ramón y Cajál in the early part of the 20th century. It was Hebb (1949), however, who proposed a theory that if two neurons are coincidentally active, the connection between them is strengthened. The strengthening of the synaptic connection was presumed to result from some type of change at the synapse, and although Hebb did not know what this change might be, he was influenced by the idea that the brain, and especially the cortex, is organized into ensembles of neurons that represent sensory events, thoughts, and so on. Such ensembles of neurons, which he called cell assemblies, could be distributed over relatively large areas of the nervous system or confined to localized areas, but the ensembles are composed of individual neurons, each of which can be modified by the activity of the ensemble. More recently, cognitive scientists have developed computer models of neuronal networks and demonstrated that they are capable of sophisticated statistical computations. The activity of individual neurons also can be correlated with behavior in physiological studies (e.g., Celebrini & Newsome, 1994). Thus, although the neurons are part of an ensemble, the activity of individual neurons is significant and, in the current context, changes in the activity of individual neurons form the basis of brain plasticity.

3. *Functions are relatively localized in the brain, a property that places constraints upon functional plasticity after injury.* Sensory information, knowledge, and the control of movement are represented at multiple levels in the nervous system, beginning in the spinal cord and sensory receptors (such as the eye and ear) and ending in the cerebral cortex. Within each level functions are found in relatively discrete regions, each of which is characterized by a unique set of inputs and a unique set of outputs (see Figure 2.1). For example, information coming to the occipital lobe travels from the eye to subcortical areas, then to visual area 1 (V1) where it is processed, and then is sent on to other visual regions such as V2. In the absence of input from the eye, there is no processing in V1. Similarly, if V1 is completely removed, there is no input to V2 and no processing in V2. This point is critical in understanding the possibility of functional restitution after injury. If a brain region, such as V1, is only partially damaged, one could imagine that some change in the property of neural networks in V1 could reorganize the function of the remaining part of V1 and possibly facilitate some type of functional improvement. But what if V1 is completely, or even substantially, absent? It follows that downstream visual areas, such as V2, will not be provided with appropriate inputs and no amount of reorganization in V2 could instantiate functional recovery. The localization of functions thus places significant constraints on recovery of function.

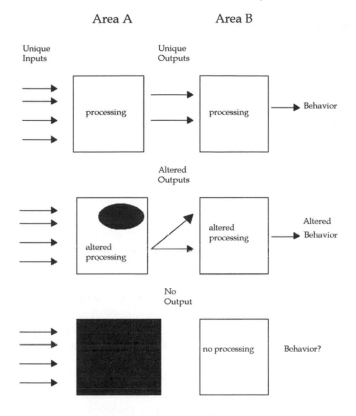

FIGURE 2.1. Unique inputs go to cerebral area A, which in turn processes the information and sends unique outputs to a second cerebral area (B). Area B sends outputs that produce some form of behavior. When Area A is partially damaged, there is a change in the inputs to Area B, which leads to a an alteration in behavior. When Area A is completely destroyed, there is no input to Area B from Area A, and thus behavior is severely disrupted.

4. *The principal mechanism of functional improvement after injury is compensation rather than recovery.* The terms "compensation" and "recovery" are often used interchangeably, but they are decidedly different. This can be illustrated by the "three-legged cat solution." Consider that cats that lose a leg to accident (and subsequent veterinary treatment) quickly learn to compensate for the lost limb and become quite mobile. In a sense the cats have shown recovery of function but the limb is still gone. The behavior of the cat has compensated for the lost limb. A similar explanation can account for most instances of apparent recovery of function after brain injury. Imagine a right-handed person who has a stroke that leads to the loss of the right hand and arm. Unable to

use the right hand to do daily activities such as turning the page of a book or writing one's name, the person switches to the left hand. This type of compensation is presumably associated with some type of change in the brain, but it would be quite different from a change that returned the use of the lost limb. The key point here is that when we look for plastic changes in the brain that could underlie functional improvement we need to know exactly what has changed. Similarly, when we design rehabilitative treatments, we need to know what the ultimate goal might be. Given our assumption about functional localization, it follows that treatments need to be aimed at changing tissue that is able to support the changes we want. This point has become clear in recent years from the work of Taub and his colleagues (e.g., Taub & Morris, 2001). They have shown that if people have impaired use of a limb after a stroke, and compensate by using the opposite limb, the loss of function in the impaired limb may actually become worse. In contrast, if people are forced to use the impaired limb rather than compensating with the normal limb, they may actually be able to initiate plastic changes in the injured hemisphere that can underlie some functional improvement. We return to this idea later.

5. *It will be difficult, but not impossible, to have functional recovery after brain injury*. I have argued that the constraints of cortical localization of function will prevent much functional recovery. Nonetheless, if lost neurons can be replaced after injury, such as in the case of transplantation or endogenous neurogenesis, it ought to be possible to generate at least some of the lost neuronal circuits and to show some functional recovery. This will be a tall order, however, and in the short run, it is an unlikely scenario. There first must be considerably more basic laboratory research on mechanisms stimulating neural generation.

CORTICAL PLASTICITY IN THE INTACT BRAIN

The capacity to change appears to be a basic characteristic of the nervous system and can be seen in even the simplest of organisms, such as the tiny worm *C. elegans*, which has only 302 neurons. When the nervous system changes, there is often a correlated behavioral change. This behavioral change is known by names such as learning, memory, addiction, maturation, and recovery of function. It follows logically that to understand processes such as functional recovery and plasticity, it is necessary to understand the nature of plastic processes in the intact brain.

Neural plasticity can be studied at many levels beginning with cerebral maps, and then becoming progressively more molecular to synaptic organization, physiological organization, molecular structure, and mitosis. This chapter considers each level in turn. (For a extensive review, see Shaw & McEachern, 2001.)

Plasticity in Cortical Maps

A basic principle of cortical organization is that the sensory systems each have multiple maps that provide a topographic representation of the external world. The motor and somatosensory cortices provide excellent examples in the homunculi. The size and organization of motor maps can be examined by stimulating the cortex either directly with microelectrodes or transcranially using magnetic stimulation to induce movements, or by using functional imaging to map the area of activation when subjects are engaged in different motor or sensory behaviors. Changes in the organization of maps can be used to infer plastic changes in the organization of the cortex.

Elbert, Heim, and Rockstroh (2001) and colleagues studied string instrument players as a model for how experience can alter the organization of the sensorimotor maps of the hand. The second through fifth digits of the left hand are continuously engaged in fingering the strings whereas the thumb, which grasps the neck of the instrument, is less active. The right hand moves the bow, which also involves much less finger movement. Neuroimaging showed not only that the fingers of the left hand occupied more space than the thumb or the fingers of the right hand but that the amount of change was proportional to the age that musical training began. The representational zone of the left-hand fingers was largest in those subjects who had begun regular practice before age 13, that is, before puberty. But, even if training began later in life, the representation of the relevant digits still exceeded subjects without musical training.

The details of the changes in the maps can be studied using more invasive techniques too, such as cortical microstimulation. Nudo, Plautz, and Frost (2001) examined the changes in motor maps directly in squirrel monkeys by training animals to grasp either small or large food objects from little wells. In the former case the animals used a pincer grasp of the digits to retrieve the food whereas in the latter case they used gross movements of the whole hand and wrist. As illustrated in Figure 2.2, when Nudo et al. (2001) mapped the motor cortex with microelectrodes, the area representing the digits was increased in the animals making digit movements, whereas the area representing the wrist was increased in animals making grosser movements involving the wrist. Kleim et al. (2002) have shown similar results in rats and, in addition, that there are large individual differences in maps—changes that correlate with behavioral capacity. Thus, those animals with large digit representations have better motor skills than do those with smaller ones.

Like motor maps, sensory maps are also modified by experience. For example, Pantev et al. (1998) showed a 25% increase in the cortical representation for the musical scale in musicians compared to nonmusicians. This enlargement was correlated with the age at which musicians began to practice music. Perhaps the extreme example of enhanced musical representations has been proposed by Rauschecker (2001). He notes that early blindness results in

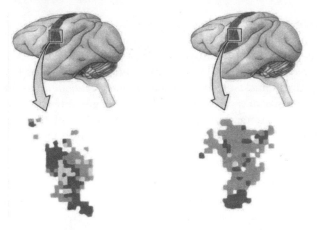

FIGURE 2.2. Differential effects of motor-skill acquisition and motor use on functional organization of the squirrel monkey motor cortex. Training procedures consisted of retrieving small pellets from either a small or large well. The monkey is able to insert the entire hand into the large well but only one or two fingers into the small well. Maps of forelimb movements were produced by microelectrode stimulation of the cortex. The maps showed systematic changes in the digit representation (dark patches) in the animals trained with the small but not the large well. Adapted from Nudo, Platz, and Milliken, 1997.

an expansion of the auditory–responsive areas in the parietal and occipital lobes—areas that would not have auditory functions in sighted people. He concludes that this finding lends credibility to the claim that blind people have greater musical abilities.

One of the best known examples of somatosensory plasticity is seen in the now extensive studies of people and monkeys with amputations. In a now classic study, Pons et al. (1991) mapped the somatosensory representation of monkeys that had been deprived of somatosensory input to one limb by a nerve transection 12 years earlier. They found that the denervated hand and arm area responded to tactile stimulation of the face on the affected side. What was most surprising, however, was that the changes in the map were very large, encompassing more than 1 cm, as shown in Figure 2.3. The major change in the map is that the face area expands to invade the denervated limb area. Parallel studies have now been done in people and show similar results (see review by Elbert et al., 2001).

Plasticity in Synaptic Organization

In the 1870s, Camillo Golgi discovered a "black reaction" that allowed him to visualize a random sample of about 5% of the neurons in the brain. This stain, which became known as a Golgi stain, was later improved by Ramón y Cajál, who used the technique to generate his now classic studies on brain development. Golgi-type stains remain valuable tools in looking at brain organization and in the past decade have provided an invaluable method of showing synaptic changes in the brain. The general assumption is that changes in the amount of synaptic space available on the dendritic field of neurons reflect changes in the synaptic organization of ensembles of neurons.

One of the most compelling sets of studies in human postmortem tissue

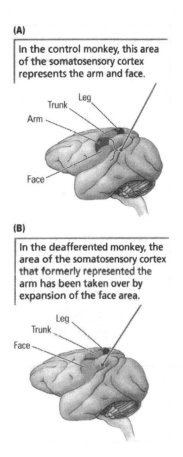

(A)

In the control monkey, this area of the somatosensory cortex represents the arm and face.

Trunk   Leg
Arm

Face

(B)

In the deafferented monkey, the area of the somatosensory cortex that formerly represented the arm has been taken over by expansion of the face area.

Leg
Trunk
Face

FIGURE 2.3. Somatosensory cortex of a control monkey (A) and a monkey that had received arm deafferentation (B). In the deafferented monkey, the area of sensory cortex that had formerly represented the hand and arm area of the body now represents the face. Thus, the area that represents the face is greatly expanded. Electrical recordings show that only the lower face has expanded. From Kolb and Whishaw (2003). Copyright 2003 by Worth Publishers. Reprinted by permission.

has been conducted by Jacobs and Scheibel (1993; Jacobs, Schall, & Scheibel, 1993). The authors began with two hypotheses. First, they suggested that there is a relationship between the complexity of dendritic arbor and the nature of the computational tasks performed by a brain area. To test this hypothesis they examined the dendritic structure of neurons in different cortical regions that involved different computational tasks. For example, when they compared the structure of neurons corresponding to the somatosensory representation of the trunk versus those for the fingers, they found the latter to have more complex cells. They reasoned that the somatosensory inputs from receptive fields on the chest wall would constitute less of a computational challenge to cortical neurons than those from the fingers and thus the neurons representing the chest would be less complex as shown in Figure 2.4. This hypothesis was correct. Similarly, when they compared the cells in the finger area to those in the supramarginal gyrus (SMG), a region of the parietal lobe that is associated with higher cognitive processes (i.e., thinking), they found the SMG neurons to be more complex.

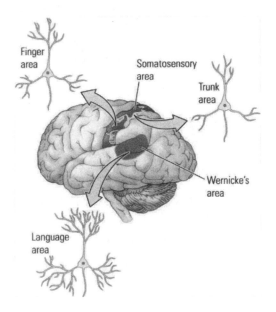

FIGURE 2.4. An illustration of Jacob & Scheibel's hypothesis that cell complexity is related to the computational demands required for the cell. Cells that represent the trunk area of the body have relatively less computational demand than that required for cells representing the finger region. In turn, cells engaged in more cognitive functions (such as language in Wernicke's area) would have greater computational demands than those engaged in higher functions. Adapted from Kolb and Whishaw (2003). Copyright 2003 by Worth Publishers. Adapted by permission.

The second hypothesis examined by Jacobs and Scheibel (1993) was that dendritic trees in all regions are subject to experience-dependent change. As a result, they hypothesized that predominant life experiences (e.g., occupation) should alter the structure of dendritic trees. Although they did not test this hypothesis directly, they did have an interesting observation. In their study comparing cells in the trunk area, finger area, and the SMG, they found curious individual differences. For example, especially large differences in trunk and finger neurons were found in the brains of people who had a high level of finger dexterity maintained over long periods (e.g., typists). In contrast, no trunk–finger difference was found in a sales representative. One would not expect a good deal of specialized finger use in this occupation and thus less complex demands on the finger neurons.

Golgi-type studies are much easier to do in studies of laboratory animals, largely because the tissue is much easier to obtain. Such studies have shown that experience-dependent changes can be seen in every species of animals tested, ranging from fruit flies and bees to rats, cats, and monkeys (for a review, see Kolb & Whishaw, 1998). The Golgi-type analyses are especially useful in studies looking at rehabilitation strategies. For example, we have seen repeatedly that animals that show good functional outcome show a significant increase in synaptic space whereas animals that fail to show functional improvement after a treatment fail to show synaptic increases.

Figure 2.5 presents an example from studies in which animals received one of two neurotrophic factors—nerve growth factor (NGF) or basic fibroblast growth factor (bFGF)—after an ischemic lesion of the motor cortex. Animals receiving NGF showed functional improvement whereas animals receiving bFGF did not, and as Figure 2.4 shows, the NGF-treated brains showed an increase in synaptic space in cortical pyramidal cells whereas the bFGF-treated brains did not (Kolb, Côté, Ribeiro-da-Silva, & Cuello, 1997). Curiously, in a later study we were able to show that although bFGF alone was ineffective in stimulating functional improvement, as was behavioral therapy, the combination of the two was effective both functionally and in stimulating synaptic change.

One of the fundamental assumptions underlying the Golgi-type studies is that an increase in synaptic space really is related to an increase in synapse numbers. Electron microscopic studies have confirmed this to be the case (e.g., Sirevaag & Greenough, 1988).

Plasticity in Molecular Structure

The demonstration of synaptic changes, either maps using or Golgi-type methods, remains phenomenological in the sense that they show that the brain changes in response to experience but what they do not show is how or why. We can assume that if a cell generates more synapses, there must be some cel-

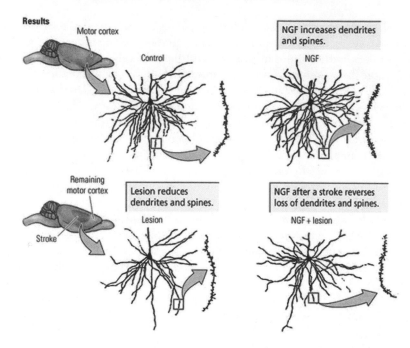

FIGURE 2.5. Cortical injury reduces dendritic branching and spine density in remaining motor cortical pyramidal neurons. The cells from NGF-treated rats show a marked increase in both dendritic branching and spine density. This plastic change is hypothesized to be responsible for the partial functional recovery in the NGF-treated rats. Adapted from Kolb and Whishaw (2003). Copyright 2003 by Worth Publishers. Adapted by permission.

lular signal that tells the cell to generate the proteins necessary to make synapses in particular locations on the dendritic field. The measurement of this presumed proteomic signal can be done in several ways, two of which are Western blot analysis and gene-chip arrays. In the former case, brain tissue is homogenized and separated into different proteins by molecular weight. Then, immunohistochemical procedures are used to identify the identity of different molecules in the tissue. Because glial cells are believed to play a major role in synaptic change, we can therefore predict that there will be more glia-related proteins in the tissue, and this is normally the case. One drawback of the Western blot technique is that it would be impractical to look at all possible proteins; thus researchers tend to focus on molecules of a particular type.

The second molecular procedure that is being used increasingly is the gene-chip array, which is a type of genetic screen. These procedures are conceptually similar to the Western blot analyses except that they analyze which genes have been affected by a particular experience. In these techniques a miniature grid (about 1 cm in diameter) that can identify up to 10,000 genes, each in a different location on the chip is reacted to a homogenate of tissue. Genes that are present in the tissue will show up in a reaction on the chip. Although such techniques are undoubtedly powerful, they have the unfortunate drawback that a lot of information about which genes change in response to, say, housing animals in complex environments versus laboratory cages can be generated, but it is far from clear what the changes actually tell us about brain function. A study by Rampon et al. (2000) provides a good example. These investigators placed rats in complex environments for different lengths of time and were able to show that there were more than 100 genes (of 11,000 genes screened) that showed a significant increase in activity in response to the experience. Of course, knowing that genes change is only a start. The real question is what the changes mean. Nonetheless, understanding how genes are altered by experience is an important step in understanding how to enhance (or reduce) plastic changes in the brain, and especially after injury.

Mitotic Activity

Changes in synaptic organization are found not only in ensembles of existing neurons but also in the generation of new neurons. The olfactory bulb provides perhaps the best example of this neurogenesis. In adulthood there is a relatively constant loss of cells in the olfactory bulb and, at the same time, a continual repopulating of the lost cells. The new cells come from a population of stem cells that line the anterior part of the subventricular zone of the lateral ventricles (Weiss et al., 1996). Cells destined to become cells in the olfactory bulb are generated here and migrate along a route known as the rostral migratory stream, ending in the bulb. Once the cells arrive in the bulb they differentiate and integrate into the existing circuitry to become functional units. The reason for this lifelong neurogenesis is not known, but we can speculate that it is related to some mechanism that allows for the loss of old olfactory memories and the generation of new ones.

A similar process also occurs in the dentate gyrus of the hippocampus and again, although the reason is not known for certain, we can speculate that it is related to functions of the hippocampus. For example, Gould and her colleagues have shown that when animals are trained in tasks that require hippocampal circuitry, there is an increase in the number of new neurons found in the hippocampus relative to the numbers found in animals that are trained in tasks not dependent on hippocampal circuits (Gould, Reeves, Graziano, & Gross, 1999). The generation of new cells in the hippocampus not only occurs when animals learn hippocampal-dependent tasks, but as Table 2.1 illustrates, the generation of new granule cells in the hippocampus is also affected by a variety of variables.

In principle, there is no reason to believe that neocortical circuits do not also incorporate new neurons, but this idea has turned out to be controversial indeed. There is little doubt that small numbers of new neurons are spontaneously produced in the injured cortex, but the issue of neurogenesis in the intact cortex is most certainly not settled. For example, although Gould, Beylin, Tanapat, Reeves, and Shor (1999) have reported evidence of new neocortical neurons in the cortex of intact monkeys, Pasko Rakic (2002) has suggested that evolution appears to have gone to great lengths to prevent the production of new neurons in most of the adult brain. He notes, for example, that although tumors made up of astrocytes (astrocytomas) are relatively common in the adult brain, there are virtually no neuron tumors (neuromas) in the adult brain, a fact that speaks to the rarity of which new neurons are produced in adults. Indeed, he has gone so far as to suggest that if we could understand why neurons are not produced more often, we might have an insight into how to stop tumorous growths of other types of body cells, including astrocytes.

The debate over whether neurogenesis actually occurs in the intact mammalian neocortex should not overshadow that fact that it most certainly occurs in the olfactory bulb and hippocampus of the intact brain and in the cerebral cortex of the injured brain. There is, therefore, the possibility that experience, including therapy after brain injury, could increase neurogenesis in the brain and that the newly formed cells could form ensembles of neurons that integrate into the brain and underlie functional improvement after injury.

TABLE 2.1. The Effect of Various Factors on Cell Proliferation and Hippocampal Granule Neuron Survival in Laboratory Rats

Factor	Proliferation	Survival
Adrenal steroids	Down	NC
Aging (rats)	Down	Down?
Adrenalectomy	Up	Up
Dentate gyrus lesions	Up	Up
Running wheel activity	Up	
High levels of estradiol	Up	Up
Serotonin agonists (e.g., Prozac)	Up	
Hippocampal-dependent learning	NC	Up
Season (short photoperiod)	Up	Up
Kindling	Up	NC
Exposure to stress	Down	Down?

Note. NC, no change. Data from Ormerod and Galea (2001).

PLASTICITY IN THE INJURED BRAIN

Just as plasticity in the normal brain can be investigated at different levels, so too can plasticity in the injured brain. To date, most work has focused on changes in maps, determined either by functional imaging or by brain stimulation, and on synaptic changes using Golgi techniques. I consider each in turn here.

Functional Imaging after Cerebral Injury

If patients can recover from stroke, despite having lost significant areas of cerebral cortex, it must mean that there has been some type of change in remaining parts of the brain. The simplest way in which to identify those parts is to do cortical mapping, either by using functional imaging techniques in human patients or by doing physiological mapping in laboratory animals. Functional imaging techniques, and especially positron emission tomography (PET), functional magnetic resonance imaging (fMRI), and transcranial magnetic stimulation (TMS), can be used repeatedly during the weeks and months after stroke to document changes in cerebral activation that might correlate with functional improvement. There have been several recent reviews of the results of functional imaging studies after stroke, which lead us to several conclusions (see especially reviews by Cramer & Bastings, 2000; Rijntjes & Weiller, 2002).

1. *Activation of the motor areas during limb movements recruits cortical areas along the rim of cortical injury.* In addition, there is often a larger area of the motor cortex activated for a given movement. For example, hand or limb movements often activate regions of the face area, possibly because of intact pyramidal tract fibers leaving the face area.

2. *If the primary sensorimotor cortex survives a stroke, there is likely to be some functional improvement over time, even if there is hemiparesis immediately after the stroke.* Although the efferent fiber tracts may be damaged, which leads to the hemiparesis, it remains possible to activate the remaining cortex. Functional improvement is correlated with the appearance of this activation. The result is that stroke patients tend to activate much larger areas of cortex, and especially parietal and premotor areas, than do control subjects making similar movements.

3. *Reorganization of maps is not restricted to one hemisphere after a unilateral injury, but similar changes occur bilaterally.* Thus, although the performance of a unilateral motor task largely activates only the contralateral cortex, after stroke there is a marked increase in bilateral activation. The increased activation in the contralateral hemisphere is not restricted to motor areas, however. Patients with disturbances of language may show activation in the complementary tissue in the opposite hemisphere.

4. *The capacity for reorganization declines with increasing size of stroke and increasing age.* The relationship to stroke size likely reflects the fact that the presence of incompletely damaged regions, such as Wernicke's area, are good predictors of functional improvement. This conclusion is in line with our assumption regarding localization of function.

5. *There is considerable variability in map changes across stroke victims.* The variability may be related to preinjury differences in map organization, which presumably reflects both genetic differences and preinjury experience. The genetic differences might be especially important in left-handers, who may already show some bilateral activation for language or movement. Rijntjes and Weiller (2002) note that the extent of activation of the right hemisphere during language tasks is highly variable and that the pattern of activation in those people who have shown recovery from Wernicke's aphasia is remarkably similar to the maximal areas of right-hemisphere activation seen in normal brains.

One basic assumption of the imaging studies is that changes in map organization are actually the basis for functional improvement. One way to test this hypothesis is to disrupt the enhanced activation that develops after injury. This can be accomplished by using TMS. Although there are few studies of this sort in stroke patients, studies of people with altered maps for other reasons are instructive. Cohen, Chen, and Celnik (1999) delivered TMS to blind and sighted subjects who were reading Braille or embossed roman letters. Stimulation of the occipital areas disrupted reading and induced phantom tactile sensations in the early blind, but not sighted, subjects. Thus, the occipital cortex had been recruited for tactile processing in the blind subjects and the TMS disrupted the expanded tactile maps. These results indicate that cortical plasticity can play a functionally compensatory role and provide a strategy for studying the basis of functional improvements in brain-injured subjects.

Physiological Mapping after Cerebral Injury

The advantage of direct electrophysiological mapping after cerebral injury is that subtle changes in map organization can be more easily shown than in imaging studies that are constrained by the limits of resolution of the techniques. Perhaps the most elegant studies have been done by Nudo, Wise, S. Fuentes, and Milliken (1996; Nudo, Plautz, & Milliken, 1997). These investigators mapped the motor cortex of monkeys to identify the hand and digit areas of the motor cortex. When they removed a portion of the digit area, they found that the monkeys showed reduced use of the contralateral hand. When they remapped the motor cortex, they found that they were unable to produce movements of the lower portion of the limb, wrist, and digits, as illustrated in Figure 2.6. That is, the hand area was gone from the cortical map, and only a stump of the upper arm remained. They subjected additional animals to the same procedure, except that following surgery

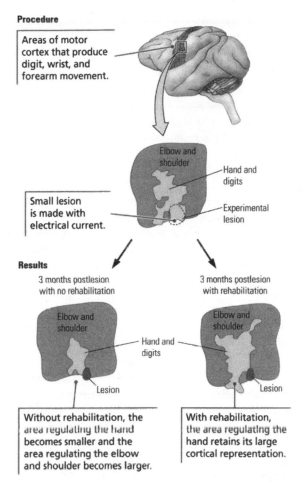

Procedure

Areas of motor cortex that produce digit, wrist, and forearm movement.

Elbow and shoulder

Hand and digits

Small lesion is made with electrical current.

Experimental lesion

Results

3 months postlesion with no rehabilitation

3 months postlesion with rehabilitation

Elbow and shoulder

Hand and digits

Elbow and shoulder

Lesion

Lesion

Without rehabilitation, the area regulating the hand becomes smaller and the area regulating the elbow and shoulder becomes larger.

With rehabilitation, the area regulating the hand retains its large cortical representation.

FIGURE 2.6. Effect of experience on the cortical representation of the forelimb in the motor cortex of a monkey after brain damage. The cortical representation of the digit, wrist, and forearm is made using microstimulation. A small lesion is then made in the area indicated by the dashed lines. When the cortex is remapped months later, the map has reduced in size much beyond the area of the lesion. Further, the map has a larger representation of the elbow and shoulder than in the pre-injury map. In monkeys that received rehabilitation, the hand area maintains its size. Adapted from Kolb and Whishaw (2003). Copyright 2003 by Worth Publishers. Adapted by permission.

they provided therapy for the affected limb, which consisted of substantial forced use. The good limb was bound so that the monkey was forced to use the affected limb. When they examined the motor map of these monkeys again, the hand and digit area was present, but the area that subserved the digits—which had had its cortical representation removed—was not restored. Nevertheless, even though the representation for the affected digits was not restored, therapy did allow some recovery of the use of those digits. Presumably, the movements made by the digits that had lost their cortical representation were mediated by the representations of the remaining digits.

The significant feature of the Nudo experiments is the importance of therapy. Therapy is necessary to maintain the functions of the undamaged cortex and the movements they represent. Therapy can also enable compensation for the affected body parts. Parallel studies have been performed in rats by Kleim et al. (2002), with the same general findings. The next step in the Nudo and Kleim studies is to use Golgi or electron microscopic techniques to examine changes in synaptic organization related to the map changes. Such studies have been completed in intact brains and are in progress for the injured brain (e.g., Kleim et al., 2002).

Synaptic Organization After Injury

As a general rule of thumb we can state that when neurons lose connections there is a retraction of dendritic processes and when neurons gain connections there is an extension of dendritic branches and/or an increase in spine density. Thus, when the brain is injured and neurons are lost there will be a decrease in connections for some neurons, and as the brain reorganizes there will be a subsequent increase. For example, when we removed frontal cortex in adult rats we found an initial drop in dendritic arborization in proximal cortical regions such as the motor cortex (see Figure 2.5). This atrophy slowly resolved and four months later there was a significant increase in dendritic morphology, which was correlated with the partial restitution of function on both motor and cognitive tasks (e.g., Kolb, 1995). This type of compensatory change has been described after injury to the both the neocortex and hippocampus (e.g., Kolb, 1995; Steward, 1991) and can likely occur after damage to subcortical regions as well.

We noted earlier that treatments such NGF can stimulate dendritic changes (Figure 2.5), which are correlated with functional recovery.

FACTORS AFFECTING RECOVERY

One characteristic of functional change after cerebral injury is its variability. I noted earlier, for example, that changes in maps shown by functional imaging studies of brain-injured subjects showed considerable variability in the extent of change and in the degree of altered activational patterns. Although we suggested that some of this difference is likely due to preinjury experience, a variety of other factors can influence functional outcome. Although space prohibits an extensive review of these factors, a general overview provides a flavor for how these factors can influence functional outcome after cerebral injury.

Age

It has been known since the time of Broca that children seem to have a better outcome after early injury than do adults, but it is only recently that it has begun to be understood why this might be so. The first systematic studies showing better recovery from brain injury during infancy than in adulthood were done by Margaret Kennard, who studied the effects of motor cortex lesion in infant monkeys. Her seminal observation was that the animals with early lesions showed better recovery of motor functions than those with injuries in adulthood (e.g., Kennard, 1942). Teuber (1975) later termed this observation the "Kennard principle." But not all studies have shown that earlier is better. Hebb (1949) postulated that brain injury early in life will, under some circumstances, result in more severe behavioral disruption than similar damage later in life. In other words, Hebb proposed essentially the opposite of the Kennard principle. He based his hypothesis on his observation that children with perinatal injuries to the frontal lobe appeared to fare worse in adulthood than did children with injuries later in life or in adulthood.

Subsequent studies with laboratory animals have shown that both Kennard and Hebb were right. Three factors turn out to be important in the apparent Kennard Hebb difference. The first factor is the exact developmental age at injury. Because different species are born at different developmental times it is possible to vary the age at injury in a systematic way (e.g., Kolb, 1995; Villablanca & Hovda, 2000; Villablanca, Hovda, Jackson, & Gayek, 1993). We can now reach the following conclusions.

1. If the cerebral cortex is damaged while neurogenesis is still ongoing, the brain is able to compensate by making more neurons and there is a relatively better functional outcome than if injury is in adulthood.
2. If there is damage during the time of neural migration, there is a poor functional outcome.
3. Injury during the peak time of synaptogenesis allows for compensatory synaptogenesis and correlated functional improvement.

In human terms, this means that injury during the third trimester, including around birth, will lead to a poor functional outcome because this is the time of maximum migration. In contrast, injury during the next 18 months or so will allow a better outcome because this is the time of peak synaptogenesis. Studies in laboratory animals, such as rats, have shown a similar pattern. Damage during the first postnatal week, which is a time of postmitotic neuronal migration allows little functional recovery, whereas damage during the second postnatal week, which is the time of maximum synaptogenesis, allows for quite remarkable recovery (e.g., Kolb, 1995).

The second and third factors influencing the effects of early injury are the location of the injury and the nature of the behavior measured. Damage to language areas in humans allow unusually complete functional recovery of language, but such children still have significant deficits on tests of executive functions (e.g., Kolb, 1995). Although few laboratories have systematically looked at the relative recovery after injury to different cortical regions on the same developmental day, Kolb and his colleagues have shown that damage to prefrontal and anterior cingulate regions in the second postnatal week allow nearly complete functional recovery. But damage to the posterior parietal region at the same time is associated with a far less favorable functional outcome (Kolb & Whishaw, 1989; Kolb & Cioe, 1998).

Although Kennard did not study anatomical change, she predicted that there would be some sort of corresponding change in the remaining cortical cells that would account for the good functional outcome, which turns out to be the case. In a series of studies, Kolb and his colleagues have shown this to be the case: Damage during the first few days of life is associated with dendritic atrophy (and thus relatively fewer synapses per neuron) in the remaining cortical neurons, whereas damaged in the second week is associated with synaptogenesis. One exception is seen in animals with posterior parietal injuries, but recall that there was less complete recovery after these lesions. Curiously, the increased synaptogenesis was associated with changes to the intrinsic circuitry of the cortex and not to the production of anomalous connections to cortical or subcortical regions (Kolb, Gibb, & van der Kooy, 1994). Rather, animals with poor functional outcomes were more likely to have anomalous connections, which presumably interfered with function.

But age is not just related to being very young: There is a gradient of severity of functional loss that is related to age during adulthood as well. For example, Teuber (1975) reported that on a number of tests, recovery by soldiers from natural lesions is greater in the 17–20 age group than in the 21–25 age group, which in turn is greater than in the age group 26 and over. Similarly, Milner (1975) reports that patients over 40 who have removals near the posterior temporal speech zone in the left hemisphere show less recovery than do younger patients. It is noteworthy that age does not always appear as a significant factor in studies of recovery, as reported by Kertesz (1988). Age is also a contributing factor to many kinds of brain damage; that is, strokes and other kinds of brain abnormality are common in older people, and these are just the people who may be showing declines in motor and cognitive function due to the normal processes of aging. Thus, recovery may tend to be obscured by aging.

Time

By time, we mean the amount of time since injury. We noted in the previous chapter that the brain undergoes a cascade of inflammatory and other changes after injury. These changes produce temporary behavioral losses that can clear in time and that are unrelated to experience or other treatments (Whishaw, 2000). In addition, studies of both human patients and laboratory animals have shown that there can be a gradual functional improvement that may continue for weeks, or in the case of humans, even months or years. Although the bases of these behavioral improvements are largely conjecture at this point, there are dendritic changes that can take months to develop, and these are correlated with functional improvement (Kolb, 1995).

Individual Differences

There are at least four types of individual differences that appear to influence cerebral plasticity and functional restitution. The first is intelligence. It is generally believed that people with superior intelligence will show better recovery than those with lower intelligence. There is no clear reason why this would be, although it is possible that whatever neural properties allow for higher intelligence may also provide an advantage after injury. For example, people of higher intelligence may have more plastic brains and thus respond better to injury, although this is not easy to prove. Recall, however, that Jacobs, Schall, and Scheibel (1993) showed that people with more education have more cortical synapses so the plasticity hypothesis appears at least superficially viable. Alternatively, people of higher intelligence may be able to generate more strategies to solve problems than less intelligent people. One complication is that although the ultimate recovery of a very intelligent individual may be excellent in relation to the recovery of others, the actual residual deficit may be equal simply because the very intelligent person would normally function at a higher level.

Handedness and sex, both for much the same reason, may influence the outcome of brain damage. A number of theories argue that female and male brains differ in both anatomy and functional organization, with less functional lateralization shown in imaging studies in the female (for a review, see Kolb & Whishaw, 2003). Given the imaging evidence in brain-injured patients discussed earlier, it seems likely that if females have more bilateral functional activation, they ought to show more functional recovery. Likewise, familial left-handers appear to be less lateralized in function than right-handers, again providing an advantage for recruiting undamaged regions after brain injury.

It is not possible to study the role of handedness in recovery in laboratory animals, but there is now a considerable literature on gonadal-hormone-dependent differences in cortical architecture in both brain-injured and intact laboratory animals. It is clear from such studies that manipulation of gonadal hormones can influence functional recovery after cerebral injury (e.g., Clark & Goldman-Rakic, 1989; Kolb & Cioe, 1996; Kolb & Stewart, 1995; Stein, 2001). The effect of gonadal hormones may vary, however, with the timing after injury. There is now good evidence that progesterone and likely estrogen afford significant advantage in the immediate postinjury period, partly because progesterone has anti-inflammatory properties and estrogen acts as a neuroprotectant (e.g., Stein, 2001). In contrast, the presence of estrogen may interfere with functional recovery as neural circuits are reorganizing. For example, estrogen appears to suppress synaptogenesis (Steward & Kolb, 1994). Indeed, the fact that estrogen is not present during the time of maximal synaptogenesis during development may provide an important clue to whether it is advantageous to have it present during periods of postinjury plasticity.

One final individual difference is personality. The role of personality in recovery is difficult to evaluate, but it is widely thought that optimistic, extroverted, and easygoing people have a better prognosis following brain injury. One reason could be that such people are more likely to comply with rehabilitation programs. One complication, of course, is that brain damage may change personality. For example, patients with postinjury depression might be expected to show poorer, or at least slower, recovery.

Experience

It would seem logical that people with brain injuries should be placed into a rehabilitation program of some sort. Surprisingly, however, the nature of the optimal program, the timing of the initiation of the program, or even the duration of the program is not well understood. Although it is often assumed that both speech and physiotherapies are effective, the role of any specific therapy is a matter of debate. Consider, for example, that patients getting speech therapy not only get speech training but also get daily contact with the therapist. Much of this interaction will be social and not strictly related to language training.

The importance of nonspecific stimulation cannot be understated. There is growing evidence that patients who are placed in a dedicated stroke unit, rather than treated on an outpatient basis, are likely to show a better outcome. A stroke unit will have a variety of professional rehabilitation therapists working together and providing stimulation for much of the waking day. Studies of laboratory animals have consistently shown that the single most successful treatment strategy for optimizing functional recovery is placing animals in complex, stimulating environments (e.g., Johansson & Belichenko, 2002). But this is not to suggest that rehabilitation therapies are not useful. Indeed, the laboratory studies showing that specific types of training can alter motor maps suggest otherwise. Consider two examples.

Edward Taub and his colleagues have developed "constraint-induced movement therapy." This therapy was based on the notion that after stroke, many patients have initial hemiparesis and develop strategies to use the unimpaired, opposite, limb. In doing so, the patients failed to attempt to use the impaired limb. The goal of constraint-induced therapy is to force patients to use the affected limb for several hours a day over a period of weeks. This use is accomplished by placing the unaffected limb in a sling and forcing the patient to perform daily activities with the impaired limb. In addition, patients are given various tasks to practice with the affected limb—tasks such as picking up objects or turning the pages of magazines. This therapy is affective in stimulating sometimes dramatic improvement in the affected limb.

One explanation for the improvement with constraint-induced therapy is that the motor training stimulates plastic changes in the brain, leading to an enlargement of the motor representation of the affected arm and hand (see also Nudo's study described earlier). In one study, Joachim Liepert and colleagues measured this increase by using TMS both before and after 12 days of constraint-induced therapy. They found that the training stimulated an increase in the area of the cortex representing the paretic hand. The increase was dramatic: There was a 50% increase in map size after 12 days of training and this increase was still present 6 months later. The location of the map expansion varied from patient to patient, presumably because the precise area of injury varied across individuals.

PHARMACOLOGICAL THERAPIES

There has been a long-standing interest in the use of pharmacological therapies for ameliorating the effects of brain damage. The general idea is to use compounds that will facilitate plastic changes in the brain. For example, psychomotor stimulants such as amphetamine or nicotine are known to stimulate changes in cortical and subcortical circuits in the normal brain (e.g., Brown & Kolb, 2001; Lena & Changeux, 1999; Robinson & Kolb, 1999). Given the power of these agents in stimulating plastic changes in the brain, it is hypothesized that administering these compounds after injury will stimulate plastic changes that support functional improvement and preliminary clinical studies support the hypothesis (e.g., Feeney & Sutton, 1987; Goldstein, 2000).

One complication of using psychomotor stimulants is that a large segment of the population has been exposed to nicotine preinjury. The question thus arises whether preinjury exposure will influence subsequent functional effects of cerebral injury. Laboratory studies by Brown, Gonzalez, and Kolb (2000; Brown, Gonzalez, Whishaw, & Kolb, 2000) have shown that preinjury treatment with nicotine is without functional benefit whereas postinjury treatment is beneficial after either frontal or hippocampal injury. We note, parenthetically, that the effect of nicotine is studied by giving animals nicotine alone and not in conjunction with smoke and other contaminants related to taking nicotine by smoking tobacco. It seems likely that postinjury smoking would not be the ideal treatment, especially after stroke.

Neurotrophic Factors

Basic neurobiological research over the past decade has shown that there are several proteins that have the property of stimulating neurogenesis as well as synaptogenesis both during development and in adulthood. Two classes of such proteins have been identified (see Table 2.2). These compounds have generated considerable interest because of their potential for treatment of dementing diseases (e.g., Hefti, Hartikka, & Knusel, 1989) as well as recovery from injuries (e.g., Hagg, Louis, & Varon, 1993). I describe herein one example of the effect of neurotrophic factors on recovery and dendritic growth.

I noted earlier that the administration of NGF stimulated functional improvement that was correlated with synaptogenesis (Kolb, Côté, Ribeiro-da-Silva, & Cuello, 1997). In subsequent studies we have examined the effect of other factors, and in particular basic fibroblast growth factor (bFGF). bFGF is particularly interesting both because psychomotor stimulants transiently increase bFGF (Flores & Stewart, 2000) and because bFGF acts to enhance synaptogenesis. Preliminary studies by Kawamata, Alexis, Dietrich, and Finklestein (1996) suggested that administration of bFGF after stroke can stimulate functional improvement, although the effects are small and task-dependent. Later studies by Witt-Lajeunesse and Kolb (2003) are intriguing because although they show that bFGF alone has a minimal effect on recovery from

TABLE 2.2. Molecules Exhibiting Neurotrophic Activities

Proteins initially characterized as neurotrophic factors
    Nerve growth factor (NGF)
    Brain-derived neurotrophic factor (BDNF)
    Neurotrophin-3 (NT-3)
    Ciliary neurotrophic factor (CNTF)

Growth factors with neurotrophic activity
    Fibroblast growth factor, acidic (aFGF or FGF-1)
    Fibroblast growth factor, basic (bFGF or FGF-2)
    Epidermal growth factor (EGF)
    Insulin-like growth factor (ILGF)
    Transforming growth factor (TGF)
    Lymphokines (Interleukin 1, 3, 6 or IL-1, IL-3, IL-6)
    Protease nexin I, II

Cholinergic neuronal differentiation factor

Note. For reviews, see Hefti et al. (1989) and Hagg et al. (1993).

motor cortex injury, given in combination with either complex housing or behavioral therapy, it was remarkably effective in stimulating functional improvement. Furthermore, this improvement was correlated with increased synaptogenesis in the remaining motor regions.

One important aspect of the actions of neurotrophic factors is that their endogenous production is potentiated by experience (e.g., Kolb, Forgie, Gibb, Gorny, & Rowntree, 1998). Thus, it is possible that one mechanism whereby experience facilitates functional recovery is by increasing the endogenous production of neurotrophic factors, which in turn stimulate synaptic changes. One experience that appears to be especially effective is exercise (Cotman & Berchtold, 2002). For example, allowing animals to spontaneously run in running wheels (or explore complex environments) can increase levels of growth factors, stimulate neurogenesis, increase resistance to brain injury, and improve learning and mental performance. The production of neurotrophic factors is presumed to be critical to this cascade of effects and suggests that exercise should be a simple means to promote brain plasticity. We must note, however, that the mere act of being exercised in the absence of the learning of a motor or mental task does not appear to produce synaptic changes (Kleim et al., 1998; Robinson & Kolb, 1999). The prediction would be that animals given exercise ought to learn faster and show more rapid changes in synaptic organization than animals not given exercise.

Brain Tissue Transplants and Stem Cell Induction

The idea of transplanting neural tissue in mammals and the techniques for doing so go back to the first decade of this century. Yet until recently, the possibility that neural transplantation had any practical application was viewed as rather remote. During the 1980s it was discovered that if fetal tissue containing immature cells from particular brain regions was dissected out and placed into the appropriate region of a recipient animal, the tissue would grow and integrate into the host brain. Although such a procedure would be impractical for repairing damage to a complex circuit such as the neocortex, it was believed that transplantation of specific cell types, such as dopaminergic cells from the brainstem, could be beneficial to patients missing these specific cells, such as Parkinson patients. There have now been more than 100 patients who have received transplants. Although there have been positive reports on individual cases, there is considerable variation across patients with some suggestions that relief from symptoms is minor or only short-lived in many patients (see Polgar, Morris, Reilly, Bilney, & Sandberg, 2003, for a review). There is, however, another approach to transplanting fetal tissue: the stimulation of stem cells within the host brain by using growth factors. The general idea is that because the brain is capable of making new neurons even in adulthood, it ought to be possible to potentiate the production of new neurons after injury. If these new neurons can be induced to migrate to the site of injury, and the right conditions are present for the cells to integrate into the host brain, functional improvement may be possible. An alternate approach is to take stem cells from a patient's brain or perhaps even from some other part of a patient's body (e.g., bone marrow), culture the cells to form thousands or millions of neurons of a particular type (e.g., dopaminergic cells) and then place these cells into the injured brain. In principle, the cells will differentiate and integrate their circuitry into the intact brain. Preliminary studies suggest that both of these procedures are viable, at least in principle.

Implications for Rehabilitation

We began the chapter by suggesting that the most perplexing question facing rehabilitation researchers and practitioners is the issue of how to repair the injured nervous system in order to restore lost functions. We have examined the nature of brain plasticity and the factors that affect plasticity, but we are still left with the question of how this knowledge might affect the development of rehabilitation strategies in the short run. Five basic principles related to rehabilitation design can be extracted from our discussion.

   1. Effective therapies will be those that stimulate morphological changes in the brain. We have seen that behavioral change is always correlated with some form of plastic change in the structure of the brain and thus for therapies to be effective, they must stimulate change.
   2. Because the brain begins to make plastic changes shortly after injury, it is advantageous for therapies to take advantage of the brain's plastic state and to shape the changes in ways that are beneficial. There are two corollaries of this conclusion. First, if therapy is delayed until the endogenous plastic changes in the brain are completed, it will be more difficult to reinitiate changes. Second, because not all endogenous changes will be beneficial, such as the changes that occur when patients disuse one side of the body after stroke, it will be necessary to reverse some changes, which may prove difficult.
   3. Because focused behavioral therapies are less effective than multidimensional behavioral therapies in laboratory studies, it seems likely that an important rehabilitation strategy is to develop multidimensional programs, such as would be found in dedicated stroke units.
   4. The brain is responsive to both behavioral and chemical therapies. The combination of these therapies is likely to be more effective than either alone. We saw an example in the facilitating effects of neurotrophic factors and behavioral therapies in stimulating functional improvement after cortical injury.
   5. The effectiveness of different therapies is likely to vary with factors such as age, sex, and education. Future work will need to identify exactly how these factors interact with different rehabilitation strategies.

REFERENCES

Brown, R., Gonzalez, C.R., & Kolb, B. (2000). Nicotine improves Morris water task performance in rats given medial frontal cortex lesions. *Pharmacology, Biochemistry and Behavior, 67*, 473–478.

Brown, R. W., Gonzalez, C. L. R., Whishaw, I. Q., & Kolb, B. (2000). Nicotine improvement of Morris water task performance after fornix lesions is blocked by mecamylamine. *Behavioral Brain Research, 119*, 185–192.

Brown, R. W., & Kolb, B. (2001). Nicotine sensitization increases dendritic length and spine density in the nucleus accumbens and cingulate cortex. *Brain Research, 899*, 94–100.

Celebrini S., & Newsome, W. T. (1994). Neuronal and psychophysical sensitivity to motion signals in extrastriate area MST of the macaque monkey. *Journal of Neuroscience, 14*, 4109–4124.

Clark, A. S., & Goldman-Rakic, P. S. (1989). Gonadal hormones influence the emergence of cortical function in nonhuman primates. *Behavioral Neuroscience, 103*, 1287–1285.

Cohen, L. G., Chen, R., & Celnik, P. (1999). Functional relevance of cortical plasticity. In J. Grafman & Y. Christen (Eds.), *Neuronal plasticity: Building a bridge from the laboratory to the clinic* (pp. 4–17). Heidelberg: Springer-Verlag.

Cotman, C. W., & Berchtold, N. C. (2002). Exercise: a behavioral intervention to enhance brain health and plasticity. *Trends in Neurosciences, 25*, 295–301.

Cramer, S. C., & Bastings, E. P. (2000). Mapping clinically relevant plasticity after stroke. *Neuropharmacology, 39*, 842–851.

Elbert, T., Heim, S., & Rockstroh, B. (2001). Neural plasticity and development. In C. A. Nelson & M. Luciana (Eds.). *Handbook of Developmental Cognitive neuroscience* (pp. 191–204). Cambridge, MA: MIT Press.

Feeney, D. M., & Sutton, R. L. (1987). Pharmacotherapy for recovery of function after brain injury. *Critical Reviews in Neurobiology, 3*, 135–197.

Flores, C., & Stewart, J. (2000). Basic fibroblast growth factor as a mediator of the effects of glutamate in the development of long-lasting sensitization to stimulant drugs: Studies in the rat. *Psychopharmacology, 151*, 152–165.

Goldstein, L. B. (2000). Effects of amphetamines and small related molecules on recovery after stroke in animals and man. *Neuropharmacology, 39*, 852–859.

Gould, E., Beylin, A., Tanapat, P., Reeves, A., & Shors, T. J. Learning enhances adult neurogenesis in the hippocampal formation. (1999). *Nature Neuroscience, 2*, 260–265.

Gould, E., Reeves, A. J., Graziano, M. S., & Gross, C. G. (1999). Neurogenesis in the neocortex of adult primates. *Science, 286*, 548–552.

Hagg, T., Louis, J. C., & Varon, S. (1993). Neurotrophic factors and CNS regeneration. In A. Gorio (Ed.), *Neuroregeneration* (pp. 265–287). New York: Raven Press.

Hebb, D. O. (1949). *Organization of behavior*. New York: McGraw-Hill.

Hefti, F., Hartikka, J., & Knusel, B. (1989). Function of neurotrophic factors in the adult and aging brain and their possible use in the treatment of neurodegenerative diseases. *Neurobiology of Aging, 10*, 515–533.

Jacobs, B., Schall, M., & Scheibel, A. B. (1993). A quantitative dendritic analysis of Wernicke's area. II. Gender, Hemispheric, and environmental factors. *Journal of Comparative Neurology, 237*, 97–111.

Jacobs, B., & Scheibel, A. B. (1993). A quantitative dendritic analysis of Wernicke's area in humans. I. Lifespan changes. *Journal of Comparative Neurology, 32,* 83–96.

Johansson, B. B., & Belichenko, P. V. (2002). Neuronal plasticity and dendritic spines: Effect of environmental enrichment on intact and post-ischemic rat brain. *Journal of Cerebral Blood Flow and Metabolism, 22,* 89–96.

Kawamata, T., Alexis, N. E., Dietrich, W. D., & Finklestein, S. P. (1996). Intracisternal basic fibroblast growth factor (bFGF) enhances behavioral recovery following focal cerebral infarction in the rat. *Journal of Cerebral Blood Flow Metabolism, 16,* 542–547.

Kennard, M. (1942). Cortical reorganization of motor function. *Archives of Neurology, 48,* 227–240.

Kertesz A. (1988). What do we learn from recovery from aphasia? *Advances in Neurology, 47,* 277–292.

Kleim, J. A., Barbay, S., Cooper, N. R., Hogg, T. M., Reidel, C. N., Remple, M. S., et al. (2002). Motor learning-dependent synaptogenesis is localized to functionally reorganized motor cortex. *Neurobiology of Learning and Memory, 77,* 63–77.

Kleim, J. A., Swain, R. A., Armstrong, K. A., Napper, R. M., Jones, T. A., & Greenough, W. T. (1998). Selective synaptic plasticity within the cerebellar cortex following complex motor skill learning. *Neurobiology of Learning and Memory, 69,* 274–289.

Kolb, B. (1995). *Brain plasticity and behavior.* Mahwah, NJ: Erlbaum.

Kolb, B., & Cioe, J. (1996). Sex-related differences in cortical function after medial frontal lesions in rats. *Behavioral Neuroscience, 110,* 1271–1281.

Kolb, B., & Cioe, J. (1998). Absence of recovery or dendritic reorganization after neonatal posterior parietal lesions. *Psychobiology, 26,* 134–142.

Kolb, B., Côté, S., Ribeiro-da-Silva, A., & Cuello, A. C. (1997). NGF stimulates recovery of function and dendritic growth after unilateral motor cortex lesions in rats. *Neuroscience, 76,* 1139–1151.

Kolb, B., Forgie, M., Gibb, R., Gorny, G., & Rowntree, S. (1998). Age, experience, and the changing brain. *Neuroscience and Biobehavioral Reviews, 22,* 143–159.

Kolb, B., Gibb, R., & van der Kooy, D. (1994). Neonatal frontal cortical lesions in rats alter cortical structure and connectivity. *Brain Research, 645,* 85–97.

Kolb, B., & Stewart, J. (1995). Changes in neonatal gonadal hormonal environment prevent behavioral sparing and alter cortical morphogenesis after early frontal cortex lesions in male and female rats. *Behavioral Neuroscience, 109,* 285–294.

Kolb, B., & Whishaw, I. Q. (1989). Plasticity in the neocortex: Mechanisms underlying recovery from early brain damage. *Progress in Neurobiology, 32,* 235–276.

Kolb, B., & Whishaw, I. Q. (1998). Brain plasticity and behavior. *Annual Review of Psychology, 49,* 43–64.

Kolb, B., & Whishaw, I. Q. (2003). *Fundamentals of human neuropsychology* (5th ed.). New York: Worth/Freeman.

Lena, C., & Changeux, T. P. (1999). Pathological mutations of nicotinic receptors and nicotine-based therapies for brain disorders. In J. Grafman & Y. Christen (Eds.), *Neuronal plasticity: Building a bridge from the laboratory to the clinic,* (pp. 1–15). Springer: Heidelberg.

Milner, B. (1975). Psychological aspects of focal epilepsy and its neurosurgical management. *Advances in Neurology, 8,* 299–321.

Nudo, R. J., Plautz, E. J., & Frost, S. B. (2001). Role of adaptive plasticity in recovery of function after damage to motor cortex. *Muscle and Nerve, 24,* 1000–1019.

Nudo, R. J., Plautz, E. J., & Milliken, G. W. (1997). Adaptive plasticity in primate motor cortex as a consequence of behavioral experience and neuronal injury. *Seminars in Neuroscience, 9,* 13–23.

Nudo, R. J., Wise, B. M., SiFuentes, F., & Milliken, G. W. (1996). Neural substrates for the effects of rehabilitative training on motor recovery after ischemic infarct. *Science, 272,* 1793.

Ormerod, B. K., & Galea, L. A. M. (2001). Mechanism and function of adult neurogenesis. In C. A. Shaw & J. C. McEachern (Eds.), *Toward a theory of neuroplasticity* (pp. 85–100). Lillington, NC: Taylor & Francis.

Pantev, C., Oostenveld, R., Engelien, A., Ross, B., Roberts, L. E., & Hoke, M. (1998). Increased auditory cortical representation in musicians. *Nature, 392,* 811–814.

Polgar, S., Morris, M. E., Reilly, S., Bilney, B., & Sanberg, P. R. (2003). Reconstructive neurosurgery for Parkinson's disease: A systematic review and preliminary meta-analysis. *Brain Research Bulletin, 60,* 1–24.

Pons, T. P., Garraghty, P. E., Ommaya, A. K., Kaas, J. H., Taum, E., & Mishkin, M. (1991). Massive cortical reorganization after sensory deafferentation in adult macaques. *Science, 272,* 1857–1860.

Rakic, P. (2002). Adult neurogenesis in mammals: an identity crisis. *Journal of Neuroscience, 22,* 614–618.

Rampon, C., Jiang, C. H., Dong, H., Tang, Y. P., Lockhart, D. J., Schultz, P. G., et al. (2000). Effects of environmental enrichment on gene expression in the brain. *Proceedings of the National Academy of Sciences (USA), 97,* 12880–12884.

Rauschecker, J. P. (2001). Cortical plasticity and music. *Annals of the New York Academy of Sciences, 930,* 330–336.

Reynolds, B. A., & Weiss, S. (1992). Generation of neurons and astrocytes from isolated cells of the adult mammalian central nervous system. *Science, 255,* 1613–1808.

Rijntjes, M., & Weiller, C. (2002). Recovery of motor and language abilities after stroke: The contribution of functional imaging. *Progress in Neurobiology, 66,* 109–122.

Robinson, T. E., & Kolb, B. (1999). Alterations in the morphology of dendrites and dendritic spines in the nucleus accumbens and prefrontal cortex following repeated treatment with amphetamine or cocaine. *European Journal of Neuroscience, 11,* 1598–1604.

Shaw, C. A., & McEachern, J. C. (Eds.). (2001). *Toward a theory of neuroplasticity.* Philadelphia: Taylor & Francis.

Sirevaag, A. M., & Greenough, W. T. (1988). A multivariate statistical summary of synaptic plasticity measures in rats exposed to complex, social and individual environments. *Brain Research, 441,* 386–392.

Stein, D. G. (2001). Brain damage, sex hormones and recovery: a new role for progesterone and estrogen? *Trends in Neuroscience, 24,* 386–891.

Steward, O. (1991). Synapse replacement on cortical neurons following denervation. In A. Peters & P. G. Jones (Eds.), *Cerebral cortex* (Vol. 9, pp. 81–132). New York: Plenum Press.

Stewart, J., & Kolb, B. (1994). Dendritic branching in cortical pyramidal cells in response to ovariectomy in adult female rats: Suppression by neonatal exposure to testosterone. *Brain Research, 654,* 149–154.

Taub, E., & Morris, D. M. (2001). Constraint-induced movement therapy to enhance recovery after stroke. *Current Atherosclerosis Reports, 3,* 279–286.

Teuber, H. L. (1975). Recovery of function after brain injury in man. In *Outcome of severe damage to the nervous system* (Ciba Foundation Symposium 34). Amsterdam: Elsevier North-Holland.

Villablanca, J. R., Hovda, D. A., Jackson, G. F., & Gayek, R. (1993). Neurological and behavioral effects of a unilateral frontal cortical lesions in fetal kittens: I. Brain morphology, movement, posture, and sensorimotor tests. *Behavioral Brain Research, 57,* 63–77.

Villablanca, J. R., & Hovda, D. A. (2000). Developmental neuroplasticity in a model of cerebral hemispherectomy and stroke. *Neuroscience, 95,* 625–637.

Weiss, S., Reynolds, B. A., Vescovi, A. L., Morshead, C., Craig, C. G., & van der Kooy, D. (1996). Is there a neural stem cell in the mammalian forebrain? *Trends in Neuroscience, 19,* 387–393.

Whishaw, I. Q. (2000). Loss of the innate cortical engram for action patterns used in skilled reaching and the development of behavioral compensation following motor cortex lesions in the rat. *Neuropharmacology, 39,* 788–805.

Witt-Lajeunesse, A., & Kolb, B. (2003). *Therapy and bFGF interact to stimulate recovery after cortical injury.* Manuscript submitted for publication.

3

■ ■ ■ ■

Rehabilitation
of Nonspatial Attention

Jennie Ponsford
Catherine Willmott

WHAT IS ATTENTION?

Despite the fact that the term "attention" has been the subject of study since the late 19th century and is still frequently used in many contexts, the meaning of this construct has long been an enigma for theorists, researchers, and clinicians in psychology and philosophy. One reason for this is the fact that attention is, in fact, a multidimensional concept. As Parasuraman (2000) points out: "Attention is not a single entity, but the name given to a finite set of brain processes that can interact, mutually, and with other brain processes, in the performance of different perceptual, cognitive, and motor tasks" (p. 4). As early as 1890 William James cogently proposed that attention was "the taking possession by the mind, in clear and vivid form, of one out of what seems several simultaneously possible objects or trains of thought. Focalization, concentration, of consciousness are of its essence. It implies withdrawal from some things in order to deal effectively with others" (James, 1890, p. 416). More recently, Cohen (1993) described attentional processes as follows:

> Metaphorically, attention is like the aperture and lens system of a camera. By changing the depth of field and the focal point, attention enables humans to direct themselves to appropriate aspects of external environmental effects and internal

59

operations. Attention facilitates the selection of salient information and the allocation of cognitive processing appropriate to that information. Therefore, attention
acts as a gate for information flow in the brain. (p. 3)

These definitions infer the presence of a number of dimensions of attention,
which are described within the theoretical models outlined in this chapter.

THEORETICAL MODELS OF ATTENTION
AND THEIR ANATOMICAL CORRELATES

Aspects of attention are mediated by diverse brain regions, which are linked by
neural networks, or functional systems. Numerous models of attentional systems have been proposed over the past two decades. These are by no means
mutually exclusive, and there are wide variations in the use of terminology, but
some common themes emerge.

Posner and his colleagues describe three attentional networks (Posner &
Peterson, 1990; Posner & Rothbart, 1992). The posterior network, which involves the superior colliculus, lateral pulvinar nucleus of the posterolateral
thalamus, and the posterior parietal lobe, is said to be responsible for visuospatial orienting (aligning attention with incoming sensory information or a
representation stored in memory) and shifting of attention, bringing attention
to a specific location in space and generating awareness. Damage to this system
causes object recognition difficulties and unilateral spatial neglect. The second
system is said to mediate alertness, vigilance, or sustained attention. This represents the ability to prepare and sustain alertness to process high-priority signals over extended periods. It involves the locus coeruleus in the brainstem
reticular formation and its norepinephrine input to the cortex. Posner and
Rothbart (1992) argued for a significant role of the right hemisphere, particularly the right lateral frontal cortex, in these processes. This system also involves the posterior attentional system, where the locus coeruleus has its
norepinephrine connections to the parietal lobe, pulvinar, and colliculi, facilitating object recognition and selection of high-priority visual information during vigilant states. The anterior attentional network mediates selective or focused attention—the detection or selection of signals for conscious processing
(target detection) and the ability to maintain attention in the presence of distraction or conflicting response tendencies. Selective attention is linked with
awareness and voluntary or conscious control over information processing.
This system is said to involve the anterior cingulate gyrus, the mid-prefrontal
cortex, and the basal ganglia (Posner & Rothbart, 1992).

An important distinction has been made by Shiffrin and Schneider (1977)
between automatic and controlled information processing systems. Automatic

processing, involved in routine, well-learned tasks, such as driving a car, can occur in parallel and has an unlimited capacity, whereas conscious or controlled processing is serial in nature and has a limited capacity and rate, limited by the short-term store. Controlled processes can eventually become automatic. They are learned by linking memory nodes in sequence, when stimuli are consistently mapped to responses. This is a potentially important factor in a rehabilitation context. Focused-attention difficulties are said to arise when an automatic response interferes with a response required in a consciously mediated task. Divided-attention difficulties arise from limitations in the speed of consciously controlled processing. They occur whenever controlled processing fails to deal with all the information that should be processed for optimal task performance. Capacity and speed of information processing are thus critical factors in determining the efficiency of divided attention.

Norman and Shallice (1980) further developed the concept of conscious control. They proposed the existence of the Supervisory Attentional System (SAS), which supervises the focusing and dividing of attention on nonroutine tasks, distributing conscious processing capacity over various tasks in a goal-directed fashion, via contention scheduling. Once tasks are practiced and become automatic, an action schema is formed that triggers when the stimulus is presented and the supervisory system is not needed. The SAS is seen as necessary for internally planned or voluntary actions, situations that require overcoming of habitual responses, or in which responses are not well learned or contain novel sequences of actions. Desimone and Duncan (1995) argue that the receptive fields of visual subprocessing systems perform selection from competing stimuli via inhibition in the local neural circuit. This can be biased by a top-down mechanism that selects objects that are important to the current behavior or goal. Burgess and Shallice (1996) have attributed the function of the SAS to the left prefrontal cortex, whereas Posner and DiGirolamo (2000) attribute it to the anterior cingulate. The involvement of these regions in a given task dissipates with practice (i.e., as the task performance becomes more routine).

Baddeley (1993) proposed the existence of a Central Executive, analogous to Shallice's SAS. This is said to incorporate working memory, as a means of temporary storage and manipulation during conscious information processing. Functional magnetic resonance imaging (fMRI) studies suggest that frontal structures play a role in devising strategies involved in conscious manipulation of information (D'Esposito et al., 1995; Jonides, Smith, Koeppe, & Awh, 1993).

Stuss and Benson (1986) described the frontal diencephalic brainstem system. This model combines the vigilance and anterior networks described by Posner and colleagues. According to this model, the ascending reticular activating system regulates tonic alertness (our continuing receptivity to incoming stimulation, which changes slowly over the course of the day), the diffuse thalamic projection system regulates phasic alertness (which changes quickly in preparation for response to an incoming stimulus), and the frontal, thalamic gating system regulates selective or directed attention.

A theoretical distinction has been proposed between selective and intensive attention (Clark, Geffen, & Geffen, 1989; Sturm & Willmes, 2001; Stuss & Benson, 1986; van Zomeren & Brouwer, 1994). Clark et al. (1989) define selective attention as "the selection of one input from an array of available inputs. Importantly, however, it may also involve selection from amongst the properties of a stimulus as well as selection of response in order to orient sense organs with stimulus objects" (p. 354). This concept incorporates the constructs of focused and divided attention. Intensive attention refers to the degree of attention underlying and affecting the efficiency of selection. It has been related to general level of arousal or wakefulness as well as to a more specific state of what has previously been termed "activation," "alertness," or "readiness to respond" (Clark et al., 1989; Sturm & Willmes, 2001). This concept thus incorporates both alertness and sustained attention. Stuss and Benson (1986) proposed that the frontal diencephalic brainstem system regulates intensity by a partial control over the brainstem and the diffuse thalamic projection system. It regulates selectivity by "gating" sensory pathways on the thalamic level. Using PET and fMRI data, Sturm and Willmes (2001) have provided further evidence for the role of the anterior cingulate gyrus and the dorsolateral frontal cortex in exerting a top-down control over the noradrenergic activation from brainstem structures, thought to be mediated by the reticular nucleus of the thalamus. They argue that the network controlling intensity processes exists mostly in the right hemisphere, but under conditions of phasic alertness there are additional activations of left-hemisphere frontal and parietal structures, thought to be related to attentional selectivity.

Cohen's (1993) theoretical framework of attention incorporates four component processes: sensory selective attention, response selection and control, capacity and focus, and sustained attention. The first two of these factors, sensory selective attention and response selection and control, are congruent with the construct of selective attention. Attentional capacity and focus and sustained attention represent elements of the intensity construct. Sensory selective attention refers to the processes whereby information is selected for additional cognitive processing. Its processes include sensory filtering, which occurs early in the process, selection and focusing, disengagement, and automatic shifting. Similar to Posner's posterior orienting system, Cohen posits that the parietal cortex mediates sensory selective attention. Two visual information-processing pathways are outlined, namely, the superior or dorsal occipito-parietal pathway, involving the inferior parietal lobe, which is involved in spatial selective attention, and the inferior or ventral occipitotemporal pathway, responsible for visual object recognition. Physiological studies have shown that neurons in areas along this pathway respond selectively to visual features relevant to object identification, such as color and shape, whereas those along the occipitoparietal pathway respond to spatial aspects of stimuli such as direction of motion (Desimone & Ungerleider, 1989). Desimone, Wessinger, Thomas, and Schneider (1990) have proposed a third pathway, directed to the cortex of the rostral superior temporal sulcus, that plays a role in either complex motion perception and/or the integration of object and spatial perception. There is also evidence that the dorsal and ventral pathways extend into the frontal lobes, such that the inferior prefrontal convexity, which receives information from the inferior temporal cortex, is important for keeping in mind what an object is, whereas the dorsolateral prefrontal cortex, which receives information from the parietal cortex, is important for keeping in mind where an object is. The inferior parietal area is seen as being responsible for attentional focusing within a broad frame of reference. The superior temporal lobe is responsible for attentional focusing within a narrow frame of reference. The thalamus is proposed as a central relay station of incoming and outgoing information.

The second component of Cohen's (1993) framework, response selection and control, involves intention. The process is more conscious and effortful than sensory selective attention, which can occur automatically. Executive functions, such as active switching and inhibition, are required. Frontal and subcortical structures are said to be involved in these processes. The orbital frontal area is involved in initiation and inhibition of responses. The medial frontal area, including the cingulate region, mediates focused attention and controlled processing.

Focused attention determines the allocation of attentional resources to a task. Attentional capacity is limited by both energetic (e.g., arousal) and structural (e.g., processing speed and working memory) constraints. Sustained attention is contingent upon the other three processes and is also influenced by reinforcement contingencies, fatigue characteristics, and vigilance. Vigilance is defined as a special form of sustained attention, "in which there is a demand for a high level of anticipatory readiness for low probability targets or stimulus events" (Cohen, Malloy, & Jenkins, 1998, p. 574). The midbrain reticular activating system plays a role in arousal. The amygdaloid and septal nuclei influence the salience of stimuli, and other limbic structures influence motivational aspects of attention. The hippocampus is involved in mediating *mnemonic* aspects of attention.

Mesulam (1985) proposed a functional asymmetry of attention. He proposed that the left hemisphere played an important role in attention to detail and focused attention. The right hemisphere is seen as mediating panoramic attention, alertness, and sustained attention. The right hemisphere is said to have the capacity to maintain awareness of both sides of space; hence individuals with left parietal lesions are less prone to exhibit unilateral spatial neglect.

Despite their differing terminology, many common themes emerge from these theoretical frameworks of attention. First, it would appear that there are several multifocal interconnected networks, each of which mediates some aspects of attention. The first of these are the midbrain reticular activating system and limbic structures, which mediate arousal, mood, motivation and the salience of stimuli in relation to past and recent memories, and readiness to respond, thus incorporating the concepts of sustained attention and vigilance. Second, a sensory selective attentional system, mediated by the parieto–temporo–occipital area, is responsible for the orienting, engaging, and disengaging of attention and object recognition processes, which may occur automatically. Third, an anterior system, mediated by the frontal lobes and the anterior cingulate gyrus and also involving the basal ganglia, is responsible for response selection and control, involving intentional control, active switching and inhibition, and imposition of strategies for conscious manipulation of information. The thalamus is seen as the relay station of incoming information and outgoing responses. Finally, the right hemisphere appears to mediate alertness and sustained attention, and the left hemisphere selective or focused attention. Neurons along each of these pathways respond selectively to the specific features of a stimulus relevant to their role.

Another important aspect of cortical organization is its hierarchical nature. Projections from lower-order areas to higher-order areas, termed "feedforward," originate mainly in layer III of cortex and terminate predominantly in layer IV, whereas projections from higher-order areas to lower-order areas, termed "feedback," originate mainly in layers V and VI of cortex and terminate both above and below but not in layer IV. These projections are thought to play a top-down role in perceptual processing, as with selective attention. Connections between areas at the same hierarchical level are termed "intermediate." The feedforward projection is essential for the functioning of higher-order areas, in that they cannot function in absence of lower-order input in that modality, whereas lower-order or primary areas can function in absence of higher-order input (Webster & Ungerleider, 2000).

PHARMACOLOGY OF ATTENTION

Neural networks mediate attentional and other cognitive functions via chemical pathways. The neurotransmitter systems most commonly implicated in attention include the noradrenergic system, the dopaminergic system, and the serotonergic system. These neurotransmitters are all biogenic amines.

The Noradrenergic System

Noradrenaline (NA) is supplied to the cerebral cortex principally by the locus coeruleus (LC), whose axons travel in the dorsal tegmental bundle. NA is released onto alpha-1, alpha-2 and beta receptors, each of which has three subtypes, with differential distributions in cortical laminae. There are three pathways:

1. *Locus coeruleus complex*. Axons from the locus coeruleus in the pons project to the cerebellum, spinal cord, and nearly all parts of the telencephalon and diencephalon through the median forebrain bundle, including the neocortex, hippocampus, amygdala, septum, thalamus, and hypothalamus.

2. *Lateral tegmental system*. Axons project caudally to the spinal cord to regulate cardiovascular and visceral functions, and rostral projections terminate in the hypothalaums and other diencephalic structures.

3. *Dorsal medullary group*. Fibers project to the nucleus of the tractus solitarius in the medulla which receives sensory inputs and relays it to the thalamus and cranial nerves.

The locus coeruleus noradrenergic pathways were initially thought to be involved in general arousal as their activity varies according to the sleep–wake cycle and some sensory stimuli increase cell firing. However, they were found to be inhibited during maintenance behaviors such as grooming and eating (and rapid eye movement [REM] sleep), when some level of arousal was required (Aston-Jones & Bloom, 1981). Aston-Jones (1985) proposed instead that this system was critical for vigilance. These neurons rest during maintenance behaviors, but when exposed to strong stimuli that elicit an alerting response, locus coeruleus neurons are strongly but briefly activated, preparing the brain for sensory processing. Clonidine is an alpha-adrenergic agonist which inhibits noradrenergic activity, discussed in relation to attention in the following section.

Dopamine

Dopamine constitutes up to 80% of total brain catecholamine content. The dopaminergic system has three main tracts:

1. *Nigrostriatal*. Cell bodies in the substantia nigra project to the corpus striatum and medial frontal lobes.
2. *Mesolimbic/mesocortical*. Cell bodies in the ventral–tegmental area (adjacent to the substantia–nigra) project to the cortex and limbic system.
3. *Tuberoinfundibular*. Cell bodies in the arcuate nucleus and periventricular area of the hypothalamus project to the infundibular and anterior pituitary.

Dopamine is released onto d1, d2, d3 and d4 receptors, each of which has two or more subtypes differentially distributed across the cortical laminae. d1 and d2 receptors are highly represented in the caudate nucleus, putamen, and nucleus accubens; d3 receptors are also expressed in the nucleus accumbens and caudate, whereas d4 receptor protein is expressed mainly in the cortex.

Dopamine appears to play a role in the integration of sensory, motivational, and motor functions. The nigrostriatal system is involved in motor function, and a lack of dopamine in this pathway is associated with Parkinson's disease. Drugs used to evaluate the role of dopamine in arousal and cognition include methylphenidate (a catecholamine agonist) and droperidol (a dopamine antagonist). The actions of dopamine are terminated in two ways: reuptake by presynaptic neurons and recycled, or metabolized. The primary metabolite of dopamine is homovanillic acid (HVA).

Serotonin

Serotonin is an indolealkylamine also known as 5-hydroxytryptamine (5-HT). Serotonergic cells are located in the dorsal raphe (DR) nucleus of the pons. These neurons are divided into a caudal and a rostral system. The caudal neurons descend to the spinal cord. The rostral system has dorsal and ventral pathways, and the dorsal and median raphe nuclei account for up to 80% of forebrain serotonin terminals.

1. *The rostral system* supplies projections to numerous parts of the diecephalon, basal ganglia, limbic system and cortex.
2. *The dorsal system* supplies the mesencephalic gray, inferior, and superior colliculi, and other fibers enter the median forebrain bundle to join the ventral pathway.
3. *Other pathways* innervate the cerebellum and structures in the pons and medulla (e.g., locus coeruleus).

Serotonin has also been established as a mediator of attention. It is released in response to arousing stimuli in order to aid attentional and perceptual functioning so that the most salient stimuli are attended to (Joseph, 1990).

The Role of Catecholamine Systems in Attention

The role of biogenic amine neurotransmitters in attention is highly complex, and the research in this area has progressed in three directions in the past two decades.

Selective Attention and Processing Capacity

Clark, Geffen, and Geffen (1986a, 1986b, 1987) investigated the role of catecholamines in selective attention and processing capacity using dichotic monitoring tasks. Participants were asked either to divide their attention equally between ears (divided) or to focus their attention to the left or right ear (focused). Poorer performance was observed, following droperidol (a dopamine antagonist), on both focused and divided attention tasks. It was concluded that the dopamine blockade had reduced general processing capacity rather than just focused selective attention. Methylphenidate, when administered after droperidol, reversed the effects, suggesting that release of dopamine improved attentional performance. Clonidine acts to dampen the noradrenergic coeruleocortical pathway, and hence the activity of central noradrenergic neurons. As with droperidol, its administration resulted in poorer target detection and target discrimination and longer reaction times for both tasks. The lack of differential effects on focused- and divided-attention tasks suggested that clonidine influenced response rather than stimulus set selectivity. The administration of methylphenidate on its own did not influence target discrimination or response time. However, it resulted in increased target detection and error rates during divided-, but not focused-attention tasks, suggesting an overall increase in response rate rather than an effect on selective attention per se. The authors concluded that noradrenergic neurons of the locus coeruleus in the upper pons, with preferential innervation of sensory neocortex, were implicated in the early processing that facilitates attention to relevant environmental information. In contrast, the dopaminergic neurons in the midbrain ventral tegmentum which innervate the association cortex and the subcortical motor structures were implicated in the later selection of appropriate responses to this environmental stimulation.

Orientation or Shifting of Attention

Clark et al. (1989) also investigated the involvement of these neurotransmitters in the orientation or switching of attention. Using Posner's (1980) covert-orientation-of-attention task, they found that both clonidine and droperidol were associated with a reduced cost linked with invalid cues but had no effect on the benefit of valid cues. The latter also resulted in slowed reaction times. It was concluded that these drugs affect the disengaging or switching of attention. Faster disengagement and switching followed a reduction in dopaminergic and noradrenergic activity. Interestingly, high concentrations of both substances are found in the inferior parietal cortex, which is involved in spatial analysis. In contrast, areas such as the inferotemporal structures associated with feature extraction were thought to have little catecholamine innervation. Thus, according to Clark et al. (1989), the inferior parietal cortex appears to play an important role in the disengagement of attention, which is facilitated by a reduction in catecholamine levels.

Rogers et al. (1999) investigated the effects of tryptophan depletion, methylphenidate, and clonidine on stimulus–reward learning and shifting attentional bias in healthy adults. Tryptophan is the dietary precursor of serotonin, and a reduction in tryptophan depletes serotonin levels. They found that a reduction of tryptophan (and thereby serotonin) was associated with impaired learning of stimulus–reward associations but did not affect shifting attention. In contrast, increasing catecholamine levels with methylphenidate facilitated the reallocation of attention toward newly relevant features of environmental stimuli, but it also slowed response times. The dorsolateral prefrontal cortex was proposed as the modulator of this change. Clonidine was found to have no effect.

Ward and Brown (1996) modified the Posner covert-orienting task for use in rats prior to and following dopamine-depleting lesions in the striatum. They found that reaction times of responses made to the side contralateral to the lesion were increased following surgical lesions. However, there was no change in the magnitude of the difference in reaction time between trials with valid versus invalid cues. They concluded that dopamine-depleting lesions of the striatum had no adverse effect on the covert orienting of attention but, rather, caused a motor impairment.

The inconsistent findings in the literature with respect to the role of neurotransmitter systems in attention appear, at least in part, to reflect a number of sources of variability. Task differences include modality assessed (e.g., visual/verbal) and indices measured (e.g., accuracy/reaction time). Drug variables include which receptors are targeted (e.g., for dopamine d1 or d2 receptors) and dosages (Arnsten, 1997). Most important, the brain regions studied have varied considerably, from the more sophisticated dorsolateral prefrontal cortex to the phylogenetically primitive locus coeruleus complex of the brain stem.

PET Scanning and Neuroanatomical Correlates of Attentional Systems

Three recent PET studies involving healthy adult subjects have evaluated the impact of methylphenidate and clonidine administration on catecholamine modulation. Using PET scanning techniques, Volkow et al. (2001) confirmed that methylphenidate increases extracellular dopamine levels in the brain. Patients with attention-deficit/hyperactivity disorder (ADHD) have been found to have increased dopamine transporters, which deplete extracellular dopamine levels. Methylphenidate causes dopamine transporter blockade, thereby increasing these levels.

Mehta et al. (2000) found that methylphenidate resulted in reduced regional cerebral blood flow (rCBF) in the dorsolateral prefrontal cortex and the posterior parietal cortex and enhanced performance on a spatial-working memory task, relative to placebo. Those with lower baseline performance scores were found to show greater improvements following drug administration. The reduction in rCBF was attributed to greater efficiency in information processing and again an increase in signal-to-noise ratio (due to increases in dopamine and noradrenaline).

Coull, Büchel, Friston, and Frith (1999) attempted to measure the role of noradrenaline in the integration of a neuroanatomical attentional network.

They studied effective connectivity in terms of rCBF, as a measure of the influence of one brain region on another. They found that, at rest, the noradrenergic system is relatively inactive, and that clonidine further reduced connectivity, particularly between the frontal cortex, thalamus, and visual system. However, in situations of high arousal (i.e., during performance of a visual-attention and working-memory task), the integration of networks from the locus coeruleus to parietal cortex, and from parietal cortex to frontal cortex and thalamus, was enhanced by clonidine. The authors proposed that noradrenaline exerts its role on attention by coordinating a dynamic network system rather than directly modulating activity within a specific brain region.

Taken together, these studies suggest that catecholamine blockade results in reduced attentional capacity and altered response selection in healthy controls. With release of dopamine and noradrenaline, via pharmacological agents, attentional capacity, speed of response, spatial working memory, and other attentional components are facilitated. Diffuse networks, including the dopaminergic and noradrenergic afferent pathways to the frontal lobes, in particular the dorsolateral prefrontal cortex, the parietal lobe, and the thalamic projection system, mediate these processes.

ATTENTION FOLLOWING TRAUMATIC BRAIN INJURY

As most rehabilitative efforts in the domains of attention have tended to focus on traumatic brain injury (TBI), attentional deficits associated with this condition will be discussed in some detail. TBI tends to be heterogeneous in nature and severity, but diffuse axonal injury and injury to the frontotemporal poles, the hippocampus, the basal ganglia, the corpus callosum, and midbrain are particularly common (Ponsford, Sloan, & Snow, 1995). All these areas play a role in mediating aspects of attention.

Neurochemical changes associated with TBI are difficult to measure as procedures tend to be invasive and findings vary depending on the time postinjury that samples are taken (Bareggi et al., 1975). Altered levels of dopamine and serotonin have been identified in lumber cerebrospinal fluid (CSF) following TBI, and these changes have been associated with severity of injury (Bareggi et al., 1975; Vecht, van Woerkom, Teelken, & Minderhoud, 1975). Findings regarding plasma norepinephrine levels have been inconsistent and results are confounded by the norepinephrine activity of the sympathetic nervous system. Norepinephrine levels have, however, been found to be associated with measures of coma depth, injury severity and level of recovery, such as Glasgow Coma Scale score (Hamill, Woolf, McDonald, Lee, & Kelly, 1987) and Glasgow Outcome Scale scores (Woolf, Hamill, Lee, Cox, & McDonald, 1987).

It has been well established that attentional deficits are among the most frequently occurring sequelae of TBI. Follow-up studies, including those of van Zomeren and van den Burg (1985); McKinlay, Brooks, and Bond (1983);

Olver, Ponsford, and Curran (1996); and Ponsford, Olver, and Curran (1995), have documented attention and concentration difficulties and slowed information processing as among the most common cognitive problems reported by individuals with TBI and their relatives. They appear to contribute significantly to ongoing disability and handicap, affecting the individual's capacity to cope with myriad daily tasks including work or study and domestic and social activities. In a study by Ponsford and Kinsella (1991), therapists most commonly observed "slowness in performing mental tasks" in their severe TBI patients. Other common difficulties included "not being able to pay attention to more than one thing at a time," "making mistakes because he/she wasn't paying attention properly," "missing important details," and "having difficulty concentrating."

Aspects of attention following TBI have been studied experimentally using a wide range of approaches. Summarizing the findings of these studies, we find strong evidence for the presence of a reduction in speed of information processing following TBI (Gronwall & Sampson, 1974; Ponsford & Kinsella, 1992; Spikman, van Zomeren, & Deelman, 1996; Stuss et al., 1989; van Zomeren & Brouwer, 1994). This reduction appears to be proportionate to the severity of injury and improves over time, although individuals with moderate or severe injuries may be left with a lasting deficit (Stuss et al., 1989; van Zomeren; 1981; Spikman et al., 1996).

Findings regarding additional problems with divided attention, or sharing of attention between tasks, are mixed. Dual tasks are performed significantly more slowly by individuals with TBI (Cicerone, 1996; Stablum, Leonardi, Mazzoldi, Umilta, & Morra, 1994; Vilkki, Virtanen, Surma-Aho, & Servo, 1996). However, the findings of Brouwer, Ponds, van Wolffelaar, and van Zomeren (1989); Spikman et al. (1996); and Veltman, Brouwer, van Zomeren, and van Wolffelaar (1996) suggest that such difficulties are proportionate to the degree of slowing, and that dividing of attention per se is not impaired. More recent findings by Azouvi, Jokic, van der Linden, Marliet, and Bussel (1996); Park, Moscovitch, and Robertson (1999); McDowell, Whyte, and D'Esposito (1997); Couillet, Leclercq, Martin, Rousseaux, and Azouvi (2000); and Withaar (2000) suggest that deficits in divided attention emerge only on more complex, strategy-driven tasks performed under high time pressure or involving substantial working-memory load (i.e., tasks requiring executive control by the anterior attentional network).

Results of a study by Tromp and Mulder (1991) suggest that task novelty has a crucial influence on speed of information processing, with less familiar tasks being performed more slowly by individuals with TBI. Indeed Schmitter-Edgecombe and Nissley (2000) have demonstrated that automatic processing in the domain of memory appears to be relatively unaffected by TBI. This finding has some significance for approaches to rehabilitation. Following from this finding, Schmitter-Edgecombe and Beglinger (2001) used a semantic category visual-search task to investigate skill acquisition and automatic process development in individuals with severe TBI. Training using consistent mapping, where responses to the same class of stimuli were always the same, resulted in dramatic performance improvements and development of an automatic attention response, whereas varied mapping training, where responses varied from one stimulus class or exposure to the next, resulted in little improvement and continued reliance on controlled processes. These results suggest that skill acquisition guidelines can be used to teach individuals with TBI new automatic skills.

In the domain of alertness, there is some electrophysiological evidence of impaired phasic alertness (Curry, 1981; Rizzo et al., 1978; Rugg et al., 1989; Segalowitz, Unsal, & Dywan, 1992), but this has not been demonstrated behaviorally (Ponsford & Kinsella, 1992; Whyte, Fleming, Polansky, Cavallucci, & Coslett, 1997). Although it has not been possible to demonstrate a vigilance decrement, or decline in accuracy of performance over time, there is a demonstrated reduction in the level of vigilance, in the form of decreased perceptual sensitivity, particularly when stimuli are degraded in some way, thereby requiring sustained effortful processing (Brouwer & von Wolffelaar, 1985; Ponsford & Kinsella, 1992; Parasuraman, Mutter, & Molloy, 1991; Robertson, Manly, Andrade, Baddeley, & Yiend, 1997; Spikman et al., 1996; Whyte, Polansky Fleming, Coslett, & Cavallucci, 1995; Zoccolotti et al., 2000). Robertson, Manly, Andrade, et al. (1997) suggested that errors on the Sustained Attention to Response Task (SART) resulted from a drift of controlled processing into automatic responding. Stuss et al. (1989), Stuss, Pogue, Buckle, and Bondar (1994) and Whyte et al. (1995) have suggested that the reaction-time (RT) performances of individuals with TBI may be characterized by greater *variability* in performance within RT tasks and target-identification tasks, although this has not been a consistent finding in other studies (van Zomeren & Brouwer, 1987; Spikman et al., 1996). Segalowitz, Dywan, and Unsal (1997) found that RT variability, rather than speed of RT, was related to P300 amplitude, reflecting the ability to allocate and sustain attention.

Individuals with TBI appear to be slower and less efficient in performing visual and auditory selective-attention tasks (Heinze, Munte, Gobiet, Niemann, & Ruff, 1992; Ponsford & Kinsella, 1992; Robertson, Ward, Ridgeway, & Nimmo-Smith, 1994; Schmitter-Edgecombe & Kibby, 1998). However, they are not necessarily more susceptible to distraction, even when there are strong conflicting response tendencies, as on the third subtest of the Stroop (Gronwall & Sampson, 1974; Miller & Cruzat, 1980; Ponsford & Kinsella, 1992; Spikman et al., 1996; Stablum et al., 1994; Stuss et al., 1989; van Zomeren, Brouwer, & Deelman, 1984). Increased sensitivity does emerge when a significant distracting load is added to the Stroop task (Elting, van Zomeren, & Brouwer, 1989; Bohnen, Jolles, & Twijnstra, 1992), or where target-distractor similarity is high (Schmitter-Edgecombe & Kibby, 1998). Simpson and Schmitter-Edgecombe (2000) found no decrease in ability to suppress irrelevant information on a negative priming task. On the other hand, Zahn and Mirsky (1999) found that individuals with TBI showed greater difficulty shifting attention to unexpected stimuli. Whyte et al. (1996; Whyte, Fleming, Polansky, Cavallucci, & Coslett, 1998) developed a naturalistic inattentiveness assessment and were able to demonstrate marked differences in performance, measured in terms of on-task behavior and fidgeting behavior in both distracting and nondistracting environments, between participants with TBI and controls.

Finally, there is evidence of inefficiency of the SAS, as measured on the Tower of London task, in the form of a general slowing in planning abilities. However, Ponsford and Kinsella (1992), Veltman et al. (1996), and Spikman, Deelman, and Van Zomeren (2000) did not find that participants with TBI made more errors on this task. Veltman et al. (1996) found that patients with severe TBI had difficulty applying strategies on a tracking task with changing task demands. Stablum et al. (1994) and Vilkki (1992) have demonstrated reduced cognitive programming and mental flexibility in subjects with TBI. The findings of Shallice and Burgess (1991), Boyd and Sautter (1993), and Spikman et al. (2000) suggest that difficulties with the goal-directed allocation of attention across a number of tasks may be more apparent when the tasks have a greater load or are performed in more complex environments. On more structured tasks, individuals with TBI appear to be able to maintain the accuracy of their performance by sacrificing speed.

This is not to say, however, that some of the more structured tests may not be sensitive to deficits in individual cases. There is clearly significant heterogeneity in pathology across individuals with TBI, so that summarized scores may mask individual differences. Trexler and Zappala (1988) found differences in the pattern of attentional performance when subjects were classified into different clinicopathological groups. Zoccolotti et al. (2000) have also suggested that there may be distinct patterns of impairment across individuals with TBI. The impact of head injuries primarily characterized by diffuse axonal injury may be quite different from those involving extensive frontal and temporal lobe contusions. Patients with diffuse axonal injury may exhibit slow information processing, whereas those with focal frontal and temporal injuries may exhibit problems with mental programming and switching, as well as working- and recent memory deficits, and some patients will exhibit both problems.

No association has been demonstrated between the nature of attentional impairments and the presence of focal contusions (Spikman et al., 2000). However, Fontaine, Azouvi, Remy, Bussel, and Samson (1999) found in a PET study that performance on attentional tasks was associated with hypometabolism at rest in prefrontal and cingulate areas. Using fMRI, McAllister et al. (1999) found modified activation in prefrontal and parietal regions during a working-memory task 1 month after mild TBI. As Leclercq and Azouvi (2002) have concluded, "defective activation or modulation of attentional/executive networks including but not limited to the prefrontal cortex" (p. 273) may be associated with attentional impairments following TBI. Clearly, due to the wide heterogeneity of pathology seen following these injuries, different patterns of attentional difficulty will emerge from one case to the next, and each needs to be assessed individually.

IMPAIRMENTS OF ATTENTION
IN CEREBROVASCULAR DISEASE

As noted by Rousseaux, Fimm, and Cantagallo (2002) in their comprehensive chapter on this subject, defining syndromes associated with different types of cerebrovascular disease is problematic for a number of reasons. First, there are difficulties in accurately defining the topography and volume of anatomical lesions resulting from cerebrovascular accident (CVA) using neuroimaging techniques. Second, CVA may have remote consequences—"diaschisis"—which also need to be taken into account. Third, there are frequently other cognitive impairments associated with aging or degenerative disease present in this population. Finally, patient groups have been studied over variable time frames. Impairments of attention will be considered in terms of the broad anatomical location of the primary lesion.

Anterior Cerebrovascular Accident

Given the importance of the dorsolateral prefrontal cortex and the cingulate gyrus in most models of attentional systems, it would be expected that anterior CVA would result in some attentional impairments. The most common syndrome is that associated with aneurysms of the anterior communicating artery. CVA affecting anterior structures appears to result in perceptuomotor slowing, as assessed by visual and auditory RT tasks (Benton & Joynt, 1958; Godefroy, Lhullier, & Rousseaux, 1996). Godefroy et al. (1996) found this slowing to be correlated with lesions in the left dorsolateral prefrontal cortex. Such slowing is also associated with posterior lesions, however. No impairments of vigilance in its classical form (i.e., a decline in performance over time on tasks lasting over 30 minutes) have been identified in patients with anterior lesions.

Impairments of focused attention are evident in the form of prolonged RT and increased errors of commission made on Go/No Go and Stroop tasks in patients with vascular frontal lesions, involving the dorsolateral prefrontal cortex and the anterior cingulate gyrus, particularly on the left side (Godefroy & Rousseaux, 1996; Godefroy et al., 1996; Rousseaux, Godefroy, Cabaret, Benaiim, & Pruvo, 1996). Increased sensitivity to distracting information has also been demonstrated (Chao & Knight, 1995). Godefroy and Rousseaux (1996); Rousseaux et al. (1996), and Leclercq et al. (2000) have found greater difficulties in dividing and switching attention between perceptual channels and between tasks in patients with vascular prefrontal lesions (aneurysms of the anterior communicating artery), again more when the lesion was on the left side.

Cerebrovascular Accident in the Thalamus

The thalamus has rich connections with the basomedial and dorsdolateral prefrontal cortex and forms part of the frontal-thalamic gating system put forward by Stuss and Benson (1986) as a regulator of selective attention. Findings regarding the impact of thalamic lesions on aspects of attention come mainly from case studies and these have been mixed. Some studies have documented perceptuomotor slowing (Rousseaux, Kassiotis, Signoret, Cabaret, & Petit, 1991) and increased errors on the Stroop, indicating focused attentional problems in patients with anterior thalamic lesions (Bogousslavsky, Regli, & Assal, 1986; Sandson, Duffner, Carvalho, & Mesulam, 1991; Pepin & Auray-Pepin, 1993), but these impairments have not always been evident (Hashimoto, Yoshida, & Tanaka, 1995; Rousseaux, Carabet, Bernati, Pruvo, & Steinling, 1998). Striatal vascular lesions do not result in slowing on simple visual or auditory RT tasks (Godefroy et al., 1992).

Posterior Cerebrovascular Accident

Posterior lesions, particularly those involving parietal lobe structures, are commonly associated with disorders of spatial attention, most notably unilateral spatial neglect. This is discussed in detail in Chapter 6 (this volume). Posner's theoretical model of attention proposed that the sustained attention system exerts a strong modulatory influence on the functioning of the spatial attention system, located posteriorly. In support of this theory, Robertson, Manly, Beschin, et al. (1997) found significant correlations between performance on a test of sustained attention (monotonous tone counting) and aspects of spatial attention (as measured by performance on visuomanual tasks) in patients with right-hemisphere lesions. As far as nonspatial attention is concerned, in the studies cited in the previous section, patients with posterior lesions were shown to exhibit perceptuomotor slowing but showed no impairments of focused or divided attention.

REHABILITATION OF NONSPATIAL ATTENTION

Computer-Assisted Attentional-Training-Directed Stimulation

While numerous techniques have been used with the aim of rehabilitating attentional impairments acquired as a consequence of brain injury, by far the most common approach has involved training, usually on computer-mediated tasks. Such training is based on the assumption that attentional impairments can be alleviated by direct stimulation of brain structures involved in attention or an aspect of attention. Subjects are given repeated but highly structured practice on tasks exercising the area of deficit. Generally these tasks involve responding selectively to shapes, colors, digits, or letters according to predetermined rules. Parameters such as complexity, quantity, speed of presentation, or the amount of cueing given are gradually altered depending on the goal of therapy. Proponents argue that it is most efficient to focus on the causes of difficulties rather than the symptoms, the aim being to restore lost function so that therapeutic gains can be applied in many facets of daily life. Indeed, this approach is congruent with the findings presented in Chapter 2 (this volume), which show that therapy or forced use of damaged structures may facilitate either synaptic regrowth/rearrangement and/or compensatory activity by adjacent, intact structures.

The studies conducted to date include those of Ben Yishay, Piasetsky, and Rattok (1987); Sohlberg and Mateer (1987); Gray and Robertson (1989); Niemann, Ruff, and Baser (1990); Sturm and Willmes (1991); Gray, Robertson, Pentland, and Anderson (1992); Ruff, Maheffey, Engel, Farrow, Cox, and Karzmark (1994); Novack, Caldwell, Duke, Bergquist, and Gage (1996); Sturm, Willmes, Orgass, and Hartje (1997); Palmese and Raskin (2000); Stablum, Umilta, Mogentale, Carlan and Guerrini (2000); Malec, Jones, Rao, and Stubbs (1984); Wood and Fussey (1987); Ponsford and Kinsella (1988); Gansler and McCaffrey (1991); and Park, Proulx, and Towers (1999). Most of these studies have demonstrated improvement on the trained tasks, where this was measured. For example, Ben-Yishay et al. (1987) applied the Orientation Remedial Module, a computerized series of five tasks forming an overlapping hierarchy in complexity to a series of patients with severe TBI. Training resulted in a progression from initially impaired performances to the average normal range. Sohlberg and Mateer (1987) and Palmese and Raskin (2000) demonstrated gains following training on a hierarchy of five sets of treatment tasks aimed at different aspects of attention and labeled "Attention Process Training." Wood and Fussey (1987) found a gradual improvement in the ability to scan moving symbols on a screen. These findings suggest that patients can learn to carry out specific tasks in the visuomotor domain or in visual search, but gains are task specific.

These studies also evaluated the impact of training on performance on neuropsychological measures. The 10 studies listed first, from Ben Yishay et al. (1987) to Palmese and Raskin (2000), have all demonstrated gains on such measures. For example, Ben Yishay et al. (1987) found gains in visual reaction time, auditory digits, and according to the Wechsler Adult Intelligence Scale (WAIS) verbal IQ; Sohlberg and Mateer (1987) demonstrated gains on the Paced Auditory Serial Addition task (PASAT); Gray and Robertson (1989) and Gray et al. (1992) found significant gains on the PASAT and WAIS Arithmetic tasks; and

Niemann et al. (1990) found gains on the Trail Making test. In all these studies the training tasks involved elements similar to these measures.

Sturm et al. (1997) focused their training on specific aspects of attention in patients with left or right focal brain damage of vascular aetiology. They evaluated the efficacy of game-like computerized training programs for intensity aspects of attention (alertness and vigilance) and selectivity aspects (selective and divided attention). Each patient received consecutive training in the two most impaired of the four attention domains. Assessment on a standardized computerized attention test battery comprising tests for the four attention functions was carried out at the beginning and after each of the two training periods of 14 1-hour sessions each. There were significant specific training effects for both intensity aspects (alertness and vigilance), and also for response time in the selective attention and error rate in the divided-attention task. For selectivity aspects of attention, RT also improved after training of basic attentional domains. The authors concluded that attentional processes were hierarchical, and that training the most basic aspects (alertness and vigilance) could have a positive impact upon higher aspects (SAS–dual task or selective-attention tasks). These findings were replicated in a subsequent multi-centre study involving TBI patients as well as stroke patients (Sturm et al., 2002). The gains were, however, confined to neuropsychological tests which bore some resemblance to the training tasks, and there was no attempt to measure the generalization or maintenance of gains. In contrast to these findings, Novack et al. (1996), in a study rated as Class I, found no significant differences between the impact of focused, structured, hierarchical computer-mediated interventions for attentional difficulties, and that of nonsequential, nonhierarchical activities focusing on a range of cognitive functions, as measured on neuropsychological measures of attention and other cognitive function, or functional skills measured on the Functional Independence Measure (FIM). Both groups, which were in the acute stages of recovery, showed improvement.

Stablum et al. (2000) conducted a study that aimed to improve dual task performance in 10 TBI patients and 9 anterior communicating artery aneurysm (ACoA) rupture patients relative to a group of 19 controls. A computer-mediated dual-task paradigm was implemented over five sessions. Although both experimental and control patients improved on the dual-task paradigm, treated patients improved at a greater rate than did controls. Treated patients' larger gains on the PASAT relative to controls indicated generalization. Dual-task performance remained stable at 3-month and, in the AcoA group, 12-month follow-up. Again, there was no measurement of generalization to daily activities, but there was anecdotal report of improved real-life functioning (e.g., card playing) in one participant.

An alternative interpretation of all these findings is put forward by Park et al. (1999). They argue that the mechanism is one of specific skill training (e.g., training in responding quickly and accurately to material presented on a computer screen), which generalizes to tasks of a similar nature rather than improved integrity of underlying damaged attention functions. In their own study they evaluated whether Attention Process Training improved the performance of participants with TBI more than controls on the PASAT. The control measure, on which no response to treatment was expected, was Consonant Trigrams. Significant improvements were evident on the PASAT in both TBI and control groups. The TBI group also improved on the Consonant Trigrams. This finding casts doubt on the findings of Sohlberg and Mateer (1987), who used improvement on the PASAT as an indication of improved attentional functions.

Following from this, Park and Ingles (2001) conducted a meta-analysis of 30 studies of efficacy of attention training, including those listed previously. They compared outcomes between studies which used pre- and posttraining scores with those that also included a control condition. Using the d_+ statistic, significant performance improvements were evident only in the pre–post studies but not in those studies using controls. They concluded that specific-skills training resulted in gains or practice effects on tests of attention similar to the training tasks but did not have a significant impact on overall outcomes in those treated.

There was one exception to this pattern, and that was the study by Kewman et al. (1985), which focused more directly on specific skills of functional significance. They attempted to improve the driving skills of a brain-injured group, using a shaping procedure. While driving a small electric-powered vehicle, the experimental group completed a number of auditory and visual monitoring tasks, designed to exercise important driving skills, such as keeping track of more than one thing at once or shifting the focus of attention from one activity to another. The brain-injured control group drove the car for a similar period but did not complete the monitoring tasks. Outcome was evaluated via on-road driving tests conducted before and after training. There was a significantly greater improvement evident in the driving performance of the experimental group relative to controls. Thus, by focusing training on the specific skills required to perform the actual daily task, functional gains were apparently made.

Relatively few of the attentional training studies have controlled adequately for spontaneous recovery, effects of practice, and concurrent therapy, or have assessed the degree to which training generalizes to aspects of everyday life, and whether gains are maintained over time. The two studies that did meet all these criteria, particularly in terms of measuring generalization of effects to everyday life, namely, those of Ponsford and Kinsella (1988) and Wood and Fussey (1987), were not able to demonstrate significant gains. Ponsford and Kinsella (1988) trained speed of information processing in 10 subjects with severe TBI 6–34 weeks postinjury. A single-case multiple-baseline-across subjects (A-B-BC-A) design was employed. Following a 3-week baseline, daily training sessions were given for 3 weeks. In the next 3 weeks, feedback and re-inforcement was added to the training before return to baseline. Dependent measures included neuropsychological measures of speed and accuracy, ratings on a rating scale of attentional behavior by therapists blind to the timing of the intervention, and a video recording of time spent directed to a clerical task in the occupational therapy department. Results on all measures indicated a grad-ual improvement across all phases, reflecting either spontaneous recovery or practice effects. Gains were not significantly greater in the intervention phases.

The lack of generalization to everyday measures of attention in these stud-ies is perhaps not surprising, given that everyday activities are inevitably more complex, involving a multitude of additional functions and considerable varia-tion in task demands and environmental conditions. The results of these atten-tion training studies lend support to Schmitter-Edgecombe and Beglinger's (2001) findings, indicating that specific training results in improved perfor-mance on tasks involving the same processes. It is arguable that some of the computer-mediated attention training tasks may be performed relatively auto-matically, at least after the first few trials, when they are no longer novel. Task performance thereby no longer places demands on the controlled processing systems, impairment of which is preventing brain-injured individuals from ef-fectively dividing their attention in more complex activities in everyday life. Because the ultimate goal of rehabilitation is to improve the ability to perform these more complex functional activities, it is arguably preferable to focus the intensive training or massed practice on specific elements of those activities di-rectly, providing training until they become automatic and no longer place de-mands on the capacity-limited controlled processing system, rather than on the more abstract elements of the attention training tasks. The findings of Schmitter-Edgecombe and Beglinger (2001) suggest that such training should be provided in a manner whereby responses to the same class of stimuli are al-ways the same. As they point out, "studies with non head-injured participants have shown that complex multiple-task performances can improve to a skilled level when one of the tasks is first practised alone and becomes 'automatic' (e.g., Schneider & Fisk, 1982)" (p. 628).

Other significant factors for consideration here are the size and location of the lesions in the patients being trained. In the foregoing studies, the majority of participants were victims of severe TBI and therefore would have had exten-sive brain lesions. As Kolb and Cioe have pointed out in Chapter 1, capacity for recovery depends on the size of the lesion. It remains feasible that individuals with less extensive or more circumscribed lesions might show a greater capac-ity for restoration of functions in response to training. The extent to which a function might be reestablished will also depend on whether those areas medi-ating basic perceptual functions at a lower level remain intact, in order to allow higher-order areas to reestablish functions (Webster & Ungerleider, 2000).

Behavioral Approaches

It would appear that some elements of attention can be shaped behaviorally, although there is no evidence to suggest a change in attentional behaviors other than those which are the focus of the shaping procedures. Deacon and Campbell (1991) evaluated the impact of feedback (green vs. red lights), and the imposition of time windows, given over three trials, on the auditory RT of 12 TBI and 12 controls. Gains in RT were maintained after the withdrawal of feedback and windows and were approximately equal to the RTs of controls prior to presentation of cues. The RTs of patients occurred at approximately the same time as the P300 wave form. Some evidence of carryover was evident on replication of the study.

Wood (1986, 1987, 1988) used contingent token reinforcement to enhance attentional behavior in a number of single cases. Baseline observations recorded at intervals over 5 days, recorded at 2 minute intervals whether the patient was attending or not attending to a therapy task. During training, patients received a token at 2-minute intervals if, and only if, they were attending to the therapy activity. Tokens could be exchanged for sweets, soft drinks, or cigarettes at the end of the session. Gains were demonstrated in terms of percentage of time spent attending to the task in three subjects described, although gains were withdrawn when the treatment was withdrawn in one of the three subjects. Wood emphasized that the treatment was aimed at "attentiveness" (behavior), which should be distinguished from the cognitive or information-processing component. There was no evidence that improving attentive behavior led to a parallel increase in information processing capacity.

Strategy Training Approaches

Strategies for Stimulating Alertness and Sustained Attention

As noted earlier, a number of lines of evidence suggest that the right hemisphere, particularly the right lateral frontal cortex, is involved in maintaining alertness and sustained attention. Robertson, Manly, Bechin, et al. (1997) have shown that patients with right-hemisphere lesions have greater difficulty than those with left-sided lesions in counting tones separated by long intervals, and that patients with visual neglect had significantly greater difficulty with tone counting than did patients without neglect. Robertson, Mattingley, Rorden, and Driver (1998) showed that playing a loud alerting tone removed the spatial bias of patients with left-sided neglect, suggesting a direct link between neglect and alertness.

Following from these findings, Robertson, Tegner, Tham, Lo, and Nimmo-Smith (1995) trained patients with persistent left unilateral neglect in self-alerting techniques as used by Meichenbaum and Cameron (1973). Initially this was prompted by the therapist banging on the table and saying, "Attend!" in a loud voice; then the therapist knocked as a prompt for the patients to say out loud to themselves, "Attend!" Then the patients were required to knock on the desk and say "Attend." The external prompting was gradually faded and the patients were cued to use self-instruction, at first out loud and then covertly. Eight neglect patients showed significant improvements in response to this training, both in terms of performance on measures of sustained attention and on measures of visual neglect. However, there was no follow-up regarding whether the patients were able to implement the self-alerting procedure and/or whether it improved their visual scanning behavior in other settings. Sturm and Willmes (2001) reported that computer-mediated alertness training resulted in improved scanning performances on letter cancellation and line bisection tasks and increased right frontal activation on fMRI. Chapter 6 outlines further strategies for rehabilitation of unilateral spatial neglect. A recent study by Manly, Hawkins, Evans, Woldt, and Robertson (2002) found that the provision of brief auditory alerting stimuli improved performance of an executive task—the Hotel test—to near normal levels. The next question that arises is whether such alerting procedures could be used successfully in patients with intact phasic alertness but impaired sustained attention, in the *absence* of neglect.

Brief Mindfulness Training

Following from his research with neglect patients, Ian Robertson, along with Tom McMillan and colleagues (McMillan, Robertson, Brock, & Chorlton, 2002), evaluated the impact of a mindfulness meditation technique on sustained attention. This technique involved training in a relaxation-like procedure, where the subject has to learn to control attention by concentrating on breathing over extended periods. Following promising results of a pilot study, 145 participants with TBI were randomly allocated to one of three groups. The attention control training (ACT) group received five 45-minute training sessions over a 4-week period using an audiotape and were asked to practice daily with the tape in the intervening periods. A second group had the same amount of therapist and audiotape contact, but this focused on physical fitness training. A third control group received no therapist contact but was assessed at the same time intervals, at pretreatment, posttreatment, and 12-month follow-up. No statistically significant differences were evident on any of the dependent measures, which included self-reported cognitive failures, performance on the Test of Everyday Attention, the PASAT, Trail Making Test and List and Story recall, Hospital Anxiety and Depression Scales, and the General Health Questionnaire. Although it was acknowledged that more intensive training by skilled therapists may have been more effective, it was considered that this was not feasible within the existing health care system.

Strategies for Dealing with Attentional Slips
When Reading

Arguably, training of this nature can only be effective if it is more intensive and specifically focused on attentional difficulties as they are manifested in the individual's daily activities. In one such single case intervention, Wilson and Robertson (1992) worked with a head-injured man who was bothered by involuntary slips of attention while reading which affected his ability to complete accountancy homework. The intervention focused on helping him understand how his difficulties came about, relaxation training, and strategies for dealing with internal and external distractions. He was asked to identify and count involuntary slips of attention when reading, defined as when he needed to reread a word or sentence or when his mind wandered from the text to a different train of thought.

After a 16-day baseline, training began. A preparation procedure involved brief relaxation and focusing on breathing for five breaths. He would then practice reading without an attention slip. If a slip occurred he was instructed to mentally "bin it" and continue reading for the prescribed duration, which was expanded after three consecutive successful trials. Results showed a steady increase in times reading novels without a slip (from 50 to 325 seconds) over 39 days. The next phase of training introduced "inoculation against distraction." Reading was conducted against a background of distraction of speech—based radio programs. Slips were dealt with by focusing on a wall and counting focused breathing for two breaths before returning to the text. After 11 days, no improvements had occurred, so the training strategy was altered such that the subject aimed at no more than two slips in a 3-minute period before expanding the duration by 15 seconds, the final goal being 5 minutes with no more than two slips. Over a period of 26 days, this resulted in some improvement. An accountancy text was read for 15 minutes per day and attentional slips recorded on a control measure. There was a significant decrease in attentional slips while reading the accountancy text only after the introduction of the second phase of intervention.

In summary, this young man increased his time of reading a novel without a slip modestly from 1.5 to 5 minutes, but this did not generalize to slips recorded reading an accountancy text. Introduction of inoculation against distraction led to a reduction in the number of without training slips and the number of test text slips also remained lower. Anecdotally he reported increased reading for pleasure and significant subjective gains. The gains from this relatively intensive intervention, although significant, were nevertheless quite modest and one could question whether the outcome justified such an intensive effort.

Webster and Scott (1983) used the self-instructional technique developed by Meichenbaum and Cameron (1973) to train a construction worker 2 years post-head injury to focus attention during reading or listening. Paragraphs from periodicals were used for training. He was taught self-instructional statements to prepare himself to listen and ask for repetition if attention had strayed, as follows: "To really concentrate, I must look at the person speaking to me"; "I also must focus on what is being said, not on other thoughts which want to intrude"; "I must concentrate on what I am hearing at any moment by repeating each word in my head as the person speaks"; and "Although it is not horrible if I lose track of conversation, I must tell the person to repeat the information if I have not attended to it." The statements were initially repeated aloud, then whispered, then subvocalized, and finally the time allowed for subvocalizing was decreased. Results showed significant gains in recall of stories and improvement was noted in other settings. Effects were reportedly still evident 18 months later.

Strategies for Improving Divided Attention or Working Memory

Cicerone (2002) trained four participants who had sustained mild TBI and had "working attentional" difficulties to more effectively allocate their attention resources when performing tasks requiring divided attention. Treatment tasks included increasingly demanding dual-task paradigms, including the n-back, random generation, and dual-task procedures. While performing these tasks during weekly training sessions conducted between 11 and 27 weeks, participants were encouraged to develop and employ strategies for more effectively allocating their attentional resources and managing the rate of information during task performance. Additional specific training tasks were also developed which bore some resemblance to the demands of their work-related tasks, and there was extensive discussion of methods of applying the strategies in their daily lives. Performances on outcome measures were compared with those of a group of untreated individuals with mild TBI. Greater gains were evident in the treated group on measures of attention, with the most clinically meaningful gains exhibited on the PASAT and continuous performance tasks. The treatment group also reported a greater reduction in their experience of attentional problems in their daily lives. Cicerone did not claim that performance of the training tasks alone brought about improvement but, rather, the discussion and implementation of management strategies for allocating working attentional resources.

Strategies for Mental Slowness: Time Pressure Monitoring

Fasotti, Kovacs, Eling, and Brouwer (2000) have developed and implemented a more specific set of compensatory strategies for dealing with reduced speed of information processing, termed "time pressure management" (TPM). A randomized pretraining versus posttraining versus follow-up group study was used to evaluate this method. Participants had sustained severe TBI more than 3 months earlier and had slowed information processing. Fasotti et al. (2000) compared the effectiveness of TPM training with more general instructions to concentrate on videotaped instructions regarding, first, directions to get somewhere and, second, the use of a computer program. TPM training involved the following steps:

1. Increasing the person's awareness of the problem—in this case the relationship between the person's mental slowness and performance on the tasks and his or her ability to discriminate between effective and ineffective performance on the task
2. Accepting and acquiring the TPM strategy, using a short variant of Meichenbaum's (1977) self-instruction method. The strategy involved four steps: recognizing the sources of time pressure in the task at hand; planning ways to reduce time pressure before starting the task; developing "managing steps" to deal with time-pressure problems experienced while performing the task as quickly as possible (e.g., turning off the tape, asking for repetition, or asking the person to slow down the delivery of information); and monitoring the implementation of the TPM strategies. First the instructor demonstrated how to perform the task with TPM, then the patient instructed himself out loud and wrote down the four TPM steps. When he forgot a step he was given a written prompt. Gradually these prompts were withdrawn and the patient used overt self-guidance to implement the steps. Earlier videotapes were repeated to demonstrate the improvement in performance using TPM strategies.
3. The final stage involved application and maintenance of strategies under more distracting and difficult conditions (e.g., with a radio playing in the background).

The experimental group ($n = 12$) had this training. A control group ($n = 10$) received the following instructions without TPM: to listen to the same tapes and to focus on and remember the main themes, to avoid being distracted by irrelevant sounds from the environment or by their own thoughts, and to try to imagine the things that are said. The effects of TPM were evaluated using two tasks similar to the training tasks, as well as measures of attention, memory, and psychosocial well-being administered before and after training and at 6-month follow-up. Both treatments improved task performance. However, following training the experimental group took significantly more TPM "managing steps" than did controls, which appeared to result in greater and more durable gains in task performance, which also generalized to other measures of speed and memory function. There was no change in measures of psychosocial well-being. Kovacs (personal communication, November 2000) has reported that there were some excellent time pressure managers who responded better than others. Factors influencing the success of the training included self-awareness (subjects must see the sense in using the strategy if they are to use it) and assertiveness to take managing steps in social situations.

Goal-Management Training

A number of studies have also focused on the facilitation of self-monitoring in patients with executive dysfunction, who have difficulty planning and following through with a course of action, generally secondary to frontal lobe impairment. These patients may also exhibit problems with efficient allocation of attentional resources where controlled processing is required, difficulty switching, or paying attention to more than one thing at a time and difficulty holding in working-memory instructions to guide performance of a task or tasks. Although all these functions may be considered under the realm of attention, they are comprehensively covered in Chapter 7 (this volume), which focuses on rehabilitation of executive function and self-awareness. Readers are referred to that chapter.

Environmental Manipulation to Maximize Attentional Performance

Clearly the use of any of these compensatory strategies to overcome attentional difficulties presupposes some level of self-awareness and some capacity for verbal self-regulation of behavior. This is not always present especially in cases in which the brain injury is very diffuse and extensive and/or when there is extensive frontal lobe impairment. In these cases there will be minimal potential for recovery and regeneration, or the use of compensatory strategies. However, there are ways in which the environment can be manipulated to minimize the impact of attentional problems. As suggested by Sloan and Ponsford (1995), the work environment might be modified to reduce distractions (e.g., work in a quiet room, facing a wall; reduce interruptions and background noise; and clear workspace). Tasks may be modified to reduce the amount of information to be processed or the speed at which they are presented.

Rest breaks could be built into the activity (e.g., 5 minutes rest for each 15 minutes). Verbal prompts may be provided to encourage the person to refocus on the task, or others may be trained to do this. Verbal or written prompts may also be provided to assist the person to move from one component of the task to the next in a logical fashion. By removing unstructured periods there is less opportunity for the person to become distracted. It can also be helpful to change activities frequently in order to maintain interest. It may be appropriate to allow for repetition of material to be remembered, such as instructions. In work or study environments a dictaphone may be useful to record and replay important material.

It is also important to allow a realistic time frame for completion of tasks to reduce time pressure and associated stress. More complex tasks should be scheduled at the time of day when fatigue levels are lowest and there are fewest competing demands. The injured person and others can be trained to identify the signs of fatigue and take appropriate action. Stress management, relaxation, or meditation techniques may also be helpful.

Pharmacological Approaches

Attention-Deficit/Hyperactivity Disorder

The most well known and robust example of effective pharmacological rehabilitation in the treatment of attention is the use of methylphenidate (Ritalin) in children with ADHD. Methylphenidate is a central nervous system stimulant, which increases activity of dopamine, noradrenaline, and, to a lesser extent, serotonin, by reducing reuptake into pre-synaptic neurons and increasing release from presynaptic stores (O'Shanick, 1991).

Improvements in accuracy and speed on measures of sustained attention, such as the continuous performance task, have been demonstrated in children with ADHD treated with methylphenidate (Keith & Engineer, 1991; Klorman et al., 1988; Sonnerville, Njiokiktjien, & Hilhorst, 1991; Solanto, Wender, & Bartell, 1997). Others show improvements in self-control and impulsivity (Malone & Swanson, 1993; O'Toole, Abramowitz, Morris, & Dulcan, 1997). Findings regarding selective attention are less consistent, and few significant medication effects have been found on neuropsychological tasks (Everett, Thomas, Cote, Levesque, & Michaud, 1991; Balthazor, Wagner, & Pelham 1991; Dalebout, Nelson, Hletko, & Frentheway, 1991). Electrophysiological studies have revealed that methylphenidate may alter P3 amplitude and latency (Klorman et al., 1990; Sunohara et al., 1999), suggesting that the pharmacological effect is to enhance selective attention, resulting in less inattention, reduced impulsivity, and faster RT (Greenham, 1998). Long-term follow-up studies have shown that these beneficial effects dissipate rapidly when treatment is ceased (Zeiner, 1999), advocating for a combined drug/therapy/educational intervention approach to the treatment of attentional disturbance in ADHD.

Traumatic Brain Injury

In contrast to the abundant research into the use of pharmacological agents in the ADHD literature, the application of this approach to attentional disturbance following TBI has been relatively limited. Again, most of the work has focused on the use of methylphenidate, typically administered at a dose of 0.3 mg per kg twice a day. Other variables, however, such as duration of treatment, time from injury to recruitment, and performance measures investigated have varied greatly. A number of the studies have not met the criteria for randomized, double-blind, placebo-controlled trials and so interpretation of the results remains tentative.

The majority of studies have found positive methylphenidate treatment effects in the domain of processing speed. Within a paediatric sample, Mahalick et al. (1998) found improved performance on the Ruff 2 and 7 test, a cancellation task designed to evaluate parallel and serial aspects of information processing, and the attentional composite score of the Woodcock–Johnson Psychoeducational Test Battery—Revised, with methylphenidate administration. Within the adult population Kaelin, Cifu, and Matthies (1996) evaluated patients within the first 3 months postinjury. Significantly faster performance on the Symbol Search subtest was evident during the drug condition compared with baseline comparisons, and gains were maintained 1 week postdiscontinuation. In a *post hoc* analysis of those deemed to be "responders" and "nonresponders," methylphenidate effects were observed on the Ruff 2 and 7 test number of correct responses (Gualtieri & Evans, 1988). Improvement on this task, and the PASAT, was also evident in a study by Plenger et al. (1996).

There has been limited evidence of improved vigilance or sustained attention in response to methylphenidate in these studies. After 30 days of drug treatment, and a 30-day drug-free follow-up, subjects treated with methylphenidate demonstrated better vigilance performance than a placebo control group on the continuous performance task (Plenger et al., 1996). Speech, Rao, Osmon, and Sperry (1993) found no statistically significant drug effects on a vigilance task from the Gordon Diagnostic System (GDS) after 1 week of treatment with methylphenidate. However, Mahalick et al. (1998) found significant drug treatment effects in a pediatric sample on the same measure. Findings from mood or behavior ratings have also been inconsistent (Gualtieri & Evans, 1988; Speech et al., 1993; Williams, Ris, Ayyangar, Schefft, & Berch, 1998).

Whyte and colleagues have provided the most convincing evidence of an effect of methylphenidate on processing speed. Whyte, Hart, et al. (1997) used a double-blind, placebo-controlled, within-subjects crossover design, whereby 19 participants with TBI—sustained 38–3,245 days previously—received methylphenidate on 3 days and placebo on 3 days alternately and were tested on all six occasions. Of 22 variables assessed, 8 results were consistent with reasonable effect sizes for the drug group, compared with placebo. Five of the eight were measures of speed of information processing. Vigilance, per se, was not significantly facilitated by methylphenidate. This study controlled for within-subjects variability and natural recovery. However, the heterogeneity of the group in terms of time since injury precluded any conclusions about the time postinjury that patients are most likely to benefit from pharmacological interventions.

In a subsequent study, Whyte, Vaccaro, Grieb-Neff, and Hart (2002) recruited 34 patients with moderate or severe TBI, sustained at least 90 days prior to evaluation. The mean time postinjury was, however, 6.7 years, limiting findings to well beyond the acute recovery stage. In a randomized, placebo-controlled crossover design participants were given methylphenidate or placebo for 6 days a week and then received the alternative on the subsequent week, and this was repeated over a 6-week program. Methylphenidate was found to significantly improve speed of information processing on computerized RT tasks. Family ratings of the participants' behavior indicated improved attention with methylphenidate, and participants demonstrated less off-task behavior in an individual setting but not in a group setting (Whyte, 2003). The drug had no effect on dual-task performance, ability to sustain attention over time, or initial accuracy. Overall, the drug was well tolerated by participants. It appears that methylphenidate does increase speed of information processing following TBI, but its impact in the acute stages of recovery when combined with behavioral therapy has not been evaluated.

The use of dopaminergic agents such as bromocriptine and levodopa-carbidopa has largely focused on augmenting arousal in patients in a vegetative state. In an unblinded, uncontrolled study, Lal, Merbitz, and Grip (1988) reported improvements in alertness, sustained attention and concentration following treatment with levodopa-carbidopa. Subjective reports of increased arousal have also followed treatment with amantadine (Gaultieri, Chandler, Coons, & Brown, 1989), and improvements in general outcome with amantadine have been found to be independent of natural recovery (Meythaler, Brunner, Johnson, & Novack, 2002). A double-blind, placebo-controlled crossover trial by McDowell, Whyte, and D'Esposito (1998) found positive treatment effects for low-dose bromocriptine on the Trail Making Test, the Wisconsin Card Sorting Test, the Controlled Oral Word Association Test, and a computerized dual task in 24 subjects with TBI. The authors concluded that the drug effect was primarily upon dual-task performance and executive processes.

Cholinergic agents have been found to enhance memory function following TBI (Blount, Nguyen, & McDeavitt, 2002), but their use has not been systematically evaluated in the domain of attention.

Cerebrovascular Disease

Studies evaluating the role of pharmacological agents in the rehabilitation of stroke patients have largely focused on recovery of motor function (e.g., Crisostomo, Duncan, Propst, Dawson, & Davis, 1988) or their role in the treatment of poststroke depression (e.g., Lingam, Lazarus, Groves, & Oh, 1988; Lazarus et al., 1992), rather than cognitive processes. In a double-blind, placebo-controlled study, Grade, Redford, Chrostowski, Toussaint, and Blackwell

(1998) found no beneficial effects of methylphenidate compared to placebo on components of the Mini-Mental State Examination. Hurford, Stringer, and Jann (1998) found that bromocriptine was associated with recovery from unilateral visual neglect in a 68-year-old gentleman, and gains were maintained following withdrawal. Although the effect of methylphenidate was superior to no drug treatment, the neglect was exacerbated when the drug was discontinued.

CONCLUSIONS

Clearly the attentional system is highly complex and multidimensional. Impairments may affect any or all of its aspects and their interactions with other functional systems. Consequently, there is and never will be any single form of attentional impairment or any single method of rehabilitating attention. Careful assessment of each aspect of attention, and the integrity of other cognitive abilities and neuronal systems, as well as the requirements of the injured person's lifestyle, should form the basis from which to plan an intervention.

Although there is no definitive evidence to show that basic attentional mechanisms can be retrained in a generalizable sense, there is evidence to suggest that it is possible to improve performance of specific skills involving attentional functions in individuals with a limited capacity for controlled attentional processing. By providing intensive practice on those tasks as they are performed in everyday life in a consistent and systematic fashion, the specific skills may be learned so that they can be performed automatically. This would bypass the need for controlled processing and dividing of attention, the capacity for which is so often limited following TBI or CVA.

For those individuals who have some degree of self-awareness and self-monitoring capacity, in whom the anterior systems modulating the capacity for controlled processing appear to be at least partially intact, there is some evidence that it may be possible to use cognitive-behavioral approaches to externally guide or modify these control processes. This may involve training in the use of self-talk to alert oneself to focus attention on the task at hand, to develop strategies to cope with time pressure or ways of dividing attention between tasks. However, there is a need for careful assessment as to suitability for such an approach. The training needs to be conducted in an intensive and systematic fashion, with application over extended periods to tasks in the person's day-to-day life if it is to be effective.

As far as pharmacological interventions are concerned, there is some evidence that speed of information processing may be enhanced by the use of methylphenidate, and that bromocriptine might enhance dual-task performance. However, the impact of these and other medications on the person's day-to-day functioning and the extent to which the effects can be maintained in the long term has not been clarified. The potential impact of methylphenidate, combined with behavioral therapy in the more acute stages of recovery, has yet to be investigated.

Sadly there will always be cases in which the damage to neural systems is so extensive that there is little prospect of recovery or remediation. For these individuals, a focus on manipulating the environments and tasks to reduce the demands on their information-processing systems would appear to be most efficacious.

REFERENCES

Arnsten, A. F. T. (1997). Catecholamine regulation of the prefrontal cortex. *Journal of Psychopharmacology, 11*(2), 151–162.

Aston-Jones, G. (1985). Behavioral functions of locus coeruleus derived from cellular attributes. *Physiological Psychology, 13*(3), 118–126.

Aston-Jones, G., & Bloom, F. E. (1981). Activity of norepinephrine-containing locus coeruleus neurons in behaving rats anticipates fluctuations in the sleep-waking cycle. *Journal of Neuroscience, 1,* 876–886.

Azouvi, P., Jokic, C., van der Linden, M., Marliet, N., & Bussel, B. (1996). Working memory and supervisory control after severe closed head injury. A study of dual task performance and random generation. *Journal of Clinical and Experimental Neuropsychology, 18,* 317–337.

Baddeley, A. D. (1993). Working memory or working attention? In A. D. Baddeley & L. Weiskrantz (Eds.), *Attention: Selection, awareness and control. A tribute to Donald Broadbent* (pp. 152–170). Oxford, UK: Oxford University Press.

Balthazor, M., Wagner, R., & Pelham, W. (1991). The specificity of the effects of stimulant medication on classroom learning-related measures of cognitive processing for attention deficit disordered children. *Journal of Abnormal Child Psychology, 19,* 149–178.

Bareggi, S. R., Porta, M., Selenati, A., Assael, B. M., Calderini, G., Collice, M., et al. (1975). Homovanillic acid and 5–hydroxyindole-acetic acid in the CSF of patients after a severe head injury. *European Neurology, 13,* 528–544.

Ben-Yishay, Y., Piasetsky, E. B., & Rattock, J. (1987). A systematic method for ameliorating disorders in basic attention. In M. J. Meier, A. L. Benton, & L. Diller (Eds.), *Neuropsychological rehabilitation* (pp. 165–181). New York: Churchill Livingstone.

Benton, A. L., & Joynt, R. J. (1958). Reaction time in unilateral cerebral disease. *Confina Neurologica, 19,* 247–256.

Blount, P. J., Nguyen, C. D., & McDeavitt, J. T. (2002). Clinical use of cholinomimetic agents: A review. *Journal of Head Trauma Rehabilitation, 17*(4), 314–321.

Bohnen, N., Jolles, J., & Twijnstra, A. (1992). Modification of the Stroop Color Word Test improves differentiation between patients with mild head injury and matched controls. *The Clinical Neuropsychologist, 6,* 178–184.

Bogousslavsky, J., Regli, F., & Assal, G. (1986). The syndrome of unilateral tuberothalamic artery territory infarction. *Stroke, 17,* 434–441.

Boyd, T. M., & Sautter, S. W. (1993). Route-finding: A measure of everyday executive functioning in the head-injured adult. *Applied Cognitive Psychology, 7,* 171–181.

Brouwer, W. H., Ponds, R. W., van Wolffelaar, P. C. van Zomeren, A. H. (1989). Divided attention 5 to 10 years after severe closed head injury. *Cortex, 25,* 219–230.

Brouwer, W. H., & van Wolffelaar, P. C. (1985). Sustained attention and sustained effort after closed head injury. *Cortex, 21,* 111–119.

Burgess, P., & Shallice, T. (1996). Response suppression, initiation and strategy following frontal lobe lesions. *Neuropsychologia, 34,* 263–273.

Chao, L. L., & Knight, R. T. (1995). Human prefrontal lesions increase distractibility to irrelevant sensory inputs. *Neuroreport, 6,* 1605–1610.

Cicerone, K. D. (1996). Attention deficits and dual task demands after mild traumatic brain injury. *Brain Injury, 10,* 79–89.

Cicerone, K. D. (2002). Remediation of "working attention" in mild traumatic brain injury. *Brain Injury, 16*(3), 185–195.

Clark, C. R., Geffen, G. M., & Geffen, L. B. (1986a). Role of monoamine pathways in the control of attention: Effects of droperidol and methylphenidate in normal adult humans. *Psychopharmacology, 90,* 28–34.

Clark, C. R., Geffen, G. M., & Geffen, L. B. (1986b). Role of monoamine pathways in attention and effort: Effects of clonidine and methylphenidate in normal adult humans. *Psychopharmacology, 90,* 35–39.

Clark, C. R., Geffen, G. M., & Geffen, L. B. (1987). Catecholamines and attention II: Pharmacological studies in normal humans. *Neuroscience and Biobehavioral Reviews, 11,* 353–364

Clark, C. R., Geffen, G. M., & Geffen, L. B. (1989). Catecholamines and the covert orienting of attention in humans. *Neuropsychologia, 27*(2), 131–139.

Cohen, R. A. (1993). *The neuropsychology of attention.* New York: Plenum Press.

Cohen, R. A., Malloy, P. F., & Jenkins, M. A. (1998). Disorders of attention. In P. J. Snyder & P. D. Nussbaum (Eds.), *Clinical neuropsychology of attention. A pocket handbook for assessment* (pp. 541–572). Washington, DC: American Psychological Association.

Couillet, J., Leclercq, M., Martin, Y., Rousseaux, M., & Azouvi, P. (2000, September 20–23). *Divided attention after severe diffuse traumatic brain injury.* Paper presented at the meeting of the European Brain Injury Association Meeting, Paris.

Coull, J. T., Büchel, C., Friston, K. J., & Frith, C. D. (1999). Noradrenergically mediated plasticity in a human attentional neuronal network. *NeuroImage, 10,* 705–715.

Crisostomo, E. A., Duncan, P. W., Propst, M., Dawson, D. V., & Davis, J. N. (1988). Evidence that amphetamine with physical therapy promotes recovery of motor function in stroke patients. *Annals of Neurology, 23,* 94–97.

Curry, S. H. (1981). Event-related potentials as indicators of structural and functional damage in closed head injury. *Progress in Brain Research, 54,* 507–515.

Dalebout, S., Nelson, N., Hletko, P., & Frentheway, B. (1991). Selective auditory attention and children with attention-deficit hyperactivity disorder: Effects of repeated measurement with and without methyphenidate. *Language, Speech and Hearing Services in Schools, 22,* 219–227.

Deacon, D., & Campbell, K. (1991). Decision-making following closed head injury: Can response speed be retrained? *Journal of Clinical and Experimental Neuropsychology, 13,* 639–651.

Desimone, R., & Duncan, J. (1995). Neural mechanisms of selective attention. *Annual Review Neuroscience, 18,* 193–222.

Desimone, R., & Ungerleider, L. G. (1989). Neural mechanisms of visual processing in monkeys. In F. Boller & J. Grafman (Eds.), *Handbook of neuropsychology* (Vol. 2, pp. 267–299). New York: Elsevier.

Desimone, R., Wessinger, M., Thomas, L., & Schneider, W. (1990). Attentional control of visual perception: Cortical and subcortical mechanisms. *Cold Spring Harbor Symposia on Quantitative Biology, 60,* 963–971.

D'Esposito, M., Detre, J. A., Alsop, D. C., Shin, R. K., Atlas, S., & Grossman, M. (1995). The neural basis of the central executive system of working memory. *Nature, 378,* 279–281.

Elting, R., van Zomeren, A. H., & Brouwer, W. H. (1989). Flexibility of attention after severe head injury. *Journal of Clinical and Experimental Neuropsychology, 11,* 370.

Everett, J., Thomas, J., Cote, F., Levesque, J., & Michaud, D. (1991). Cognitive effects of psychostimulant medication in hyperactive children. *Child Psychiatry and Human Development, 22,* 79–89.

Fasotti, L., Kovacs, F. Eling, P. A. T. M., & Brouwer, W. H. (2000). Time Pressure Management as a compensatory strategy after closed head injury. *Neuropsychological Rehabilitation, 10*(1), 47–65.

Fontaine, A., Azouvi, P., Remy, P., Bussel, B., & Samson, Y. (1999). Functional anatomy of neuropsychological deficits after severe traumatic brain injury. *Neurology, 53,* 1963–1968.

Gansler, D. A., & McCaffrey, R. J. (1991). Remediation of chronic attention deficits in traumatically brain injured patients. *Archives of Clinical Neurospsychology, 6,* 335–353.

Godefroy, O., Lhullier, C., & Rousseaux, M. (1996). Non-spatial attention disorders in patients with frontal or posterior brain damage. *Brain, 119,* 191–202.

Godefroy, O., & Rousseaux, M. (1996). Divided and focused attention in patients with lesions of the prefrontal cortex. *Brain and Cognition, 30,* 155–174.

Godefroy, O., Rousseaux, M., Leys, D., Desree, A., Scheltens, P., & Pruvo, J. P. (1992). Frontal lobe dysfunction in unilateral lenticulostriate infarcts. *Archives of Neurology, 49,* 1285–1289.

Grade, C., Redford, B., Chrostowski, J., Toussaint, L., & Blackwell, B. (1998). Methylphenidate in early post-stroke recovery: A double-blind, placebo-controlled study. *Archives of Physical Medicine and Rehabilitation, 79,* 1047–1050.

Gray, J. M., & Robertson, I. (1989). Remediation of attentional difficulties following brain injury: Three experimental case studies. *Brain Injury, 3,* 163–170.

Gray, J. M., Robertson, I. H., Pentland, B., & Anderson, S. J. (1992). Microcomputer based cognitive rehabilitation for brain damage. A randomized group controlled trial. *Neuropsychological Rehabilitation, 2,* 97–116.

Greenham, S. L. (1998). Attention deficit hyperactivity disorder and event-related potentials: Evidence for deficits in allocating attentional resources to relevant stimuli. *Child Neuropsychology, 4*(1), 67–80.

Gronwall, D., & Sampson, H. (1974). *The psychological effects of concussion.* Auckland, New Zealand: Auckland University Press/ Oxford University Press.

Gualtieri, C. T., Chandler, M., Coons, T. B., & Brown, L. T. (1989). Amantadine: A new clinical profile for traumatic brain injury. *Clinical Neuropharmacology, 12,* 258–270.

Gualtieri, C. T., & Evans, R. W (1988). Stimulant treatment for the neurobehavioural sequelae of traumatic brain injury. *Brain Injury, 2*(4), 273–290.

Hamill, R. W., Woolf, P. D., McDonald, J. V., Lee, L. A., & Kelly, M. (1987). Catecholamines predict outcome in traumatic brain injury. *Annals of Neurology, 21*(5), 438–443.

Hashimoto, R., Yoshida, M., & Tanaka, Y. (1995). Utilization behaviour after right thalamic infarction. *European Neurology, 35,* 58–62.

Heinze, H. J., Munte, T. F., Gobiet, W., Niemann, H., & Ruff, R. M. (1992). Parallel and serial visual search after closed head injury: Electrophysiological evidence for perceptual dysfunctions. *Neuropsychologia, 30,* 495–514.

Hurford, P., Stringer, A. Y., & Jann, B. (1998). Neuropharmacologic treatment of hemineglect: A case report comparing bromocriptine and methylphenidate. *Archives of Physical Medicine and Rehabilitation, 79,* 346–349.

James, W. (1890). *The principles of psychology.* New York: Dover.

Jonides, J., Smith, E. E., Koeppe, R. A., & Awh, E. (1993). Spatial working memory in humans as revealed by PET. *Nature, 363,* 623–625.

Joseph, R. (1990). *Neuropsychiatry, neuropsychology, and clinical neuroscience* (2nd ed.). New York: Plenum Press.

Kaelin, D. L., Cifu, D. X., & Matthies, B. (1996). Methylphenidate effect on attention deficit in the acutely brain-injured adult. *Archives of Physical Medicine and Rehabilitation, 77,* 6–9.

Keith, R., & Engineer, P. (1991). Effects of methylphenidate on the auditory processing abilities of children with attention deficit hyperactivity disorder. *Journal of Learning Disabilities, 24,* 630–636.

Kewman, D. G., Seigerman, C., Kintner, H., Chu, S., Henson, D., & Reeder, C. (1985). Simulation training of psychomotor skills: Teaching the brain-damaged to drive. *Rehabilitation Psychology, 30,* 11–27.

Klorman, R., Brumaghim, J., Salzman, L., Strauss, J., Borgstedt, A., McBride, M., et al. (1988). Effects of methylphenidate on attention deficit hyperactivity disorder with and without aggressive/noncompliant features. *Journal of Abnormal Child Psychology, 97,* 413–422.

Klorman, R., Brumaghim, J., Salzman, L., Strauss, J., Borgstedt, A., McBride, M., et al. (1990). Effects of methylphenidate on processing negativities in patients with attention-deficit hyperactivity disorder. *Psychophysiology, 27,* 328–337.

Lal, S., Merbitz, C. P., & Grip, J. C. (1988). Modification of function in head-injured patients with sinemet. *Brain Injury, 2,* 225–233.

Lazarus, L. W., Winemiller, D. R., Lingam, V. R., Neyman, I., Hartman, C., Abassian, M., et al. (1992). Efficacy and side effects of methylphenidate for post-stroke depression. *Journal of Clinical Psychiatry, 53,* 447–449.

Leclercq, M., & Azouvi, P. (2002). Attention after traumatic brain injury. In M. Leclercq & P. Zimmerman (Eds.), *Applied neuropsychology of attention* (pp. 257–279). London: Psychology Press.

Leclercq, M., Couillet, J., Marlier, N., Azouvi, P., Martin, Y., Stypstein, E., et al. (2000). Dual task performance after severe diffuse traumatic brain injury or vascular prefrontal damage. *Journal of Clinical and Experimental Neuropsychology, 22,* 339–350.

Lingam, V. R., Lazarus, L. W., Groves, L., & Oh, S. H. (1988). Methylphenidate in treating post-stroke depression. *Journal of Clinical Psychiatry, 49,* 151–153.

Mahalick, D. M., Carmel, P. W., Greenberg, J. P., Molofsky, W., Brown, J. A., Heary, R. F., et al. (1998). Psychopharmalogic treatment of acquired attention disorders in children with brain injury. *Paediatric Neurosurgery, 29*(3), 121–126.

Malec, J., Jones, R., Rao, N., & Stubbs, K. (1984). Video-game practice effects on sustained attention in patients with cranio-cerebral trauma. *Cognitive Rehabilitation, 2*(4), 18–23.

Malone, M., & Swanson, J. (1993). Effects of methylphenidate on impulsive responding in children with attention deficit hyperactivity disorder. *Journal of Child Neurology, 8,* 157–163.

Manly, T., Hawkins, K., Evans, J., Woldt, K., & Robertson, I. H. (2002). Rehabilitation of executive function: Facilitation of effective goal management on complex tasks using periodic auditory alerts. *Neuropsychologia, 40,* 271–281.

McAllister, T. W., Saykin, A. J., Flashman, L. A., Sparling, M. B., Johnson, S. C., Guerin, S. J., et al. (1999). Brain activation during working memory 1 month after mild traumatic brain injury. A functional MRI study. *Neurology, 53,* 1300–1308.

McDowell, S., Whyte, J., & D'Esposito, M. (1997). Working memory impairments in traumatic brain injury: Evidence from a dual-task paradigm. *Neuropsychologia, 35,* 1341–1353.

McDowell, S., Whyte, J., & D'Esposito, M. (1998). Differential effect of a dopaminergic agonist on prefrontal function in traumatic brain injury patients. *Brain, 121,* 1155–1164.

McKinlay, W. W., Brooks, D. N., & Bond, M. R. (1983). Post-concussional symptoms, financial compensation and outcome of severe blunt head injury. *Journal of Neurology, Neurosurgery, and Psychiatry, 46,* 1084–1091.

McMillan, T., Robertson, I. H., Brock, D., & Chorlton, L. (2002). Brief mindfulness training for attentional problems after traumatic brain injury: A randomised control treatment trial. *Neuropsychological Rehabilitation, 12*(2), 117–125.

Meichenbaum, D. (1977). *Cognitive behavior modification: An integrative approach.* New York: Plenum Press.

Meichenbaum, D., & Cameron, B. (1973). Training schizophrenics to talk to themselves: A means of developing attentional control. *Behaviour Therapy, 4,* 513–534.

Mehta, M. A., Owen, A. M., Sahakian, B. J., Mavaddat, N., Pickard, J. D., & Robbins, T. W. (2000). Methylphenidate enhances working memory by modulating discrete frontal and parietal lobe regions in the brain. *Journal of Neuroscience, 20*(RC65), 1–6.

Mesulam, M-M. (1985). *Principles of behavioural neurology.* Philadelphia: Davis.

Meythaler, J. M., Brunner, R. C., Johnson, A., & Novack, T. A. (2002). Amantadine to improve neurorecovery in traumatic brain injury-associated diffuse axonal injury: A pilot double-blind randomized trial. *Journal of Head Trauma Rehabilitation, 17*(4), 300–313.

Miller, E., & Cruzat, A. (1980). A note on the effects of irrelevant information on task performance after mild and severe head injury. *British Journal of Social and Clinical Psychology, 20,* 69–70.

Niemann, H., Ruff, R. M., & Baser, C. A. (1990). Computer-assisted attention retraining in head-injured individuals: A controlled efficacy study of an outpatient program. *Journal of Consulting and Clinical Psychology, 58,* 811–817.

Norman, D. A., & Shallice, T. (1980). Attention to action: Willed and automatic control of behaviour. *Center for Human Information Processing Technical Report No. 99.*

Novack, T. A., Caldwell, S. G., Duke, L. W., Bergquist, T. F., & Gage, R. J. (1996). Focused versus unstructured intervention for attention deficits after traumatic brain injury. *Journal of Head Trauma Rehabilitation, 11,* 52–60.

Olver, J. H., Ponsford, J. L., & Curran, C. (1996). Outcome following traumatic brain injury: A comparison between 2 and 5 years after injury. *Brain Injury, 10,* 841–848.

O'Shanick, G. J. (1991). Cognitive function after brain injury: pharmacologic interference and facilitation. *Neurorehabilitation, 1,* 44–49.

O'Toole, K., Abramowitz, A., Morris, R., & Dulcan, M. (1997). Effects of methylphenidate on attention and non-verbal learning in children with attention deficit hyperactivity disorder. *Journal of the American Academy of Child and Adolescent Psychiatry, 27,* 60–69.

Palmese, C. A., & Raskin, S. A. (2000). The rehabilitation of attention in individuals with mild traumatic brain injury, using the APT-II programme. *Brain Injury, 14*(6), 535–548.

Parasuraman, R. (2000). *The attentive brain.* Cambridge, MA: MIT Press.

Parasuraman, R., Mutter, S. A., & Molloy, R. (1991). Sustained attention following mild closed-head injury. *Journal of Clinical and Experimental Neuropsychology, 13,* 789–811.

Park, N. W., & Ingles, J. L. (2001). Effectiveness of attention rehabilitation after an acquired brain injury: A meta-analysis. *Neuropsychology, 15*(2), 199–210.

Park, N., Moscovitch, M., & Robertson, I. H. (1999). Divided attention impairments after traumatic brain injury. *Neuropsychologia, 37,* 1119–1133.

Park, N. W., Proulx, G., & Towers, W. (1999). Evaluation of the Attention Process training programme. *Neuropsychological Rehabilitation, 9,* 135–154.

Pepin, E. P., & Auray-Pepin, L. (1993). Selective dorsolateral frontal lobe dysfunction associated with diencephalic amnesia. *Neurology, 43,* 733–741.

Plenger, P. M., Dixon, C. E., Castillo, R. M., Frankowski, R. F., Yablon, S. A., & Levin, H. S. (1996). Subacute methylphenidate treatment for moderate to moderately severe traumatic brain injury: A preliminary double-blind placebo-controlled trial. *Archives of Physical Medicine and Rehabilitation, 77,* 536–540.

Ponsford, J. L., & Kinsella, G. (1988). Evaluation of a remedial programme for attentional deficits following closed head injury. *Journal of Clinical and Experimental Neuropsychology, 10,* 693–708.

Ponsford, J. L., & Kinsella, G. (1991). The use of a rating scale of attentional behaviour. *Neuropsychological Rehabilitation, 1,* 241–257.

Ponsford, J. L., & Kinsella, G. (1992). Attentional deficits following closed-head injury. *Journal of Clinical and Experimental Neuropsychology, 14,* 822–838.

Ponsford, J. L., Olver, J. H., & Curran, C. (1995) A profile of outcome: Two years after traumatic brain injury. *Brain Injury, 9,* 1–10.

Ponsford, J. L., Sloan S., & Snow P. (1995). *Traumatic brain injury: Rehabilitation for everyday adaptive living.* London: Erlbaum.

Posner, M. I. (1980). Orienting of attention. *Quarterly Journal of Experimental Psychology, 32,* 3–25.

Posner, M. I., & DiGirolamo, G. J. (2000). Executive attention: Conflict, target detection and cognitive control. In R. Parasuraman (Ed.), *The attentive brain* (pp. 401–423). Cambridge, MA: MIT Press.

Posner, M. I., & Peterson, S. E. (1990). The attention system of the human brain. *Annual Review of Neurosciences, 13,* 25–42.

Posner, M. I., & Rothbart, M. K. (1992). Attentional mechanisms and conscious experience. In A. D. Milnes & M. D. Rugg (Eds.), *The neuropsychology of consciousness* (pp. 91–112). London: Academic Press.

Rizzo, P., Amabile, C., Caporali, M., Spadaro, M., Zanasi, M. & Morocutti, C. (1978). A CNV study in a group of patients with traumatic brain injuries. *Electroencephalography and Clinical Neurophysiology, 45,* 281–285.

Robertson, I. H., Manly, T., Andrade, J., Baddeley, B. T., & Yiend, J. (1997). Oops!: performance correlates of everyday attentional failures in traumatically brain injured and normal subjects. *Neuropsychologia, 35*(12), 1527–1532.

Robertson, I. H., Manly, T., Beschin, N., Haeske-Dewick, H., Homberg, V., Jebkonen, M., et al. (1997). Auditory sustained attention is a marker of unilateral spatial neglect. *Neuropsychologia, 35,* 1527–1532.

Robertson, I. H., Mattingley, J. M., Rorden, C., & Driver, J. (1998). Phasic alerting of neglect patients overcomes their spatial deficit in visual awareness. *Nature, 395,* 169–172.

Robertson, I. H., Tegner, R., Tham, K., Lo, A., & Nimmo-Smith, I. (1995). Sustained attention training for unilateral neglect: Theoretical and rehabilitation implications. *Journal of Clinical and Experimental Neuropsychology, 17,* 416–430.

Robertson, I. H., Ward, T., Ridgeway, V., & Nimmo-Smith, I. (1994). *The Test of Everyday Attention.* Cambridge, UK: MRC Applied Psychology Unit.

Rogers, R. D., Blackshaw, A. J., Middleton, H. C., Matthews, K., Hawtin, K., Crowley, C., et al. (1999). Tryptophan depletion impairs stimulus-reward learning while methylphenidate disrupts attentional control in healthy young adults: Implications for the monoaminergic basis of impulsive behaviour. *Psychopharmacology, 146,* 482–491.

Rousseaux, M., Cabaret, M., Bernati, T., Pruvo, J. P., & Steinling, M. (1998). Deficit residuel du rappel verbal après un infarctus de la veine cerebrale interne gauche. *Revue Neurologique, 154,* 401–407.

Rousseaux M., Fimm, B., & Cantagallo, A. (2002) Attention disorders in cerebrovascular disease. In M. Leclerq & P. Zimmerman (Eds.), *Applied neuropsychology of attention* (pp. 280–304). London: Psychology Press.

Rousseaux, M., Godefroy, O., Cabaret, M., Benaiim, C., & Pruvo, J. P. (1996). Analyse at evolution des deficits cognitifs après rupture des aneurysms de l'artere communicante anterieure. *Revue Neurologique, 152,* 678–687.

Rousseaux, M., Kassiotis, P., Signoret, J. L., Cabaret, M., & Petit, H. (1991). Syndrome amnesique par infarctus restraint du thalamus anterieur droit. *Revue Neurologique, 147,* 809–818.

Ruff, R., Mahaffey, R., Engel, J., Farrow, C., Cox, D., & Karzmark, P. (1994). Efficacy of THINKable in the attention and memory retraining of traumatically head-injured patients. *Brain Injury, 8,* 6–14.

Rugg, M. D., Cowan, C. P., Nagy, M. E., Milner, A. D., Jacobson, I., & Brooks, D. N. (1989). CNV abnormalities following closed head injury. *Brain, 112,* 489–506.

Sandson, T. A., Duffner, K. R., Carvalho, P. A., & Mesulam, M. M. (1991). Frontal lobe dysfunction following infarction of the left-sided medial thalamus. *Archives of Neurology, 48,* 1300–1303.

Schmitter-Edgecombe, M., & Beglinger, L. (2001). Acquisition of skilled visual search performance following severe closed head injury. *Journal of the International Neuropsychological Society, 7*(5), 615–630.

Schmitter-Edgecombe, M., & Kibby, M. (1998). Visual selective attention after severe closed head injury. *Journal of the International Neuropsychological Society, 4,* 144–159.

Schmitter-Edgecombe, M., & Nissley, H. M. (2000). Effects of divided attention on automatic and controlled components of memory after severe closed-head injury. *Neuropsychology, 14,* 559–569.

Schneider, W., & Fisk, A. D. (1982). Degree of consistent training: Improvements in search performances and automatic process development. *Perception and Psychophysics, 31,* 160–168.

Segalowitz, S. J., Dywan, J., & Unsal, A. (1997). Attentional factors in response time variability after traumatic brain injury: An ERP study. *Journal of the International Neuropsychological Society, 3,* 95–107.

Segalowitz, S. J., Unsal, A., & Dywan, J. (1992). CNV evidence for the distinctiveness of frontal and posterior neural processes in a traumatically brain-injured population. *Journal of Clinical and Experimental Neuropsychology, 14,* 545–565.

Shallice, T., & Burgess, P. W. (1991). Deficits in strategy application following frontal lobe damage in man. *Brain, 114,* 727–741.

Shiffrin, R. M., & Schneider, W. (1977). Controlled and automatic human information processing: II. Perceptual learning, automatic attending and a general theory. *Psychological Review, 84,* 127–190.

Simpson, A., & Schmitter-Edgecombe, M. (2000). Intactness of inhibitory attentional mechanisms following severe closed head injury. *Neuropsychology, 14*(2), 1–10.

Sloan, S., & Ponsford, J. L. (1995). Managing cognitive problems. In J. L. Ponsford, S. Sloan, & P. Snow (Eds.), *Traumatic brain injury: Rehabilitation for everyday adaptive living* (pp. 103–135). London: Erlbaum.

Sohlberg, M. M., & Mateer, C. A. (1987). Effectiveness of an attention-training program. *Journal of Clinical and Experimental Neuropsychology, 9,* 117–130.

Solanto, M., Wender, E., & Bartell, S. (1997). Effects of methylphenidate and behavioral contingencies on sustained attention in attention deficit hyperactivity disorder: A test of the reward dysfunction hypothesis. *Journal of Child and Adolescent Psychopharmacology, 7,* 123–136.

Sonnerville, L., Njiokiktjien, C., & Hilhorst, R. (1991). Methylphenidate-induced changes in ADHD information processors. *Journal of Child Psychology and Psychiatry, 32,* 285–295.

Speech, T. J., Rao, S. M., Osmon, D. C., & Sperry, L. T. (1993). A double-blind controlled study of methylphenidate treatment in closed head injury. *Brain Injury, 7*(4), 333–338.

Spikman, J. M., Deelman, B. G., & van Zomeren, A. H. (2000). Executive functioning, attention and frontal lesions in patients with chronic CHI. *Journal of Clinical and Experimental Neuropsychology, 22,* 325–338.

Spikman, J. M., van Zomeren, A. H., & Deelman, B. G. (1996). Deficits of attention after closed-head injury: Slowness only? *Journal of Clinical and Experimental Neuropsychology, 18,* 755–767.

Stablum, F., Leonardi, G., Mazzoldi, M., Umilta, C., & Morra, S. (1994). Attention and control deficits following closed head injury. *Cortex, 30,* 603–618.

Stablum, F., Umilta, C., Mogentale, C., Carlan, M., & Guerrini, C. (2000). Rehabilitation of executive deficits in closed head injury and anterior communicating artery aneurysm patients. *Psychological Research, 63*(3–4), 265–278.

Sturm, W., Fimm, B., Cantagallo, A., Cremel, N., North, P., Passadori, A., et al. (2002). Computerized training of specific attention deficits in stroke and traumatically brain-injured patients. In M. Leclercq & P. Zimmerman (Eds.), *Applied neuropsychology of attention* (pp. 365–380). London: Psychology Press.

Sturm, W., & Willmes, K. (1991). Efficacy of a reaction training on various attentional and cognitive functions in stroke patients. *Neuropsychological Rehabilitation, 1,* 259–280.

Sturm, W., & Willmes, K. (2001). On the functional neuroanatomy of intrinsic and phasic alertness. *Neuroimage, 14*(1, Pt. 2), S76–S84.

Sturm, W., Willmes, K., Orgass, B., & Hartje, W. (1997). Do specific attention deficits need specific training? *Neuropsychological Rehabilitation, 7,* 81–103.

Stuss, D. T., & Benson, D. F. (1986). *The frontal lobes.* New York: Raven Press.

Stuss, D. T., Pogue, J., Buckle, L., & Bondar, J. (1994). Characterization of stability of performance in patients with traumatic brain injury: Variability and consistency on reaction time tests. *Neuropsychology, 8,* 316–324.

Stuss, D. T., Stethem, L. L., Hugenholtz, H., Picton, T., Pivik, J., & Richard, M. T. (1989). Reaction time after head injury: fatigue, divided and focused attention, and consistency of performance. *Journal of Neurology, Neurosurgery, and Psychiatry, 52,* 742–748.

Sunohara, G. A., Malone, M. A., Rovet, J., Humphries, T., Roberts, W., & Taylor, M. J. (1999). Effect of methylphenidate on attention in children with attention deficit hyperactivity disorder: ERP evidence. *Neuropsychopharmacology, 21*(2), 218–228.

Trexler, L., & Zappala, G. (1988). Neuropathological determinants of acquired attention disorders in traumatic brain injury. *Brain and Cognition, 8,* 291–302.

Tromp, E., & Mulder, T. (1991). Slowness of information processing after traumatic head injury. *Journal of Clinical and Experimental Neuropsychology, 13,* 821–830.

van Zomeren, A. H. (1981). *Reaction time and attention after closed head injury.* Lisse: Swets and Zeitlinger.

van Zomeren, A. H., & Brouwer, W. H. (1987). Head injury and concepts of attention. In H. S. Levin, J. Grafman, & H. M. Eisenberg (Eds.), *Neurobehavioral recovery from head injury* (pp. 398–415). New York: Oxford University Press.

van Zomeren, A. H., & Brouwer, W. H. (1994). *Clinical neuropsychology of attention.* New York: Oxford University Press.

van Zomeren, A. H., Brouwer, W. H., & Deelman, B. G. (1984). Attentional deficits: The riddles of selectivity, speed, and alertness. In N. Brooks (Eds.), *Closed head injury* (pp. 74–107). New York: Oxford University Press.

van Zomeren, A. H., & van den Burg, W. (1985). Residual complaints of patients two years after severe head injury. *Journal of Neurology, Neurosurgery and Psychiatry, 48,* 21–28.

Vecht, C. J., van Woerkom, T. C. A. M., Teelkem, A. W., & Minderhoud, J. M. (1975).

Homovanillic acid and 5–hydroxyindoleaetic acid cerebrospinal fluid levels: A study with and without probenecid administration of their relationship to the state of consciousness after head injury. *Archives of Neurology, 32,* 792–797.

Veltman, J. C., Brouwer, W., van Zomeren, A. H., & van Wolffelaar, P. C. (1996). Central executive aspects of attention in subacute severe and very severe closed head injury patients: Planning, inhibition, flexibility, and divided attention. *Neuropsychology, 10,* 357–367.

Vilkki, J. (1992). Cognitive flexibility and mental programming after closed head injuries and anterior or posterior cerebral excisions. *Neuropsychologia, 30*(9), 807–814.

Vilkki, J., Virtanen, S., Surma-Aho, O., & Servo A. (1996). Dual task performance after focal cerebral lesions and closed head injuries. *Neuropsychologia, 34,* 1051–1056.

Volkow, N. D., Wang, G-J., Fowler, J. S., Logan, J., Gerasimov, M., Mynard, L., et al. (2001). Therapeutic doses of oral methylphenidate significantly increase extracellular dopamine in the human brain. *Journal of Neuroscience, 21*(RC121), 1–5.

Ward, N. M., & Brown, V. J. (1996). Covert orienting of attention in the rat and the role of striatal dopamine. *Journal of Neuroscience, 16*(9), 3082–3088.

Webster, J. S., & Scott, R. R. (1983). The effects of self-instructional training on attentional deficits following head injury. *Clinical Neuropsychology, 5*(2), 69–74.

Webster, M. J., & Ungerleider, L. G. (2000). Neuroanatomy of visual attention. In R. Parasuraman (Ed.), *The attentive brain* (pp. 19–34). Cambridge, MA: MIT Press.

Whyte, J. (2003, April 3–5). *Pharmacological treatment of attention deficits after traumatic brain injury: Results of a randomised placebo controlled trial of methylphenidate* (Abstract). Proceedings of the 26th annual Brain Impairment Conference, Sydney, Australia.

Whyte, J., Fleming, M., Polansky, M., Cavallucci, C., & Coslett, H. B. (1997). Phasic arousal in response to auditory warnings after traumatic brain injury. *Neuropsychologia, 35,* 313–324.

Whyte, J., Fleming, M., Polansky, M., Cavallucci, C., & Coslett, H. B. (1998). The effects of visual distraction following traumatic brain injury. *Journal of the International Neuropsychological Society, 4,* 127–36.

Whyte, J., Hart, T., Schuster, K., Fleming, M., Polansky, M., & Coslett, H. B. (1997). Effects of methylphenidate on attentional function after traumatic brain injury: A randomized, placebo-controlled trial. *American Journal of Physical Medicine and Rehabilitation, 76*(6), 440–450.

Whyte, J., Polansky, M., Cavallucci, C., Fleming, M., Lhulier, J., & Coslett, H. B. (1996). Inattentive behaviour after traumatic brain injury. *Journal of the International Neuropsychological Society, 2,* 274–281.

Whyte, J., Polansky, M., Fleming, M., Coslett, H. B., & Cavallucci, C. (1995). Sustained arousal and attention after traumatic brain injury. *Neuropsychologia, 33,* 797–813.

Whyte, J., Vaccaro, M., Grieb-Neff, P., & Hart, T. (2002). Psychstimulant use in the rehabilitation of individuals with traumatic brain injury. *Journal of Head Trauma Rehabilitation, 17*(1), 284–299.

Williams, S. E., Ris, M. D., Ayyangar, R., Schefft, B. K., & Berch, D. (1998). Recovery in pediatric brain injury: Is psychostimulant medication beneficial? *Journal of Head Trauma Rehabilitation, 13*(3), 73–81.

Wilson, C., & Robertson, I. H. (1992). A home-based intervention for attentional slips during reading following head injury: A single case study. *Neuropsychological Rehabilitation, 2*, 193–205.

Withaar, F. K. (2000). *Divided attention and driving: the effects of aging and brain injury*. Unpublished doctoral dissertation, Riiksuniversiteit, Groningen.

Wood, R. L. (1986). Rehabilitation of patients with disorders of attention: From research to treatment. *Journal of Head Trauma Rehabilitation, 3*, 43–53.

Wood, R. L. (1987). *Brain injury rehabilitation: A neurobehavioural perspective*. London: Croom Helm.

Wood, R. L. (1988). Attention disorders in brain injury rehabilitation. *Journal of Learning Disabilities, 21*(6), 327–332.

Wood, R. L., & Fussey, I. (1987). Computer-based cognitive retraining: A controlled study. *International Disability Studies, 9*(4), 149–153.

Woolf, P. D., Hamill, R. W., Lee, L. A., Cox, C., & McDonald, J. V. (1987). The predictive value of catecholamines in assessing outcome in traumatic brain injury. *Journal of Neurosurgery, 66*, 875–882.

Zahn, T. P., & Mirsky, A. F. (1999). Reaction time indicators of attention deficits in closed head injury. *Journal of Clinical and Experimental Neuropsychology, 21*, 352–367.

Zeiner, P. (1999). Do the beneficial effects of extended methylphenidate treatment in boys with attention-deficit hyperactivity disorder dissipate rapidly during placebo treatment? *Nordic Journal of Psychiatry, 53*(1), 55–60.

Zoccolotti, P. Matano, A., Deloche, G., Cantagallo, A., Passadori, A., Leclerq, M., et al. (2000). Patterns of attentional impairment following closed head injury: A collaborative European study. *Cortex, 36*, 93–107.

4

Disorders of Memory

Elizabeth L. Glisky

Memory disorders are perhaps the most pervasive and debilitating of the consequences of neurological insult and among the most resistant to rehabilitation. Because of their impact, not only on virtually all aspects of everyday life but also on many facets of the rehabilitation process itself, their effective treatment is essential to the overall success of rehabilitation programs. Most theorists would agree that a learning or relearning process must be at the heart of cognitive rehabilitation, but in the case of memory impairment, it is precisely this learning mechanism that appears to be compromised. This may be, at least partly, why learning and memory problems have been so intractable. Furthermore, until recently, models of memory have been rather poorly specified cognitively and neurally, and thus rehabilitation specialists have often been forced to rely on fuzzy guidelines and clinical intuitions when designing and implementing treatments for memory disorders. Although there are still few certainties with respect to appropriate interventions for memory deficits, in recent years the choice of well-tested, theoretically derived treatments has considerably expanded. The purpose of this chapter is to describe these rehabilitation methods and to outline the cognitive and neurobiological rationale that motivates their use and the conditions under which they are most likely to be effective.

NEUROPSYCHOLOGICAL THEORIES OF NORMAL MEMORY

Since the early 1980s, substantial progress has been made in the development of memory theory and in our understanding of the cognitive and neural mechanisms of normal memory. Much of that understanding came initially from a merging of the disciplines of cognitive psychology and neuropsychology, and more recently has come from developments in basic and cognitive neuroscience, particularly the growth of neuroimaging technologies. Two complementary conceptualizations of memory, which have developed from studies of both normal and brain-injured individuals, will be discussed in this section, one that focuses on memory systems and the other on memory processes. Both models include cognitive and neuroanatomical components and both have influenced the development of memory rehabilitation techniques and in all likelihood will continue to do so.

Memory Systems

Probably the most important theoretical development in the field of memory in the past 20 years has been the conceptualization of memory not as a unitary construct subject to a single set of principles and reliant on a single underlying brain structure or system but as a set of systems, each governed by different rules and supported by different neural substrates. This proposal was based on early findings showing that, although amnesic patients could not recall or recognize recently presented materials, they could nevertheless produce those items in response to partial cues (Warrington & Weiskrantz, 1970), and on the subsequent demonstration with normal individuals that their ability to complete word fragments with recently presented words was independent of their ability to retrieve those words consciously in a recognition memory test (Tulving, Schacter, & Stark, 1982). These findings, along with many others that followed, strongly implied that memory was composed of at least two independent systems, only one of which was damaged by amnesia. Importantly for rehabilitation, these results also suggested that it might be possible to take advantage of the intact memory system to compensate for the system that was damaged. Indeed, several of the most successful rehabilitation methods have attempted to capitalize exactly on this possibility.

As empirical evidence mounted in support of the idea of multiple independent memory systems subserving different kinds of memory, contemporary researchers began to formulate models to capture the most important distinctions (Schacter & Tulving, 1994a). Among these models, one of the most comprehensive was a model described by Schacter and Tulving (1994b), which included five independent memory systems. Since its original formulation in 1994, the five-system model has been elaborated and updated to take into account not only findings from cognitive studies of normal individuals and neuro-psychological investigations of focal lesion patients but also information from more recent functional neuroimaging studies (Schacter, Wagner, & Buckner, 2000). The model has now been supported by considerable empirical evidence documenting the hypothesized brain–behavior relations and provides a relevant theoretical base from which to develop rehabilitation strategies for neurological patients.

Schacter and Tulving Five-System Model

In Schacter and Tulving's (1994b) model (see Table 4.1), five major memory systems were proposed: (1) working memory, a system designed to maintain and manipulate small amounts of information in the short term; (2) semantic memory, a long-term permanent memory system for the storage of general knowledge about the world; (3) episodic memory, a context-dependent system that retains information about specific events that occur in a person's life at a particular time and place; (4) the perceptual representation system (PRS), a system encompassing several modality specific modules that code and store information about the perceptual characteristics of words and objects; and (5) procedural memory, a system enabling the learning and retention of motor and cognitive skills. Each system was hypothesized to operate on a different type of information according to a unique set of rules. Although systems were able to operate independently, such that damage to one system could leave another

TABLE 4.1. Memory Systems

System	Function	Neural correlates
Working memory	Storage and manipulation of small amounts of information in the short term	Storage in posterior parietal cortex; maintenance and manipulation in prefrontal
Semantic memory	Permanent context-free store of general knowledge	Storage in posterior neocortex; retrieval in left prefrontal
Episodic memory	Memory for personal events that occurred in a specific spatial and temporal context	Encoding and retrieval in left and right inferior prefrontal; consolidation in medial temporal; storage in neocortex
Perceptual representation system (PRS)	Presemantic, modality specific modules that support implicit memory and priming	Visual priming in extrastriate visual cortex
Procedural memory	Memory for motor and cognitive skills	Frontostriatal and frontocerebellar circuits

system wholly intact, the operation of any one system might nevertheless be fa-cilitated by its interaction with another system. Thus, for example, the learning of a new word might involve initial coding of its perceptual features by the PRS, maintenance in working memory while related information was retrieved from semantic memory, the indexing in episodic memory of the contextual de-tails of the learning experience, and the ultimate representation of the new vo-cabulary item in the knowledge system. Although several systems might be in-volved in the acquisition of new information such as a vocabulary item, according to this model it should still be possible for such knowledge to be ac-quired, although perhaps somewhat less efficiently, if, for example, the episodic memory system was damaged but the semantic memory system was still intact.

Neural Correlates of the Five Memory Systems

Focal lesion patients and neuroimaging studies have provided evidence that these different memory systems are represented in different neural circuits, al-though such circuits may overlap and have neural components in common. This commonality may be attributable to shared processes across systems and may enable the kinds of interactions among systems that are suggested above. Alternatively, other models of memory have focused on different distinctions and have carved up the memory pie along different lines and so may view these commonalities as evidence for a different taxonomy. Squire (1987), for example, considers episodic and semantic memory as subsystems of the same declarative memory system and might see the shared neural circuitry as supportive of his model. The following summary of the neuroanatomical evidence is organized according to the five-system model, but the brain regions identified may repre-sent the operation of systems, subsystems, processes, or all of these.

The working memory system (Baddeley, 1994; Baddeley & Hitch, 1974) has been characterized as consisting of a content-independent central execu-tive, which controls and manipulates information stored in a set of material-specific subsystems. These slave systems, which store information only tempo-rarily, are thought to be represented in posterior parietal cortex, with verbal and object information primarily on the left and spatial information on the right. Maintenance of information in working memory occurs via a rehearsal mechanism involving posterior ventrolateral prefrontal cortex (i.e., Broca's area) and premotor regions on the left for verbal material and homologous re-gions on the right for spatial tasks. The central executive, which acts as an attentional controller, coordinating and manipulating the various sources of in-formation in working memory and monitoring the outcome, appears to depend on dorsolateral prefrontal cortex. (For reviews of neuroimaging evidence, see Cabeza, Dolcos, Graham, & Nyberg, 2002; D'Esposito & Postle, 2002; Fletcher & Henson, 2001; Nyberg, Forkstam, Petersson, Cabeza, & Ingvar, 2002.) Working-memory deficits are often observed following frontal damage or frontal atrophy, such as might occur in normal aging, and are likely related to executive dysfunction. A small number of cases have been reported of left inferior parietal lesions resulting in sharply reduced verbal short-term storage capacity (i.e., digit span) and right parietal damage associated with reduced visuospatial span (for reviews, see McCarthy & Warrington, 1990; Vallar & Papagno, 2002).

Semantic memory (Tulving, 1972) is a context-free permanent memory system that represents one's general knowledge about the world—facts, concepts, and the meaning of words. Knowledge is thought to be stored in domain-specific neocortical regions, primarily in anterolateral temporal cortex, with different categories of knowledge stored in distinct regions near the same areas that originally processed them (Schacter et al., 2000). Damage to these posterior neocortical regions, which occurs in late-stage Alzheimer's disease and in semantic dementia, is associated with impairments in naming, identifying, and describing the properties of objects. Patients with semantic dementia, however, although severely impaired in a range of semantic memory tasks, exhibit normal working memory and episodic memory (Hodges, 2000). Retrieval from the semantic memory system appears to be mediated by the same left inferior prefrontal regions as are involved in working memory (Fletcher & Henson, 2001; Nyberg et al., 2002; Wagner, 2002).

The episodic memory system (Tulving, 1983) is required for the acquisition and retention of personally experienced events that occur at a particular time and place. It has traditionally been associated with the hippocampus and other structures located in the medial temporal lobes, and also with the diencephalon and other limbic structures. More recently, however, mainly as a result of neuroimaging evidence, prefrontal cortex has also been implicated in episodic memory, with encoding processes assigned primarily to left inferior prefrontal cortex and episodic retrieval processes more often involving right prefrontal cortex. The left prefrontal regions overlap with areas involved in semantic memory retrieval and working memory, suggesting that these three memory systems share common frontally mediated processes. Regions in the parietal lobes (similar to those involved in working memory) are also activated during episodic memory retrieval and may mediate processes shared between those two systems (for discussion of these similarities, see Cabeza et al., 2002; Cabeza & Nyberg, 2000; Fletcher & Henson, 2001; Nyberg et al., 2002). Damage to medial temporal/diencephalic structures has been associated with an amnesic syndrome, whereas damage to prefrontal regions has usually caused more subtle memory impairments. Episodic memory deficits will be discussed in greater detail later.

The PRS (Tulving & Schacter, 1990) is thought to consist of a set of domain-specific modules that process and represent perceptual information about the form and structure but not the meaning of objects and words. This system is thought to underlie perceptual priming, a form of implicit memory that enables a stimulus to be processed more fluently as a result of its prior presentation. Priming can occur in the absence of conscious recollection (or explicit memory) of the prior encounter with the stimulus. Lesion studies and neuroimaging studies converge on the conclusion that regions of extrastriate visual cortex subserve perceptual priming in the visual domain (Cabeza & Nyberg, 2000; Gabrieli, Fleischman, Keane, Reminger, & Morrell, 1995). Conceptual priming, which involves facilitated *semantic* processing of repeated materials, can also be found in the absence of explicit memory for prior occurrence and is associated with reduced activation in left inferior prefrontal cortex (Gabrieli et al., 1996; Schacter & Buckner, 1998). Conceptual priming has been dissociated from perceptual priming in that patients with Alzheimer's disease, who have damage to association cortices, show impaired conceptual priming but intact perceptual priming (Keane, Gabrieli, Fennema, Growdon, & Corkin, 1991), whereas patients with damage to extrastriate regions of occipital cortex show the opposite dissociation (Gabrieli et al., 1995). Whether conceptual priming is dependent on yet another memory system remains to be determined (Gabrieli, 1999). Importantly for our purposes in this chapter, the PRS does not depend on the brain regions that support episodic or explicit memory and thus perceptual priming is usually intact in amnesic patients.

Procedural memory (Cohen & Squire, 1980) supports the acquisition and maintenance of cognitive and motor skills. Learning of skills proceeds gradually and incrementally over time and after large amounts of practice the skilled behavior becomes relatively resistant to forgetting and can be executed automatically. Often, the components of the skill are not accessible to conscious retrieval. Brain regions implicated in skill learning include the striatum (caudate and putamen), the cerebellum, and motor regions of the cortex (Doyon & Ungerleider, 2002). Frontal regions with connections to the basal ganglia also contribute to the learning of cognitive skills (Knowlton, 2002). As skills become well learned, evidence suggests that the pathways supporting them change; in particular there appears to be a reduction in the contribution of prefrontal and premotor cortices as behaviors become overlearned. Patients with Huntington's and Parkinson's disease, which involve damage to frontal–striatal circuits, show deficits in skill learning.

This brief overview of the neuroanatomical correlates of memory systems suggests that different systems share processing components and are mediated by overlapping neural circuits. Processes such as retrieval, for example, may be represented by general processing mechanisms that are frontally based and common to several systems (e.g., working memory, episodic and semantic memory, and perhaps even the PRS and procedural memory under some conditions). Similarly, neocortical representations may be at least partially shared among all systems. At the same time, each system appears to include neural components that are unique. The nature of a memory deficit will be critically dependent on which regions of the brain are damaged and the extent to which they are uniquely involved in one system or more generally involved in multiple systems. Further, the possibilities for rehabilitation will also hinge on what components of a system are damaged, how complete the damage is, and the extent to which other systems are preserved.

The rest of this chapter is concerned, for the most part, with the episodic memory system, the system that depends uniquely on medial temporal lobe and diencephalic brain structures. Damage to this system is implicated in most cases of clinically significant learning and memory impairment, and severe damage results in an amnesic syndrome. To gain a better understanding of the workings of this system, we need to examine more closely the processes involved in episodic memory.

Memory Processes

Traditionally, memory theory has postulated three general processes involved in episodic memory: encoding, storage, and retrieval. Although over the years theorists have debated the extent to which a good memory depends on the integrity of one or the other of these processes, more recent theorizing has taken a more comprehensive view of memory and considered how these processes might interact to influence long-term retention. In addition, processes have been decomposed further. Thus, for example, not only are the retrieval processes involved in recall and recognition tasks thought to be different but, according to several theorists, recognition itself may be further subdivided into two subprocesses—a relatively automatic familiarity process and a more consciously controlled recollection process (Kelley & Jacoby, 2000). Evidence from both neuroimaging and lesion studies has bolstered these distinctions by identifying separable brain regions associated with different processes, and although the precise mapping of function to structure is not yet certain, these studies have added much to our understanding of the ways in which memory may break down. In the next section, we consider these processes, their neural substrates, and how they may work together within the context of a general neuropsychological process model similar to one proposed by Moscovitch (1994, 1995).

Encoding and Retrieval

For years it has been known that the way in which information is processed at input (i.e., encoded) will, to a large extent, determine how well it will be subsequently remembered (i.e., retrieved). In general, the more meaningful the analysis of material and the more it is related to information already in the knowledge system, the better the memory (Craik & Lockhart, 1972; Craik & Tulving, 1975). It is also clear, however, that this statement is not true in any absolute sense because the probability of successful retrieval will always be dependent on the nature of the retrieval environment—the type and number of cues and the type of memory test—and the extent to which the information and processes engaged at retrieval overlap those at encoding (Morris, Bransford, & Franks, 1978; Tulving & Thomson, 1973). The initiation of appropriate encoding processes, which may include selective attention, formation of organizational strategies, integration of an event with its context, and access to related prior knowledge, has been found to depend primarily on left inferior prefrontal cortex. Specifically, it is this brain region that appears to be responsible for initiating and controlling these processes at encoding. Retrieval processes, on the other hand, which include the adoption and maintenance of a "retrieval mode," the generation of retrieval cues, the initiation of search strategies, and the monitoring of output, have been localized primarily to right inferior prefrontal cortex. Moscovitch has suggested that these encoding and retrieval processes "work with memory" rather than represent memory per se. The processes are, in a sense, nonmnemonic and might better be characterized as executive control or decision processes that assist with memory under certain demanding conditions.

Damage to the frontal lobes does not result in an amnesic syndrome. Instead, deficits are sometimes seen in more difficult memory tests such as free recall, which may require strategic retrieval processes, but not usually in less demanding tests such as recognition (Wheeler, Stuss, & Tulving, 1995). Recently, in a list discrimination task, we demonstrated that the frontal lobes were involved when conscious recollection was required to perform the task but not when judgments could be made on the basis of familiarity (Davidson & Glisky, 2002). Even more complex memory tasks such as remembering where or when something occurred or who told you about it (i.e., source memory; Glisky, Rubin, & Davidson, 2001; Janowsky, Shimamura, & Squire, 1989), and tasks where there is potential for interference among competing responses (Shimamura, 1994), also require the frontal lobes. They also appear to play a role in monitoring memory output to prevent false-recognition responses (e.g., Rapcsak, Nielsen, Glisky, & Kaszniak, 2002).

Storage or Consolidation

Once the components of an event have been processed by neocortical perceptual and semantic processors, according to Moscovitch (1994), if given full attention they will be delivered to consciousness. The elements of the conscious experience are then obligatorily processed by the medial temporal lobe/hippocampal complex (MTL/H) and other limbic structures, which bind the elements together in a memory trace, along with a marker in MTL/H that acts as an index to locations in neocortex where various aspects of the experience are represented. In some models, the hippocampus is viewed as having an additional role in providing the spatial context for an event and linking it to the other elements of the memory (Nadel & Moscovitch, 1997). This initial rapid binding process, which Moscovitch (1995) calls cohesion, is followed by a longer, slower consolidation process, which ensures the long-term preservation of the memory trace. In some models of memory (e.g., Squire, 1992), the neocortical memory trace ultimately (after years perhaps) becomes independent of the MTL/H and can be accessed without MTL/H assistance. In other models, such as multiple trace theory (Fujii, Moscovitch, & Nadel, 2000; Nadel & Moscovitch, 1997), the MTL/H continues to be necessary for the access of episodic memories, but semantic memories, which lack a spatiotemporal context, can be retrieved independently of the MTL/H.

Damage to structures in the MTL/H produces a profound amnesia, characterized by an inability to acquire new episodic memories (i.e., anterograde amnesia) and a difficulty in retrieving old autobiographical memories (i.e., retrograde amnesia), although overlearned semantic information about one's personal history is often available, as are memories for past public events and famous people. General knowledge of the world is usually preserved. The various regions of the MTL/H and associated limbic areas almost certainly contribute differently to consolidation and retrieval of episodic memories, either in terms of the kind of memory they subserve (e.g., object vs. spatial) or the particular process or task involved (e.g., recognition vs. recall and familiarity vs. recollection) (Aggleton & Brown, 1999; for review, see Mayes, 2000). Although the specific functions of these various regions remain controversial, it is certain that larger lesions will result in more severe and complete amnesias. Continued investigation of the contributions of these various structures to memory will be important for the future of memory rehabilitation, enabling more appropriate selection of rehabilitation techniques depending on the specific brain regions involved and the specific processes or tasks affected.

How do the encoding, storage and retrieval processes interact? The frontal lobes may become involved at encoding in organizing the conscious input to the MTL/H system, ensuring that all aspects (or the most important aspects) of an experience are encoded, elaborated, and integrated so that they will be bound together in a neocortical-MTL/H ensemble—the memory trace. Retrieval of the memory trace will occur either when cue information automatically accesses the stored memory representation (e.g., on a recognition test) or when the frontal lobes direct a strategic search for required information (e.g., on a difficult free recall or source memory task). Frontal lobes will then monitor the output from the MTL/H and decide how to act on it. Damage to the frontal lobes, as noted previously, results in deficits only on memory tasks that require these complex strategic processes.

NEUROPHYSIOLOGY AND NEUROCHEMISTRY OF NORMAL MEMORY

To gain some understanding of how rehabilitation might be possible at a neural level, some review of the basic neurophysiology and neurochemistry of normal memory might be helpful. Some of the relevant neurophysiology is covered in chapters by Kolb (Chapter 2; Kolb & Cioe, Chapter 1, this volume) and thus is summarized only briefly here (for more detailed discussions, see Eichenbaum, 2002; Kolb, 1995).

Perhaps the most important aspect of the brain's structure and function, from a rehabilitation perspective, is "plasticity." Plasticity refers to the brain's capacity to change its structure and function with experience. Thus it provides a mechanism for learning, and although the brain appears most malleable during development, it is clear that learning is possible throughout life. Plasticity results from changes that occur in synapses, the space between the axonal ending of one neuron and an element of another neuron, usually the dendrite, across which information is transmitted in the form of chemical messengers called neurotransmitters. After neurotransmitters are released from the presynaptic neuron into the synaptic space, they bind to receptors on the postsynaptic neuron that either induce that neuron to fire or inhibit it from doing so. The likelihood of firing is determined by a variety of chemical processes that control the release of the neurotransmitter and affect the sensitivity of the receptors, and by other inputs arriving at the neuron at the same time. The summation of all inputs ultimately determines the action of the receiving neuron. Learning is reflected in increased synaptic efficacy (i.e., in the likelihood of transmission) following repeated stimulation.

In mammalian brains, long-term potentiation (LTP), which reflects an increase in the responsiveness of an associated group of neurons that persists over time and results in long-lasting synaptic changes, is a mechanism considered to be a likely candidate for the formation of long-term permanent memories. Importantly, LTP has been observed most prominently in brain structures important for memory, particularly the hippocampus, and although LTP still remains a hypothesized rather than a confirmed mechanism of long-term memory, it seems to possess many of the characteristics that a process such as consolidation would have to have.

A number of neurotransmitters play a role in learning and memory and contribute to plasticity (for review, see Wenk, 2003). One of the most important is acetylcholine (Baxter & Murg, 2002), which has been implicated in learning, memory, and attention. Acetylcholine is produced in neurons in the medial septal area of the basal forebrain, which send axons to the hippocampus, and in neurons of the nucleus basalis, which innervate the amygdala and neocortex. If the cholinergic function of these neurons is interrupted by a drug such as scopolamine, memory is impaired; conversely, drugs such as physostigmine, which enhance cholinergic function, have been found to improve memory. Pharmacological treatments of memory deficits have been used in patients with Alzheimer's disease (AD), whose memory dysfunction may be partly attributable to a loss of cholinergic cells in the basal forebrain. Drug treatments currently being offered, such as tacrine and donepezil (Aricept), act to increase acetylcholine in the brain. So far, however, these drugs have produced only modest and somewhat variable effects. Although they appear to slow the rate of cognitive decline in some patients in the early stages of AD, they have minimal, if any, effects in other patients. Recent research suggests that the benefits may reflect alterations in attentional function rather than in memory per se and may differ across the various subtypes of AD (Curran, 2000). Other neuro-transmitters that may play a role in memory include norepinephrine, which plays an arousal function that probably contributes to many aspects of brain function including memory; serotonin, which may stimulate the production of new neurons in the dentate gyrus, part of the hippocampal formation (Gould, 1999); glutamate, a major excitatory transmitter, that has been implicated in LTP and plasticity; and GABA (gamma-aminobutyric acid), a major inhibitory neurotransmitter. Pharmacological treatments, involving manipulation of these neurochemicals, are still for the most part experimental and have yet to be tested in humans.

What about the growth of new synapses or neuronal elements in the nor-mal brain? A number of the early animal studies demonstrated that rats raised in enriched environments have greater numbers of dendrites and synapses, among other changes, than rats raised in isolation. Later studies have found that at least some of these changes are highly specific, occurring only in the particular regions of the brain that are stimulated by the experience (Kolb, 1995). There is also evidence of neurogenesis in the hippocampal formation of human adults (Eriksson et al., 1998), which in animal studies has been linked to the learning of hippocampally dependent associative memory tasks (Gould, Beylin, Tanapat, Reeves, & Shors, 1999).

There are now compelling reasons to believe that the same kind of plastic-ity that has been observed in normal brains can be demonstrated in damaged brains (see Kolb, Chapter 2, this volume), and that when a brain is damaged there remains significant potential for changes in dendritic morphology and synaptic connectivity, both as a result of spontaneous recovery and as a result of experience. Importantly, evidence from studies with lesioned animals suggests that these dendritic and synaptic changes have behavioral consequences in both motor and cognitive domains. Most of the evidence for plasticity in adult humans, however, involves reorganization in sensory and motor cortex, and it remains to be determined to what extent the same principles of reorganization apply to higher-level cognitive functions, particularly episodic memory, which relies on complex interactions between limbic and neocortical brain structures. Evidence is beginning to appear, however, from functional neuroimaging stud-ies that suggest, at least at a cortical level, that the brain is capable of reorgani-zation following injury or atrophy in ways that affect cognitive function. For ex-ample, Buckner, Corbetta, Schatz, Raichle, and Petersen (1996) showed that, in a patient with damage to an area of left prefrontal cortex that resulted in a lan-guage problem, the homologous region of right frontal cortex was able to take over the function, and Grady and colleagues (Cabeza et al., 1997; Cabeza, An-derson, Locantore, & McIntosh, 2002; Grady et al., 1995) have reported data suggestive of functional reorganization of frontal systems in older adults, which may support compensatory memory processes. An important goal for rehabilitation will be to find ways to stimulate cerebral reorganization as well as neural generation so that the changes that occur have adaptive functional consequences.

The balance of this chapter focuses on memory disorders and their rehabilitation. The rehabilitation approaches and techniques are evaluated against the cognitive and neurobiological background outlined previously and in the context of individual impairments and disabilities. First, I consider briefly the general characteristics of the amnesic syndrome, along with its various etiologies and neuropathology.

ETIOLOGY, NEUROPATHOLOGY, AND COGNITIVE CHARACTERISTICS OF MEMORY DISORDERS

Memory impairment can be caused by a range of neurological disorders that result in damage to the principal brain structures involved in memory—the medial temporal lobes, diencephalon, frontal lobes, and basal forebrain (for review, see O'Connor, Verfaellie, & Cermak, 1995). The importance of the hippocampus and other medial temporal lobe structures (MTL/H) in memory came initially from reports of patient H.M. who, after bilateral excision of the hippocampus and surrounding structures to control his epilepsy, was left globally amnesic, unable to acquire any new memories in either the verbal or nonverbal domain (Milner, 1966). His anterograde amnesia was accompanied by a retrograde amnesia, characterized by an inability to retrieve events that had occurred in the preceding 11 years (Corkin, 1984). H.M. also had what appeared to be a sparing of the ability to acquire new motor skills—what is now called procedural memory. His short-term or working memory was intact, as was his general intellectual function and knowledge of the world. A similar pattern of deficits has now been observed in numerous other individuals with bilateral damage to the MTL/H, which may occur following herpes simplex encephalitis, anoxic or ischemic episodes, Alzheimer's disease, or head trauma. For obvious reasons, bilateral resections of the MTL/H are no longer performed. Unilateral temporal lobectomies, which remain a treatment for intractable epilepsy, are not usually associated with a global amnesia, although material-specific memory problems often occur following surgery—verbal memory difficulties associated with left temporal lobectomy and nonverbal memory problems following right-hemisphere excisions.

Damage to midline diencephalic structures, which may occur as a result of third ventricle tumors or stroke, are also associated with amnesia. The exact structures responsible for the amnesia are somewhat controversial but include the dorsomedial and anterior nuclei of the thalamus, the mammillary bodies and the mammilothalamic tract. Patients with lesions in these areas usually have a severe anterograde amnesia with a retrograde amnesia of variable duration. They often have other cognitive deficits as well, which may be attributable to the extensive connections between the thalamus and other brain regions. Korsakoff syndrome, a neurological disorder associated with chronic alcohol abuse and thiamine deficiency that results in a severe global amnesia, is one of the most carefully documented disorders of damage to this brain region (Butters & Cermak, 1980; Talland, 1965). In addition to mammillary body and dorsomedial nucleus damage, however, people with Korsakoff syndrome also have damage to frontal regions that likely accounts for some of the unique characteristics of this patient group, such as false recognition and confabulation, which are not common in other amnesic patients.

Damage to basal forebrain regions, which may be caused by aneurysms of the anterior communicating artery (ACAA) or anterior cerebral artery and also by AD, has also been associated with a global amnesia. Reasons for the memory loss may be related to the cholinergic functions of the basal forebrain region or to a disconnection of neocortical regions from the MTL/H. People who have had ACAAs often have damage to ventromedial frontal regions as well, which may account for the particular characteristics of their memory disorders, which (like patients with Korsakoff syndrome) often include false recognition and confabulation.

Finally, as noted previously, patients with frontal lobe damage frequently show memory deficits in complex tasks such as source memory or memory for temporal order, or in difficult recall tasks that require strategic processes. They also have working-memory and executive function deficits that could impact episodic memory (Glisky, 1998). Frontal damage is a frequent sequel of traumatic brain injury (TBI), although in many head injury cases, brain damage may be widespread, affecting MTL/H regions as well as fiber tracts throughout the brain. Patients with TBI, therefore, may have a global amnesia, often have frontal-like symptoms, and could have a range of other cognitive deficits depending on the loci and extent of their injuries.

With the exception of those patients with frontal lobe damage and those with AD, all the aforementioned patient groups have an amnesic deficit that selectively impairs episodic memory, leaving the other memory systems relatively untouched and general intellectual function preserved. Of particular note are the numerous findings of normal performance on procedural memory tasks and tests of implicit memory, particularly perceptual priming, although several studies have now reported normal priming on conceptual implicit tasks as well (for reviews, see Gabrieli, 1999; Schacter, Chiu, & Ochsner, 1993; Verfaellie & Keane, 2002). These results demonstrate that although patients may be completely unable to recall the prior presentation of words or pictures, they can nevertheless respond normally in implicit tasks such as perceptual identification or word-stem completion. Importantly, although their performance on various implicit tasks reflects the influence of prior experience, they have no conscious recollection of that experience. We will see shortly how this particular characteristic of amnesia has been used to benefit patients in rehabilitation.

THEORIES OF REHABILITATION

The field of cognitive rehabilitation has often been criticized for lacking a comprehensive theory that can explain the mechanisms underlying successful interventions or dictate the methods by which such successes might best be achieved (Caramazza & Hillis, 1993). Although the latter problem is still a long way from being solved in the field of memory, as has been noted, significant progress has been made at a neural level in demonstrating that the brain can and does change in response to experience and injury, and in specifying the mechanisms involved (e.g., regeneration, sprouting, reactive synaptogenesis, and neurogenesis) and the boundary conditions under which such plasticity is most likely to be observed (Kolb & Cioe, Chapter 1, this volume). One challenge for rehabilitation research, then, is to figure out how the plasticity of the injured brain may be enhanced through intervention, under what conditions such enhancement is most likely to occur (e.g., should the timing of the intervention be soon after injury or some time later?), and how to ensure that the changes that occur are behaviorally adaptive.

At a neuropsychological level, models of memory have become more elaborated and integrated, considering both cognitive constructs and their neurobiological underpinnings. Most theorists agree that memory consists of multiple systems and processes that depend on different neural circuitry; thus, memory can break down in a variety of ways. Documentation of the nature of the memory impairment and its neural correlates through a comprehensive neuropsychological assessment and neuroimaging is essential for constructing treatment plans that target the precise disorder of each individual patient and have the highest likelihood of success. It is also important for the clinician to consider the functional consequences of patients' impairments and to try to find behavioral adaptations that will help them deal with the particular problems they are experiencing in their everyday lives. In the sections that follow, I evaluate the approaches and methods of rehabilitation from both neuropsychological and behavioral perspectives, recognizing that although the neural machinery may place limitations on what can be accomplished, the findings of plasticity make it clear that interventions can affect both brain function and behavior.

APPROACHES TO REHABILITATION

Approaches to the rehabilitation of memory disorders have usually focused on one of two goals: (1) *restitution*, which implies reliance on the same cognitive and neural processes that were used for memory premorbidly, or (2) *compensa-*

tion, which involves the use of alternate processes or methods for remembering than used normally (Robertson & Murre, 1999). The first goal is concerned with the repair or optimal use of damaged memory processes, and thus targets memory impairment. It assumes that if damaged processes are restored or can be made more efficient, across-the-board improvements in memory should occur. The second goal is concerned with finding the means to bypass damaged memory processes. This approach usually targets disability and assumes that the cognitive and neural mechanisms normally involved in memory cannot be restored but that memory tasks can still be accomplished by means of other intact processes or systems or through the use of external aids. In this case, outcomes tend to be more limited, focused on achieving particular behaviors in everyday life; broad general improvements in memory are neither assumed nor expected. Restitution is only a realistic goal if damage to a particular brain system is incomplete so that remaining neurons within a neural circuit have the potential to reconnect. If lesions are large, involving the death of many neurons and the loss of many neural connections, restitution is unlikely and the system will have to rely either on compensation from other intact neural circuits or on external support (Robertson & Murre, 1999). To date, most successful rehabilitation in the area of memory disorders has been achieved within the context of a compensation approach, whereby people have been helped to overcome some of the disabilities associated with their memory impairment and to achieve some degree of independence in their everyday lives. So far, the goal of restitution has remained elusive.

METHODS OF REHABILITATION

Within each of the two broad approaches to rehabilitation outlined previously, a number of remedial techniques have been attempted with varying degrees of success. To a large degree, treatments have been prescribed without much regard for lesion location or the nature and severity of the disorder. However, with the sophisticated assessment instruments now available along with more elaborate neuropsychological models of memory and sensitive neuroimaging techniques, rehabilitation specialists can be much more discriminating in choosing available treatments and in designing new interventions according to each individual's needs. The next section describes and evaluates the most commonly used existing rehabilitation methods.

Practice and Rehearsal Techniques

One of the oldest and most commonly used methods to improve memory is practice, and there is little question that practice should be an essential component of all treatment plans. It is also clear, however, that drill-like practice of meaningless pieces of information such as arbitrarily chosen words, digits, shapes, locations, and so forth provides no general benefits to memory. The effects of practice are highly specific; thus although people may remember the useless information they practiced, their memory in any general sense is not improved; the effects do not generalize to other materials or contexts (e.g., Berg, Koning-Haanstra, & Deelman, 1991). It is therefore important in rehabilitation to focus practice on information that is meaningful and relevant.

These findings appear at first glance to argue against the possibility that repetitive drills will be able to restore function and seem to be inconsistent with the positive effects of practice that have been found with sensory and motor disorders. However, most of the studies showing regeneration of nerve fibers following cortical injury have been in animals. Furthermore, the sensory and motor effects that have been demonstrated have also been very specific (Nudo, Barbay, & Kleim, 2000). Importantly, Nudo et al. have shown that rehabilitation in the motor domain is not effective if it involves merely simple repetitive movements. For benefits to be obtained, practice needs to be directed toward the learning of a particular functional skill. Although this finding was obtained in the context of motor learning and thus falls in the domain of procedural memory, it nevertheless seems to fit well with the cognitive data showing, in much the same way, that no benefits are achieved from repetitive practice of arbitrary materials. If practice is to be effective, it needs to be directed toward functionally appropriate and meaningful activities; under these conditions, new factual information can be acquired. It seems likely that this acquisition of new information occurs at the neocortical level and possibly reflects a relative preservation of the semantic memory system. Consistent with this view are reports of children with hippocampal pathology who, despite a dense amnesia for the episodes in their lives, have nevertheless been able to acquire considerable semantic information in school, which has enabled them to perform normally on a range of language, comprehension, and general knowledge tests (Vargha-Khadem et al., 1997).

Although people with memory disorders appear to be able to acquire new semantic information with practice, such knowledge lacks episodic tags. The addition of episodic detail, defining the time and place of occurrence of an experience, appears to require the hippocampus, either to supply the information directly (particularly the spatial context) or to link the contextual details with the content. Although, as reported earlier, there is now evidence of hippocampal neurogenesis in humans as well as in animals, whether and how those new neurons will function (i.e., adaptively, maladaptively, or not at all) and under what conditions remain speculative (Kempermann, 2002). What seems clear, however, is that boring, repetitive, meaningless exercises provide no benefits for memory. Perhaps, as in nonhuman animals, stimulating, enriched real-life environments may encourage neurogenesis or neural reorganization in humans and ultimately lead to functional improvements in memory (Ogden, 2000). This possibility remains a challenge for future research.

Given that practice is important in the acquisition of new information, it makes sense to apply principles from cognitive psychology to optimize its beneficial effects. It has long been known that rote rehearsal is ineffective for long-term memory (Craik & Watkins, 1983), and that making information meaningful by relating it to other information in the knowledge system is much more likely to improve retention. In addition, short periods of distributed practice rather than long periods of massed practice are more effective (Baddeley, 1990), and overlearning enhances retention still further (Butters, Glisky, & Schacter, 1993). A distributed practice technique that has been used effectively even for severely impaired individuals is "spaced retrieval" or "retrieval practice" (Landauer & Bjork, 1978). This method involves repeated practice at retrieving to-be-learned information at gradually increasing retention intervals and has been used successfully to teach memory-impaired individuals, including those with AD, important information in their everyday lives, including name–face associations and locations of objects (Camp & McKitrick, 1992; Schacter, Rich, & Stampp, 1985). The method may rely on residual memory function or it may tap into other preserved memory systems. Camp and McKitrick have noted in patients with AD, that acquisition of new information using this method seems to occur relatively effortlessly and so they have hypothesized that it may depend on intact implicit memory processes.

Mnemonic Strategies

A variety of mnemonic strategies, drawn from the cognitive psychology literature, have been attempted with neurological patients with varying degrees of success (for reviews, see Butters, Soety, & Glisky, 1998; Glisky & Glisky, 2002). These strategies, which include such things as visual imagery, semantic elaboration, chaining, and a variety of other organizational techniques, are essentially encoding strategies that help people organize information at input into meaningful groupings that can then serve as retrieval cues at time of remembering. For the most part, mnemonic strategies seem to benefit only people with mild to moderate memory disorders, consistent with the idea that strategies depend on the use of residual function (Wilson, 1987). People with severe memory disorders have difficulty learning the more complex techniques, and even those who can learn them, fail to use them spontaneously in their everyday lives. Thus, as with practice, some people are able to use mnemonic strategies to acquire new information, particularly associative relations such as name–face pairings (Thoene & Glisky, 1995; Wilson, 1987), but for most people these strategies provide no general mnemonic benefits.

As outlined earlier, current theory suggests that encoding strategies are constructed and implemented by the frontal lobes, which then send an organized packet of information on to the MTL/H for storage. If MTL/H damage is severe, it will not matter how good the encoding strategies are; the information will not be consolidated. On the other hand, if the MTL/H is only partially damaged, effective use of strategic frontal lobe processes may be able to optimize the functioning of residual consolidation processes in the MTL/H and perhaps stimulate recovery. Alternatively, a mild memory problem may result from damage only to frontal lobe structures. In this case, training in the use of organizational strategies may improve the quality of the information delivered to the MTL/H and thereby improve memory. Such benefits have been observed among normally aging individuals, who may experience declining frontal lobe function as they age, and have sometimes been found to persist over long periods, although benefits tend to be task-specific rather than general (Neely & Bäckman, 1995). It is possible that continued use of such strategies, particularly for learning information that is relevant and important in an individual's life, may stimulate frontal or MTL/H brain regions, encouraging synaptic growth and recovery of function. Although generalized memory benefits as a result of mnemonic strategy training beyond the specific training context have been infrequently reported (for two examples, see Berg et al., 1991; Lindgren, Hagstadius, Åbjörnsson, & Ørbæk, 1997), such training is usually not begun with neurological patients until well into the posttrauma period, and it has seldom been maintained for long periods (but see Benedict, Brandt, & Bergey, 1993). These and other variables may affect the likelihood that strategy training will facilitate the restitution or reorganization of neural structures and have lasting benefits for memory.

Mnemonic strategies have also been used successfully in a compensatory way for individuals with unilateral lesions in the temporal lobe, who are taught to use techniques that optimize the functioning of the intact hemisphere. For example, verbal strategies are taught to people who have had right temporal lobectomies and retain relatively preserved left-hemisphere function, and visuospatial strategies are encouraged for those who have left-sided damage.

Vanishing Cues and Errorless Learning

Among the most successful recent approaches to memory rehabilitation are those that have focused on developing new learning techniques to help memory-impaired individuals acquire new information and skills important in their everyday lives. Unlike repetitive drills and the learning of mnemonic strategies, which attempt to improve the efficiency of memory processes that were used premorbidly, these new methods were developed to tap into intact memory systems and processes not normally engaged for the purposes of episodic memory. Specifically, these methods were originally thought to rely primarily on implicit memory function.

Many experiments have demonstrated that amnesic patients have a preserved ability to produce recently presented information in response to partial cues—what has been called perceptual priming (for review, see Schacter et al., 1993). The method of vanishing cues (Glisky, Schacter, & Tulving, 1986b) was designed specifically to take advantage of this form of implicit memory to help people acquire new information. For example, to teach memory-impaired individuals that the various parts of a computer are collectively referred to as "hardware," Glisky et al. (1986b) presented them with as many letters of the target word as they needed to generate the correct response (e.g., "hardw_____") and then gradually withdrew the remaining letters over trials (e.g., "hard, har, ha, and h,"). Eventually, when asked what the various parts of a computer were collectively called, patients were able to produce the word "hardware" without any letter cues. Using this method, people with even severe memory impairments were able to learn a range of complex tasks, including computer operation (Glisky, Schacter, & Tulving, 1986a), computer data entry (Glisky & Schacter, 1987), and word processing (Glisky, 1995), and retain them over long periods, despite having no explicit memory for the occasions of learning. Evidence of generalization across contexts was also found; patients were able to apply what they had learned from their laboratory training to the home or work environment. Although this learning was originally believed to be a function of the PRS, it later became clear that a presemantic system such as the PRS could not easily support the kinds of responses to semantic cues that people were able to make after perceptual cues had been withdrawn. However, the findings that such learning was highly dependent on the specific form of conceptual queries appears to be consistent with more recent findings of normal conceptual priming in amnesic patients. Other findings—for example, those indicating that with overlearning, hyperspecificity declines and generalization to related cues occurs (Butters et al., 1993)—suggest a role for semantic memory late in the learning process. Thus, learning by the method of vanishing cues may involve the PRS early in learning, enabling responses to perceptual cues, but when those cues are withdrawn other semantically based memory systems may come into play.

The vanishing cues method may achieve at least part of its success by constraining possible responses to those that fit the cues, thus reducing errors. Baddeley and Wilson (1994) proposed that memory-impaired individuals, who rely on implicit memory to learn new information, may have particular difficulty eliminating errors because they lack the explicit memory to recall them. They devised a technique, "errorless learning," that essentially prevents the intrusion of incorrect responses. Rather than allowing people to guess in response to partial cues, they provided the correct response and told them to write it down, thus eliminating the possibility that people would produce errors. Performance in this errorless condition was then contrasted with performance in an errorful condition in which people were given partial letter information and, without any other constraints, were told to guess the words, virtually ensuring the generation of errors. The results showed that amnesic patients showed faster learning and less forgetting in the errorless than in the errorful condition. In numerous experiments, Wilson and her colleagues have since demonstrated that, using errorless learning methods, people with a range of memory disorders, including those with AD (Clare, Wilson, Breen, & Hodges, 1999), have been able to learn various kinds of information useful in everyday life—for example, names, the use of an electronic memory aid, the use of a memory notebook, and other pieces of general knowledge (Evans et al., 2000; Kalla, Downes, & van den Broek, 2001; Komatsu, Mimura, Kato, Wakamatsu, & Kashima, 2000; Squires, Hunkin, & Parkin, 1996; Wilson, Baddeley, Evans, & Shiel, 1994). Although there are few direct comparisons of errorless learning with other training techniques, the evidence suggests that for many tasks an errorless method is clearly superior to one that permits errors. Nevertheless, findings have not been entirely consistent, and some studies (e.g., Evans et al., 2000) have failed to find advantages for errorless learning, particularly on tasks that require explicit recall of arbitrary associations (e.g., learning routes and name–face pairs). These findings have led some researchers to speculate that errorless-learning and vanishing-cues methods may be most beneficial for those with severe memory disorders, who presumably must rely on preserved implicit memory to learn new information (Evans et al., 2000; Thoene & Glisky, 1995). More recent evidence, however, suggests that errorless learning also provides benefits for moderately impaired individuals, who likely rely on residual explicit memory function (Hunkin, Squires, Parkin, & Tidy, 1998; Wilson, 2002). Further research is needed to explore the limits of this methodology, particularly the characteristics of tasks that are most amenable to errorless methods, the characteristics of individual patients most likely to benefit, ways to enhance the method, and the extent to which such learning can be maintained over time (e.g., Clare, Wilson, Carter, Hodges, & Adams, 2001).

External Support

When brain damage and memory impairments are severe and the ability to function in everyday life is seriously compromised, it is necessary to intervene directly at the behavioral level to alleviate patients' functional disabilities and help them achieve some degree of independence. In such cases, remediation consists mainly of the provision of environmental restructurings and supports that direct behavior from an external source, bypassing the need for internally generated mnemonic processes or compensatory neural changes. Although they may provide the only treatment appropriate for those with severe impairments, external aids are often an integral part of interventions for those with milder memory deficits where they are often used in combination with other more cognitively demanding methods.

External aids can be used to satisfy a variety of everyday needs, some quite simple and others complex (for review, see Kapur, Glisky, & Wilson, 2002). At the simplest level, they can include labels and signage placed in clearly visible locations to identify the contents of cupboards, provide instructions for the use of equipment, and offer directional information to places in the proximal environment. At a more advanced level, aids such as calendars and notebooks, alarm watches and timers, and, most recently, electronic organizers have been incorporated into treatment plans to help people with prospective memory tasks—remembering appointments, birthdays, medications, and other daily events—and to provide a means for people to keep track of information important in their personal lives. Most of these devices, however, require active involvement on the part of the individual and extensive training before they can be used effectively (Sohlberg & Mateer, 1989); thus they may not be useful for people with severe memory disorders who cannot learn how to use them or those with executive deficits who may have difficulty initiating actions. Recently, however, electronic devices such as pagers and voice recorders that require little training on the part of the patient (i.e., they are programmed by caregivers or external agencies) have become available and have been used to deliver reminders and messages at preselected times during the day to help people remember their activities and appointments (Hersh & Treadgold, 1994; Kim, Burke, Dowds, & George, 1999; Kim, Burke, Dowds, Boone, & Park, 2000; Van den Broek, Downes, Johnson, Dayus, & Hilton, 2000). Wilson and colleagues (Wilson, Emslie, Quirk, & Evans, 2001; Wilson, Evans, Emslie, & Malinek, 1997) have done extensive testing of one such system and have found it to be effective even for people with severe memory impairment and executive dysfunction.

CONCLUDING COMMENTS AND FUTURE DIRECTIONS

In the past 15–20 years, memory rehabilitation has focused primarily on achieving functional outcomes that might allow people to compensate for their disabilities and gain greater independence in their everyday lives. In this respect, the field has been moderately successful: The development of new technologies has had a significant impact on rehabilitation by making available inexpensive electronic devices that have provided an acceptable form of external assistance to facilitate the performance of many everyday activities. In addition, people with memory disorders have been able to learn a range of complex materials that have allowed them in some cases to return to work, to manage their personal lives, and to achieve some sense of personal worth—goals that in the past had been thought to be unattainable. At least some of this success is attributable to the development of theoretical models of memory, which have encouraged attempts to make use of intact memory systems and processes to compensate for those that are damaged or lost.

There has also been an explosion of research in the past 10 years in the field of cognitive neuroscience driven largely by technological advances that have enabled the imaging of the functioning brain. This work, combined with more basic neuroscience research in animals, has hugely advanced our understanding of the neural processes underlying memory function. At the systems level, we have learned that prefrontal cortex has a significant and previously unappreciated supportive role to play in episodic memory as well as in other forms of memory, and we are beginning to discover that the various structures in the medial temporal lobes may serve very different functions in memory. These findings suggest that the remedial techniques that might be effective for lesions in one brain region might be ineffective for lesions in other regions. For example, many studies that have taught mnemonic strategies to memory-impaired individuals have found little in the way of long-term benefits even when such techniques were continued for long periods (e.g., Benedict et al., 1993). Given our current knowledge of the roles of different regions in memory, we might expect this negative outcome if brain damage was severe and confined to the MTL/H, whereas we might expect a more positive outcome if damage was mild and involved frontal brain regions. In recent work in my laboratory, we compared memory-impaired patients with MTL/H damage and frontal lobe damage in a task requiring the learning of new associative information. We found that error reduction was particularly important for those people with frontal lesions, whereas a training process that provided explicit links between to-be-learned information and related information in the knowledge system resulted in preferential benefits for those with MTL/H damage.

Neuroimaging studies have also suggested that the damaged brain may undergo reorganization following injury, and animal research has demonstrated plasticity in both neocortex and hippocampus that appears to be stimulated by functional exercises and enriched environments and associated with behavioral changes. These results suggest that there may be new ways that exercise and practice techniques can be adapted to encourage regeneration of neural processes or the growth of new neurons in ways that are functionally beneficial. To date, however, such attempts have met with little success in the area of memory. It may be that a combination of behavioral and pharmacological therapies will ultimately prove useful, but these are for the most part as yet untested. Still further in the future are transplants and genetic manipulations, which could eventually benefit brain-damaged individuals.

For the present, research and practice suggest that the most effective approach to rehabilitation of memory disorders is one that focuses directly on the alleviation of functional problems and derives its methods from the growing empirical and theoretical base provided by cognitive psychology, neuropsychology, and cognitive neuroscience. Continuing efforts to find ways to capitalize on preserved cognitive and neural mechanisms, and careful consideration of lesion location and the specific characteristics of each memory disorder, should lead to the development of even more effective rehabilitation methods in the future.

ACKNOWLEDGMENT

Preparation of this chapter was supported by Grant No. RO1 AG14792 from the National Institute on Aging.

REFERENCES

Aggleton, J. P., & Brown, M. W. (1999). Episodic memory, amnesia, and the hippocampal-anterior thalamic axis. *Behavioral and Brain Sciences, 22,* 425–489.

Baddeley, A. D. (1990). *Human memory.* Boston: Allyn & Bacon.

Baddeley, A. D. (1994). Working memory: The interface between memory and cognition. In D. L. Schacter & E. Tulving (Eds.), *Memory systems 1994* (pp. 351–367). Cambridge, MA: MIT Press.

Baddeley, A. D., & Hitch, G. J. (1974). Working memory. In G. A. Bower (Ed.), *The psychology of learning and motivation* (Vol. 8, pp. 47–89). New York: Academic Press.

Baddeley, A. D., & Wilson, B. A. (1994). When implicit learning fails: Amnesia and the problem of error elimination. *Neuropsychologia, 32,* 53–68.

Baxter, M. G., & Murg, S. L. (2002). The basal forebrain cholinergic system. In L. R. Squire & D. L. Schacter (Eds.), *Neuropsychology of memory* (3rd ed., pp. 425–436). New York: Guilford Press.

Benedict, R. H. B., Brandt, J., & Bergey, G. (1993). An attempt at memory retraining in severe amnesia: An experimental single-case study. *Neuropsychological Rehabilitation, 3,* 37–51.

Berg, I. J., Koning-Haanstra, M., & Deelman, B. G. (1991). Long-term effects of memory rehabilitation. *Neuropsychological Rehabilitation, 1,* 97–111.

Buckner, R. L., Corbetta, M., Schatz, J., Raichle, M. E., & Petersen, S. E. (1996). Preserved speech abilities and compensation following prefrontal damage. *Proceedings of the National Academy of Sciences USA, 93,* 1249–1253.

Butters, M. A., Glisky, E. L., & Schacter, D. L. (1993). Transfer of new learning in memory-impaired patients. *Journal of Clinical and Experimental Neuropsychology, 15*(2), 219–230.

Butters, M. A., Soety, E. M., & Glisky, E. L. (1998). Memory rehabilitation. In P. J. Snyder & P. D. Nussbaum (Eds.), *Clinical Neuropsychology* (pp. 450–466). Washington, DC: American Psychological Association.

Butters, N., & Cermak, L. S. (1980). *Alcoholic Korsakoff's syndrome: An information processing approach.* New York: Academic Press.

Cabeza, R., Anderson, N. D., Locantore, J. K., & McIntosh, A. R. (2002). Aging gracefully: Compensatory brain activity in high-performing older adults." *NeuroImage, 17,* 1394–1402.

Cabeza, R., Dolcos, F., Graham, R., & Nyberg, L. (2002). Similarities and differences in the neural correlates of episodic memory retrieval and working memory. *Neuro-Image, 16,* 317–330.

Cabeza, R., Grady, C. L., Nyberg, L., McIntosh, A. R., Tulving, E., Kapur, S., et al. (1997). Age-related differences in neural activity during memory encoding and retrieval: A positron emission tomography study. *Journal of Neuroscience, 17*(1), 391–400.

Cabeza, R., & Nyberg, L. (2000). Imaging cognition II: An empirical review of 275 PET and fMRI studies. *Journal of Cognitive Neuroscience, 12*(1), 1–47.

Camp, C. J., & McKitrick, L. A. (1992). Memory interventions in Alzheimer's-type dementia populations: Methodological and theoretical issues. In R. L. West & J. D. Sinnott (Eds.), *Everyday memory and aging: Current research and methodology* (pp. 155–172). New York: Springer.

Caramazza, A., & Hillis, A. (1993). For a theory of remediation of cognitive deficits. *Neuropsychological Rehabilitation, 3*(3), 217–234.

Clare, L., Wilson, B. A., Breen, K., & Hodges, J. R. (1999). Errorless learning of face–name associations in early Alzheimer's disease. *Neurocase, 5,* 37–46.

Clare, L., Wilson, B. A., Carter, G., Hodges, J. R., & Adams, M. (2001). Long-term maintenance of treatment gains following a cognitive rehabilitation intervention in early dementia of Alzheimer type: A single case study. *Neuropsychological Rehabilitation, 11,* 477–494.

Cohen, N. J., & Squire, L. R. (1980). Preserved learning and retention of pattern-analyzing skill in amnesia: Dissociation of knowing how and knowing that. *Science, 210,* 207–209.

Corkin, S. (1984). Lasting consequences of bilateral medial temporal lobectomy: Clinical course and experimental findings in H.M. *Seminars in Neurology, 4,* 249–259.

Craik, F. I. M., & Lockhart, R. S. (1972). Levels of processing: A framework for memory research. *Journal of Verbal Learning and Verbal Behavior, 11,* 671–684.

Craik, F. I. M., & Tulving, E. (1975). Depth of processing and the retention of words in episodic memory. *Journal of Experimental Psychology: General, 104,* 268–294.

Craik, F. I. M., & Watkins, M. J. (1983). The role of rehearsal in short-term memory. *Journal of Verbal Learning and Verbal Behavior, 12,* 599–607.

Curran, H. V. (2000). Psychopharmacological perspectives on memory. In E. Tulving & D. L. Schacter (Eds.), *The Oxford handbook of memory* (pp. 539–554). Oxford, UK: Oxford University Press.

Davidson, P. S. R., & Glisky, E. L. (2002). Neuropsychological correlates of recollection and familiarity in normal aging. *Cognitive, Affective and Behavioral Neuroscience, 2,* 174–186.

D'Esposito, M., & Postle, B. R. (2002). The neural basis of working memory storage, rehearsal, and control processes. In L. R. Squire & D. L. Schacter (Eds.), *Neuropsychology of memory* (3rd ed., pp. 215–224). New York: Guilford Press.

Doyon, J., & Ungerleider, L. G. (2002). Functional anatomy of motor skill learning. In L. R. Squire & D. L. Schacter (Eds.), *Neuropsychology of memory* (3rd ed., pp. 225–238). New York: Guilford Press.

Eichenbaum, H. (2002). *The cognitive neuroscience of memory.* Oxford, UK: Oxford University Press.

Eriksson, P. S., Perfilieva, E., Bjork-Eriksson, T., Alborn, A. M., Nordbord, C., Peterson,

D. A., et al. (1998). Neurogenesis in the adult human hippocampus. *Nature Medicine, 4,* 1313–1317.

Evans, J. J., Wilson, B. A., Schuri, U., Andrade, J., Baddeley, A., Bruna, O., et al. (2000). A comparison of "errorless" and "trial-and-error" learning methods for teaching individuals with acquired memory deficits. *Neuropsychological Rehabilitation, 10*(1), 67–101.

Fletcher, P. C., & Henson, R. N. A. (2001). Frontal lobes and human memory. Insights from functional neuroimaging. *Brain, 124,* 849–881.

Fujii, T., Moscovitch, M., & Nadel, L. (2000). Memory consolidation, retrograde amnesia, and the temporal lobe. In L. S. Cermak (Ed.), *Handbook of neuropsychology* (2nd ed., Vol. 2, pp. 223–250). Amsterdam: Elsevier.

Gabrieli, J. D. E. (1999). The architecture of human memory. In J. K. Foster & M. Jelicic (Eds.), *Memory: Systems, process, or function?* (pp. 205–231). Oxford, UK: Oxford University Press.

Gabrieli, J. D. E., Desmond, J. E., Demb, J. B., Wagner, A. D., Stone, M. V., Vaidya, C. J., et al. (1996). Functional magnetic resonance imaging of semantic memory processes in the frontal lobes. *Psychological Science, 7,* 278–283.

Gabrieli, J. D. E., Fleischman, D. A., Keane, M. M., Reminger, S. L., & Morrell, F. (1995). Double dissociation between memory systems underlying explicit and implicit memory in the human brain. *Psychological Science, 6,* 76–82.

Glisky, E. L. (1995). Acquisition and transfer of word processing skill by an amnesic patient. *Neuropsychological Rehabilitation, 5*(4), 299–318.

Glisky, E. L. (1998). Differential contribution of frontal and medial temporal lobes to memory: Evidence from focal lesions and normal aging. In N. Raz (Ed.), *The other side of the error term: Aging and development as model systems in cognitive neuroscience* (pp. 261–317). Amsterdam: Elsevier.

Glisky, E. L., & Glisky, M. L. (2002). Learning and memory impairments. In P. J. Eslinger (Ed.), *Neuropsychological interventions* (pp. 137–162). New York: Guilford Press.

Glisky, E. L., Rubin, S. R., & Davidson, P. S. R. (2001). Source memory in older adults: An encoding or retrieval problem? *Journal of Experimental Psychology: Learning, Memory, and Cognition, 27,* 1131–1146.

Glisky, E. L., & Schacter, D. L. (1987). Acquisition of domain-specific knowledge in organic amnesia: Training for computer-related work. *Neuropsychologia, 25,* 893–906.

Glisky, E. L., Schacter, D. L., & Tulving, E. (1986a). Computer learning by memory-impaired patients: Acquisition and retention of complex knowledge. *Neuropsychologia, 24,* 313–328.

Glisky, E. L., Schacter, D. L., & Tulving, E. (1986b). Learning and retention of computer related vocabulary in memory-impaired patients: Method of vanishing cues. *Journal of Clinical and Experimental Neuropsychology, 8,* 292–312.

Gould, E. (1999). Serotonin and hippocampal neurogenesis. *Neuropsychopharmacology, 21,* 46S–51S.

Gould, E., Beylin, A., Tanapat, P., Reeves, A., & Shors, T. J. (1999). Learning enhances adult neurogenesis in the hippocampal formation. *Nature Neuroscience, 2,* 260–265.

Grady, C. L., McIntosh, A. R., Horwitz, B., Maisog, J. M., Ungerleider, L. G., Mentis, M.

J., et al. (1995). Age-related reductions in human recognition memory due to impaired encoding. *Science, 269,* 218–221.

Hersh, N., & Treadgold, L. (1994). NeuroPage: The rehabilitation of memory dysfunction by prosthetic memory and cueing. *NeuroRehabilitation, 4,* 187–197.

Hodges, J. R. (2000). Memory in the dementias. In E. Tulving & F. I. M. Craik (Eds.), *The Oxford handbook of memory* (pp. 441–459). Oxford, UK: Oxford University Press.

Hunkin, N. M., Squires, E. J., Parkin, A. J., & Tidy, J. A. (1998). Are the benefits of errorless learning dependent on implicit memory? *Neuropsychologia, 36,* 25–36.

Janowsky, J. S., Shimamura, A. P., & Squire, L. R. (1989). Source memory impairment in patients with frontal lobe lesions. *Neuropsychologia, 27,* 1043–1056.

Kalla, T., Downes, J. J., & van den Broek, M. (2001). The preexposure technique: Enhancing the effects of errorless learning in the acquisition of face–name associations. *Neuropsychological Rehabilitation, 11,* 1–16.

Kapur, N., Glisky, E. L., & Wilson, B. A. (2002). External memory aids and computers in memory rehabilitation. In A. D. Baddeley, M. D. Kopelman, & B. A. Wilson (Eds.), *Handbook of memory disorders* (2nd ed., pp. 757–783). Chichester, UK: Wiley.

Keane, M. M., Gabrieli, J. D. E., Fennema, A. C., Growdon, J. H., & Corkin, S. (1991). Evidence for a dissociation between perceptual and conceptual priming in Alzheimer's disease. *Behavioral Neuroscience, 105,* 326–342.

Kelley, C. M., & Jacoby, L. L. (2000). Recollection and familiarity. In E. Tulving & F. I. M. Craik (Eds.), *The Oxford handbook of memory* (pp. 215–228). Oxford, UK: Oxford University Press.

Kempermann, G. (2002). Why new neurons? Possible functions for adult hippocampal neurogenesis. *Journal of Neuroscience, 22,* 635–638.

Kim, H. J., Burke, D. T., Dowds, M. M., Jr., Boone, K. A. R., & Park, G. J. (2000). Electronic memory aids for outpatient brain injury: Follow-up findings. *Brain Injury, 14,* 187–196.

Kim, H. J., Burke, D. T., Dowds, M. M., & George, J. (1999). Utility of a microcomputer as an external memory aid for a memory-impaired head injury patient during inpatient rehabilitation. *Brain Injury, 13*(2), 147–150.

Knowlton, B. J. (2002). The role of the basal ganglia in learning and memory. In L. R. Squire & D. L. Schacter (Eds.), *Neuropsychology of memory* (3rd ed., pp. 143–153). New York: Guilford Press.

Kolb, B. (1995). *Brain plasticity and behavior.* Mahwah, NJ: Erlbaum.

Komatsu, S., Mimura, M., Kato, M., Wakamatsu, N., & Kashima, H. (2000). Errorless and effortful processes involved in learning of face–name associations by patients with alcoholic Korsakoff's syndrome. *Neuropsychological Rehabilitation, 10*(2), 113–132.

Landauer, T. K., & Bjork, R. A. (1978). Optimum rehearsal patterns and name learning. In M. M. Gruneberg, P. E. Morris, & R. N. Sykes (Eds.), *Practical aspects of memory* (pp. 625–632). London: Academic Press.

Lindgren, M., Hagstadius, S., Åbjörnsson, G., & Ørbæk, P. (1997). Neuropsychological rehabilitation of patients with organic solvent-induced chronic toxic encephalopathy. A pilot study. *Neuropsychological Rehabilitation, 7,* 1–22.

Mayes, A. R. (2000). Effects on memory of Papez circuit lesions. In L. S. Cermak (Ed.), *Handbook of neuropsychology* (Vol. 2, pp. 111–131). Amsterdam: Elsevier.

McCarthy, R. A., & Warrington, E. K. (1990). *Cognitive Neuropsychology*. San Diego: Academic Press.

Milner, B. (1966). Amnesia following operation on the temporal lobes. In C. W. M. Whitty & O. L. Zangwill (Eds.), *Amnesia* (pp. 109–133). London: Butterworths.

Morris, C. D., Bransford, J. P., & Franks, J. J. (1978). Levels of processing versus transfer appropriate processing. *Journal of Verbal Learning and Verbal Behavior, 16*, 519–533.

Moscovitch, M. (1994). Memory and working with memory: Evaluation of a component process model and comparisons with other models. In D. L. Schacter & E. Tulving (Eds.), *Memory systems 1994* (pp. 269–310). Cambridge, MA: MIT Press.

Moscovitch, M. (1995). Recovered consciousness: A hypothesis concerning modularity and episodic memory. *Journal of Clinical and Experimental Neuropsychology, 17*, 276–290.

Nadel, L., & Moscovitch, M. (1997). Memory consolidation, retrograde amnesia and the hippocampal complex. *Current Opinion in Neurobiology, 7*, 217–227.

Neely, A. S., & Bäckman, L. (1995). Effects of multifactorial memory training in old age: Generalizability across tasks and individuals. *Journal of Gerontology: Psychological Sciences, 50B*(3), P134–P140.

Nudo, R. J., Barbay, S., & Kleim, J. A. (2000). Role of neuroplasticity in functional recovery after stroke. In J. Grafman (Ed.), *Cerebral reorganization of function after brain damage* (pp. 168–197). Oxford, UK: Oxford University Press.

Nyberg, L., Forkstam, C., Petersson, K. M., Cabeza, R., & Ingvar, M. (2002). Brain imaging of human memory systems: Between-systems similarities and within-system differences. *Cognitive Brain Research, 13*, 281–292.

O'Connor, M., Verfaellie, M., & Cermak, L. S. (1995). Clinical differentiation of amnesic subtypes. In A. D. Baddeley, B. A. Wilson, & F. N. Watts (Eds.), *Handbook of memory disorders* (pp. 53–80). Chichester, UK: Wiley.

Ogden, J. A. (2000). Neurorehabilitation in the third millenium: New roles for our environment, behaviors, and mind in brain damage and recovery? *Brain and Cognition, 42*, 110–112.

Rapczak, S. Z., Nielsen, L., Glisky, E. L., & Kaszniak, A. W. (2002). The neuropsychology of false facial recognition. In L. R. Squire & D. L. Schacter (Eds.), *Neuropsychology of memory* (3rd ed., pp. 130–142). New York: Guilford Press.

Robertson, I. H., & Murre, J. M. J. (1999). Rehabilitation of brain damage: Brain plasticity and principles of guided recovery. *Psychological Bulletin, 125*, 544–575.

Schacter, D. L., & Buckner, R. L. (1998). Priming and the brain. *Neuron, 20*, 185–195.

Schacter, D. L., Chiu, C. Y. P., & Ochsner, K. N. (1993). Implicit memory: A selective review. *Annual Review of Neuroscience, 16*, 159–182.

Schacter, D. L., Rich, S. A., & Stampp, M. S. (1985). Remediation of memory disorders: Experimental evaluation of the spaced-retrieval technique. *Journal of Clinical and Experimental Neuropsychology, 7*, 79–96.

Schacter, D. L., & Tulving, E. (Eds.). (1994a). *Memory systems 1994*. Cambridge, MA: MIT Press.

Schacter, D. L., & Tulving, E. (1994b). What are the memory systems of 1994? In D. L. Schacter & E. Tulving (Eds.), *Memory systems 1994* (pp. 1–38). Cambridge, MA: MIT Press.

Schacter, D. L., Wagner, A. D., & Buckner, R. L. (2000). Memory systems of 1999. In E.

Tulving & F. I. M. Craik (Eds.), *The Oxford handbook of memory* (pp. 627–643). Oxford, UK: Oxford University Press.

Shimamura, A. P. (1994). Memory and frontal lobe function. In M. S. Gazzaniga (Ed.), *The cognitive neurosciences* (pp. 803–813). Cambridge, MA: MIT Press.

Sohlberg, M. M., & Mateer, C. A. (1989). Training use of compensatory memory books: A three stage behavioral approach. *Journal of Clinical and Experimental Neuropsychology, 11*, 871–887.

Squire, L. R. (1987). *Memory and brain.* New York: Oxford University Press.

Squire, L. R. (1992). Memory and the hippocampus: A synthesis from findings with rats, monkeys, and humans. *Psychological Review, 99*(2), 195–231.

Squires, E. J., Hunkin, N. M., & Parkin, A. J. (1996). Memory notebook training in a case of severe amnesia: Generalising from paired associate learning to real life. *Neuropsychological Rehabilitation, 6*, 55–65.

Talland, G. A. (1965). *Deranged memory.* New York: Academic Press.

Thoene, A. I. T., & Glisky, E. L. (1995). Learning of name-face associations in memory impaired patients: A comparison of different training procedures. *Journal of the International Neuropsychological Society, 1*(1), 29–38.

Tulving, E. (1972). Episodic and semantic memory. In E. Tulving & W. Donaldson (Eds.), *Organization of memory* (pp. 381–403). New York: Academic Press.

Tulving, E. (1983). *Elements of episodic memory.* Oxford, UK: Clarendon Press.

Tulving, E., & Schacter, D. L. (1990). Priming and human memory systems. *Science, 247*(4940), 301–306.

Tulving, E., Schacter, D. L., & Stark, H. A. (1982). Priming effects in word-fragment completion are independent of recognition memory. *Journal of Experimental Psychology: Learning, Memory and Cognition, 8*(4), 336–342.

Tulving, E., & Thomson, D. M. (1973). Encoding specificity and retrieval processes in epsodic memory. *Psychological Review, 80*, 352–373.

Vallar, G., & Papagno, G. (2002). Neuropsychological impairments of verbal short-term memory. In A. D. Baddeley, M. D. Kopelman, & B. A. Wilson (Eds.), *Handbook of memory disorders* (pp. 135–165). Chichester, UK: Wiley.

Van den Brock, M. D., Downes, J., Johnson, A., Dayus, B., & Hilton, N. (2000). Evaluation of an electronic memory aid in the neuropsychological rehabilitation of prospective memory deficits. *Brain Injury, 14*(5), 455–462.

Vargha-Khadem, F., Gadian, D. G., Watkins, K. E., Connelly, A., Van Paesschen, W., & Mishkin, M. (1997). Differential effects of early hippocampal pathology on episodic and semantic memory. *Science, 277*, 376–380.

Verfaellie, M., & Keane, M. M. (2002). Impaired and preserved memory processes in amnesia. In L. R. Squire & D. L. Schacter (Eds.), *Neuropsychology of memory* (3rd ed., pp. 35–46). New York: Guilford Press.

Wagner, A. D. (2002). Cognitive control and episodic memory. In L. R. Squire & D. L. Schacter (Eds.), *Neuropsychology of memory* (3rd ed., pp. 174–192). New York: Guilford Press.

Warrington, E. K., & Weiskrantz, L. (1970). Amnesic syndrome: Consolidation or retrieval? *Nature, 228*, 628–630.

Wenk, G. L. (2003). Neurotransmitters. In L. Nadel (Ed.), *Encyclopedia of cognitive science* (Vol. 3, pp. 361–367). London: Macmillan Press.

Wheeler, M. A., Stuss, D. T., & Tulving, E. (1995). Frontal lobe damage produces episodic memory impairment. *Journal of the International Neuropsychological Society, 1*(6), 525–536.

Wilson, B. (1987). *Rehabilitation of memory*. New York: Guilford Press.

Wilson, B. A. (2002). Memory rehabilitation. In L. R. Squire & D. L. Schacter (Eds.), *Neuropsychology of memory* (3rd ed., pp. 263–272). New York: Guilford Press.

Wilson, B. A., Baddeley, A. D., Evans, J., & Shiel, A. (1994). Errorless learning in the rehabilitation of memory impaired people. *Neuropsychological Rehabilitation, 4,* 307–326.

Wilson, B. A., Emslie, H. C., Quirk, K., & Evans, J. J. (2001). Reducing everyday memory and planning problems by means of a paging system: A randomised control crossover study. *Journal of Neurology, Neurosurgery and Psychiatry, 70,* 477–482.

Wilson, B. A., Evans, J. J., Emslie, H., & Malinek, V. (1997). Evaluation of NeuroPage: A new memory aid. *Journal of Neurology, Neurosurgery and Psychiatry, 63,* 113–115.

5

Rehabilitation
of Language Disorders

Stephen E. Nadeau
Leslie J. Gonzalez Rothi

Rehabilitation after brain injury depends on two processes: (1) the endogenous responses of neural tissues (reactive plasticity), which include reactive neurogenesis, neural migration, axonal sprouting and extension to target structures, and synaptogenesis (see Kolb, Chapter 2, this volume); and (2) the replacement of knowledge lost due to injury through behavioral therapy. Although we are at the scientific threshold of manipulating reactive plasticity to therapeutic advantage, the clinical data so far are inconclusive and bear little on the rehabilitation of language processes specifically. Therefore, this chapter focuses mainly on behavioral therapies.

The efficacy of many behavioral therapies for language impairment has been demonstrated in a large number of studies, some providing level I evidence. Effectiveness—that is, the impact of these therapies as delivered in routine practice on the communicative lives of patients, is not so clear. These studies have been reviewed in recent texts (Chapey, 2001; Nadeau, Rothi, & Crosson, 2000), but we take a somewhat different approach: We consider the treatment of aphasia not from the perspective of clinical scientific standards but, rather, from the perspective of neural science. A fully neuroscientific ap-

129

proach to behavioral therapy for language impairment must ask the following questions: What types of knowledge are being replaced? and How are they represented in the brain? The answers to these questions are not known with certainty in any cognitive domain, but we probably know more about language than any other cognitive function. In fact, we have sufficient knowledge about the neural basis of language processes to propose some reasonable hypotheses about therapeutic strategies. Because we know more about language and the treatment of its disorders than we do about any other cognitive process, language and aphasiology provide a particularly broad portal to the neural principles underlying cognitive processes. Thus, the ideas discussed in this chapter may be of some value in developing neural-network-based approaches to rehabilitation in other cognitive domains.

Although a number of approaches explain language processing (e.g., linguistic, cognitive and neuropsychological), this chapter focuses on parallel distributed process modeling (PDP), or connectionist modeling, a science that enables us to link neural-network architecture to complex behavior. We begin with a brief introduction to this approach then discuss a specific PDP model of language in order to frame some hypotheses about the domains of knowledge represented. We then inquire into the nature of each of these domains of knowledge and the processes by which they are altered in order to understand the types of behavioral therapy that might best be employed to reconstruct them after injury. For unfamiliar linguistic terminology, see the glossary of common terms at the end of the chapter.

PARALLEL DISTRIBUTED PROCESSING

There are three major reasons that linguistic theories have not yet provided a satisfactory account for the language errors made by normal subjects or the language disorders observed in aphasic patients:

1. Linguistic theories have been founded on the concept of serial processing, whereas abundant data suggest that language production incorporates parallel processing (Stemberger, 1985).
2. These serial-processing-based theories of linguistic function have difficulty capturing effects that are easily explained by bottom-up and top-down processing interactions, such as the occurrence of paraphasias (speech errors) that have both semantic and phonological similarity to the target (Dell & Reich, 1981; Dell, Schwartz, Martin, Saffran, & Gagnon, 1997; Harley, 1984).
3. Linguistic theories have failed to account for how linguistic behavior might emerge from neural structure.

Cognitive neuropsychological theories incorporate, to one extent or another, information-processing models—the "box and arrow" models that date back to Wernicke and Lichtheim. As we shall see, PDP models may be quite consistent with information-processing models with respect to the topography of language processes. As an added value, PDP models provide specificity regarding the nature of the representations in the boxes and the nature of the processes symbolized by the arrows, about which information-processing models are agnostic.

PDP (connectionist) models are neural-like in that they incorporate large arrays of simple units that are heavily interconnected with each other, like neurons in the brain (Nadeau, 2000). Their processing sophistication stems from the simultaneous interaction of the large numbers of units (hundreds or even thousands) in these arrays. PDP models also incorporate explicitly defined assumptions that are "wired" into them in the mathematical details of their computer implementation. They exhibit properties of graceful degradation and probabilistic selection. That is, when they are damaged or fed noisy input, they do not produce novel or bizarre output unachievable by an intact network with good input but, rather, tend to produce output that is not so reliably correct but is rule-bound—reminiscent of many of the observations that have been made about phonological selection errors. When computer simulations are run using PDP models, large numbers of specific predictions are generated that can be (and have been) empirically tested through observations of normal subjects and patients.

A key feature of PDP models is that memories are represented in the same networks that support processing. Thus, in PDP models of language, memories of language units (e.g., stored knowledge of phonemes, joint phonemes, syllables, words, and sentence constituents) are represented in the same neural networks that support linguistic processing. This fundamental difference (one of the many) between PDP and all other approaches drastically simplifies the structure of PDP models and, in addition, emulates the organization of the brain. One direct consequence of this property is that PDP models of language are able to accommodate the phenomenon of shifts and exchanges affecting phonological selection without the need for postulating the separate identity of linguistic units and time slots into which those units are placed, as is frequently done in the psycholinguistic literature (e.g., Shattuck-Hufnagel, 1979).[1] The temporally shifting pattern of activity in the system of neural networks supporting language automatically defines, at any one instant, both a temporal interval of opportunity and a repertoire of variously suitable word (lexical) or sublexical candidates to fill that temporal interval. The latency of activity pattern shifts, related ultimately to the slowness of neural physiology, provides one potential basis for the sequential nature of language in general and phonological processing in particular. The incorporation of short- and long-term memory in the same neural networks that are responsible for processing, in conjunction with processes underlying the engagement of working memory (Goldman-Rakic, 1990), also eliminates the need to posit buffers (which are a digital computer concept). PDP models are particularly appealing in the context of language processing because they involve simultaneous processing at a number of levels and locations, apparently mimicking what is going on in the brain. Finally, and perhaps most important, pure PDP models (models without incorporated digital devices) implicitly learn the rules governing the data they process in the course of their experience with that data (e.g., Plaut, McClelland, Seidenberg, & Patterson, 1996). Thus, for example, in a pure PDP model of phonology, there is no need to build in specific structures to account for specific phonological phenomena. The structure of the model is defined entirely in terms of the domains of information accessible to it and the necessary topographical relationship of these domains to each other. The model learns the rest. The absence of specific, ad hoc devices motivated by models (e.g., linguistic) designed to account for particular phonological phenomena in an orderly fashion is also crucial to the maintenance of neurological plausibility (architectural faithfulness to neural structure). In humans, as in PDP models, the linguistic phenomena we observe reflect entirely the emergent behavior of the networks.

Finally, PDP models invoke a scientific and philosophical paradigm shift in that they reflect chaotic order rather than deterministic order. Chaotic order (Gleick, 1987) is system order deriving from the ordered behavior of the individual units of the system, whereas deterministic order reflects the impact of an overall guiding force or principle.[2] Neural-network brains, whether in Drosophila (100,000 neurons) or in human beings (100 billion neurons), also operate by chaotic principles. Because in PDP order emerges naturally from network properties and topography, rather than being defined primarily by the structure of the model, neurological plausibility replaces the goal of choosing the simplest of competing theories (i.e., Occam's razor) as the guiding force in the design of these models (see O'Reilly, 1998). Although the precise details of the organization of neural networks in the brain still largely elude us, it is now quite clear and well accepted that the brain incorporates PDP principles, and the related scientific field, computational neuroscience, is burgeoning (Rolls & Deco, 2002; Rolls & Treves, 1998).[3]

PDP models provide the means to understand how complex behavior might emerge from neural networks, which are now accepted as the fundamental unit of cortical function (Buonomano & Merzenich, 1998). No model represents a final answer to how the brain handles a domain of cognitive function. Rather, a particular model represents a specific hypothesis about the topographic organization of neural processes underlying a given function and the mathematical properties of the units and connections comprising the neural networks involved; it presumes the now well-established faithfulness of the PDP concept to the essential features of neural-network processing; and to the extent that it successfully replicates behavior of human subjects in health and disease it accommodates empirical data on brain function. The dialectic in the PDP literature between principles of neural-network topography and mathematical function on the one hand and empirical data on language behavior on the other has proven particularly fruitful in advancing the science of language and the brain. The next section presents a specific model of phonological processing, linked to semantics (meaning) and considers how grammatic function might emerge from this model and its links to other brain systems.

A PARALLEL DISTRIBUTED PROCESSING MODEL OF LANGUAGE

Phonological Processing

Figure 5.1 depicts a PDP (connectionist model) of phonological processing. It is little more than the original model of Lichtheim (1885) dressed up with "hidden units." This model enables repetition, comprehension, naming, and internally generated language. Thus, assembling a PDP version of Lichtheim's model has little impact on its basic form. Rather, it provides specificity about what is represented by the "boxes" and "arrows." Here, the boxes (ovals) represent very large numbers of units.[4] Particular patterns of activity involving subsets of these units define the represented entities. For example, the repre-

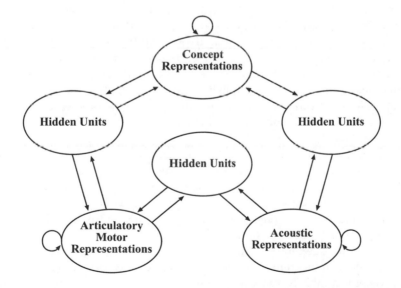

FIGURE 5.1. A PDP model of language processing that incorporates the essential substrate for repetition, comprehension, naming, and internally generated language.

sentation of the concept of "house" might correspond to activation of units representing features of houses such as visual attributes, construction materials, contents (physical and human), and so on. The exact nature of the feature units that are activated in various aggregates to define articulatory motor representations and acoustic representations is not important to our discussion, as long as they are discrete. For example, the feature units of articulatory motor representations might correspond to phonemic distinctive features. Thus, the model is explicitly phonological rather than phonetic. The model employs left–right position in acoustic and articulatory motor representations as a surrogate for temporal order in precisely the same way as the reading model of Plaut et al. (1996). Thus, articulatory motor representations would feature positions for each output phoneme or distinctive feature, ordered as they are in the phonological word form. Acoustic representations would involve an analogous representational scheme. The use of left-to-right sequential order in lieu of temporal order is a device of convenience, but there is evidence of this temporal–geographic transform in the brain (Cheung, Bedenbaugh, Nagarajan, & Schreiner, 2001).

Each arrow in the model represents the entire set of connections between every unit in one representational field and every unit in the connected field (e.g., between all the units in concept representations and all the hidden units between concept representations and articulatory motor representations). Most PDP networks have multiple layers. The units in the input and output layers are typically defined in behaviorally recognizable terms (e.g., in a reading model) as input graphemes (letter units) and output phonological distinctive features, respectively. The units interposed between input and output layers— the hidden units—have functions that depend on the connectivity of the network. These functions cannot be described in behavioral terms. Rather, studies of the activity *patterns* exhibited by the hidden units can provide insight into regularities in the knowledge implicit in the connectivity of the network. For example, in a network trained to learn the features of various living things, the patterns of activity over the hidden units reveal the network's knowledge (acquired through experience and not explicitly taught) that plants are different from animals, trees from flowers, and birds from fish (McClelland, McNaughton, & O'Reilly, 1995). Most important, hidden units in conjunction with nonlinear unit properties enable the establishment of a functional linkage between representations that have an arbitrary relationship to each other (e.g., word meaning and word phonology). They also provide the basis for much of the computational power of PDP models.

The knowledge represented in the model lies in the strengths of the connections between the units. One could set these connection strengths by hand. However, given models with connections numbering in the hundreds of thousands or millions, it makes much more sense to have models develop their own connection strengths through learning. In the most widely employed algorithm in PDP modeling, *back propagation*, a particular pattern of input (e.g., acoustic representations) is allowed to generate a stable pattern of activation in a linked representational field of interest (e.g., articulatory motor representations). The actual pattern of activity in articulatory motor representations is compared with the desired or target pattern of activity. To the extent that there is a discrepancy between actual output and target output, the connection strengths between acoustic representations and hidden units, and between hidden units and articulatory motor representations, are adjusted slightly (in proportion to their contribution to the error) such that the discrepancy is slightly reduced. With repeated cycling through the entire learning corpus, the model eventually develops the set of connection strengths that enables it to generate the correct pattern of activity within articulatory motor representations (within some defined error criterion) given a particular input to acoustic representations.

Where are the lexicons (the neural representations of word forms) in this model? In the most general neural network conceptualization, a lexicon is defined by any pattern associator network in which one of the patterns instantiates declarative memory (i.e., memory of discrete, consciously accessible "facts"). A pattern associator network translates one modality of distributed representations into another modality. Thus, the model in Figure 5.1 incorporates three pattern associator networks, but only two of them, the concept-to-articulatory-motor-representations pathway (the phonological output lexicon), and the acoustic-representations-to-concept-representations pathway (the phonological input lexicon), instantiate lexicons because only these two pathways (or pattern associator networks) incorporate the one type of representation that is declarative—concepts. Acoustic and articulatory motor representations derive meaning and conscious accessibility only by virtue of their links to concept representations. There are two lexicons in this system because the neural substrates, articulatory and acoustic, are fundamentally different and are located in different parts of the brain (Broca's area/opercular premotor cortex and auditory association cortex, respectively). This conceptualization of a lexicon as a pattern of connectivity rather than a locus of discrete pieces of knowledge is at substantial odds with the intuitive way of thinking about lexicons that has been engendered by information processing and linguistic models. However, it is well accepted in the connectionist literature and it is the only way of conceptualizing the instantiation (the representation in neural structure) of a lexicon in a computational device such as the brain in which the knowledge is represented in the connections.

All the connections in the model in Figure 5.1 are two way. Thus, it emulates the two-way connectivity generally seen in the brain. This reciprocal connectivity also provides the basis for some of the computational power of the model. As McClelland and Rumelhart (1981; Rumelhart & McClelland, 1982) showed over 20 years ago, and as was amply borne out in Dell's studies (e.g., Dell, 1986; Dell et al., 1997), much of the ability of network models to account for observed behavior derives from the combination of top-down *and bottom-up* flow of activation.

The model in Figure 5.1 also incorporates recurrent connections within each of its representational fields (symbolized by the loops at concept, articulatory motor and acoustic representations). This feature, which is neurologically plausible, enables the network to deal with the situation that arises when a pattern of input does not precisely correspond to one of the patterns on which the model was trained, either because the input pattern is novel or because input is noisy. In such circumstances, a model without recurrent connections might generate a pattern of activity in the output representational field that does not correspond to any recognizable entity. Clearly the brain has the capability for creating meaning for novel distributed representations. However, equally clearly, we derive great advantage from the ability to translate very noisy and degraded input into something we recognize. This ability corresponds to a network capacity for adjusting near-miss distributed representations until they correspond to the nearest meaningful representation ("nearest" corresponding literally to the distance in n-dimensional space between the near miss and the closest meaningful distributed representation, where n is the number of units in the representational field and "meaningfulness" is defined by the knowledge structure, latent in the network, that was acquired during the training period). This capacity is achieved by creating connections between every unit within the representational field and every other unit in that field. The field is thereby transformed into an "autoassociator" network, which is a network that tends to settle into stable states corresponding to meaningful distributed representations, as defined during the training period (Rumelhart, Smolensky, McClelland, & Hinton, 1986). This feature gives the entire network "attractor" properties, referring to the tendency of the network to settle into "attractive" stable states. Attractor properties convey another very useful property in computer simulations of network behavior: The time it takes a network to "settle" into an attractor state corresponds to the response latency of that network. In this way, the attractor feature endows the network with a performance measure, response latency, that precisely coincides with one of the most common dependent variables used in behavioral studies of human subjects.

At this point it is worth inquiring more deeply into the nature of the processes subsumed in the links between representational fields and hidden unit fields. We begin with a focus on the acoustic to articulatory motor pathway. Specifically, what is the nature of the knowledge represented in this pathway? A reading model developed by Plaut et al. (1996) provides crucial insight into this question (see also Seidenberg & McClelland, 1989). This model fundamentally recapitulates the acoustic–articulatory motor pathway of Figure 5.1, the major difference (inconsequential to this discussion) being that in place of acoustic representations, it incorporated orthographic (printed letter) representations. The model was trained, using the back-propagation algorithm (see earlier) by successively presenting, in pairs, the orthographic representation of 3,000 English single-syllable words and the desired phonological output. Ultimately, it learned to produce the correct pronunciation of all the words. One of the most striking things about the trained model is that it also was able to produce correct pronunciations of plausible English nonwords (i.e., orthographic sequences it had never encountered before). How was this possible?

One might have inferred that the model was simply learning the pronunciation of all the words by rote. If this had been the case, however, the model would have been incapable of applying what it had learned to novel words. In fact, what the model learned was the relationships between *sequences* of graphemes and *sequences* of phonemes that are characteristic of the English language. To the extent that there is a limited repertoire of such sequences, the model was able to learn it and then apply that knowledge to novel forms that incorporated some of the sequential relationships in this repertoire. The information the model acquired through its long experience with English orthographic–phonological sequential relationships went considerably beyond this, however. Certain sequences, those most commonly found in English single-syllable words, were more thoroughly etched in network connectivity. The model encountered difficulty (reflected in prolonged reading latency) only with low-frequency words, and only to the extent that it incorporated different, competing pronunciations of the same orthographic sequence. Thus, it was slow to read "pint" because in every case but "pint," the sequence "int" is pronounced /Int/ (e.g., mint, tint, flint, and lint). It was also slow, though not quite so slow, to read words such as "shown" because there are two equally frequent alternatives to the pronunciation of "own" (gown, down, town vs. shown, blown, flown). This behavior precisely recapitulates the behavior of normal human subjects given reading tasks.

To be more precise, the knowledge the model acquires reflects competing effects of type frequency and token frequency. If a single word is sufficiently common (high token frequency), the model acquires enough experience with it that competing orthographic–phonological sequential relationships have a negligible impact on naming latency. However, if a word is relatively uncommon (e.g., "pint"), its naming latency will be significantly affected by the knowledge of other words that, though equally uncommon, together belong to a competing type (e.g., mint, flint, tint, and sprint).

The capacity of the model to read nonwords reflects its ability to capture patterns in the sequential relationships between orthographic and articulatory word forms and to apply this knowledge to novel word forms. Plaut et al. (1996), as well as Seidenberg and McClelland (1989), in their earlier work on this reading model, focused on differences in rhyme components of single syllable words (the nucleus plus the coda, e.g., b*at*) because these are the major determinants of whether a word is orthographically regular (e.g., "mint") or irregular (e.g., "pint"). However, as Seidenberg and McClelland point out, the

network architecture in these models is capable of capturing any kind of regu-
larity in the orthographic and phonological sequences it is exposed to, limited
only by the extent of exposure. Such regularities would include joint phonemes
other than rhymes (e.g., "str" of stream, street, stray and strum), and, in a
multisyllabic version, syllables and morphemes (affixes and the root forms of
nouns and verbs), as well as functors (e.g., articles, auxiliary verbs, conjunctions, certain prepositions).

The acoustic–articulatory motor pathway in the model of Figure 5.1 would
capture analogous patterns in the sequential relationships between acoustic
and articulatory word forms (actually somewhat more redundant, because in
English, acoustic–articulatory correspondences are substantially more consistent than are orthographic–articulatory correspondences). These sequential relationship patterns potentially involve sequences of varying length, from phoneme pairs (joint phonemes) and syllables up to and including whole words
and, possibly, multiple word compounds. These patterns represent the repository of knowledge about subword (sublexical) entities in general, as well as our
knowledge of phonotactic constraints (the rules that determine whether or not
a given phonemic sequence is permissible in a particular language). This repository of sequence knowledge also provides the basis for "neighborhood" effects
(Vitevitch, 1997). Neighborhood effects reflect the influence of variously competing pieces of sequence knowledge on the ultimate phonological sequence
selection and the tendency to produce near-miss phonological sequence errors
that correspond to one of the close neighbors.

The acoustic–articulatory pathway of the model depicted in Figure 5.1 has
the capacity for representing sequence knowledge, and hence, knowledge of
sublexical entities, because it is a pattern associator that links representational
domains that are *both* intrinsically sequential. In the process of learning, this
network captures the sequence regularities that are common to the two representational domains. In contrast, the pattern associator linking concept representations to articulatory motor representations in this model provides
relatively little basis for sequence knowledge because only one of the representational domains (articulatory) is sequential. In contrast, a semantic representation is defined by a *configuration* of activity over concept features,
not a sequence. It elicits an articulatory motor representation as a single
compound—in effect the reverse of the process by which an orthographic
whole-word image elicits a concept when one reads via the semantic route (i.e.,
reads silently for meaning). Even though the ultimate output of the concept–
articulatory motor pattern associator is a sequence of movements, the network
architecture provides a poor substrate for capturing the regularities of phonological sequences because there are no regularities to be captured between a
configurational field (concepts) and a sequential field (articulatory motor representations). Therefore, the fact that in the process of engaging articulatory motor representations from concept representations, normal subjects experience

slips of the tongue and aphasic subjects produce phonemic paraphasias in naming and internally generated language quite comparable to those produced during repetition (which engages the acoustic–articulatory motor pathway) tells us that this model cannot be correct. There must be a means by which concept representations access the sublexical, phoneme sequence knowledge within the acoustic–articulatory motor pathway. Thus we arrive at the model depicted in Figure 5.2.

In this model, concept representations interface with the domain of sequence knowledge at the hidden units of the acoustic–articulatory-motor-pattern associator. Although this semantic input constrains the sequence knowledge in the latter, it tends to bind phonological sequences only to the extent that they are linked to words known to the person rather than to the extent that they instantiate phonotactic relationships (implicit knowledge about the likelihood of particular phoneme sequences gained from language experience). Thus, in all that follows, we refer to this as lexical semantic input and reserve the term "sequence knowledge" for the phonotactic knowledge in the acoustic-to-articulatory-motor-pattern associator.

If one accepts the logic of these arguments, one might well ask why, in

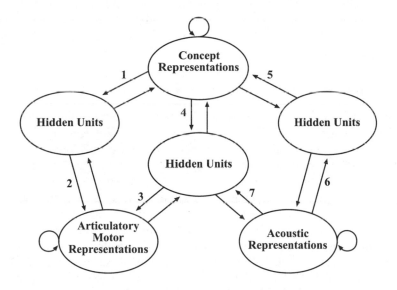

FIGURE 5.2. The PDP model of Figure 5.1, modified by the addition of two-way connectivity between concept representations and the hidden units of the acoustic–articulatory motor pattern associator. This link provides the explanation for phonological slips in language production by normal subjects, phonemic paraphasias in language production by aphasic subjects, as well as the convergence of lexical semantic and sequence knowledge in phonological processing.

the model of Figure 5.2, we also posit a direct, concept-representations-to-articulatory-motor-representations pathway (pathway 1-2). The single most important reason is that many studies of language in aphasic patients demonstrate anomia in internally generated language or during naming to confrontation that cannot be adequately accounted for by semantic or phonological dysfunction or some combination thereof. The results of these studies suggest that yet another pathway must exist, instantiating another domain of knowledge, dysfunction of which yields pure anomia. Pathway 1-2 meets this requirement. In addition, the two pathways, direct (1-2) and indirect (4-3), posited in this model offer a convenient explanation for certain phenomena such as data on verb past tense formation)(Nadeau, 2001). Finally, the existence of pathway 1-2 finds direct support in observations of patients with repetition conduction aphasia and deep dysphasia; these patients appear to lack all phonological sequence function but can repeat words and apparently do so using this pathway because they do not make phonemic paraphasias during repetition.

This model represents a hypothesis about the topography of neural network structure underlying phonology. Its many potential limitations have been discussed at length elsewhere (Nadeau, 2001). The model has not been subjected to simulation studies; thus its current appeal is mainly theoretical. It does appear to provide a cogent explanation for a very large number of observations of phonological phenomenology in normal subjects producing slips of the tongue and in aphasic patients. In a later section, we consider implications of this model for therapeutic strategies.

Semantics

In the model elaborated in the previous section, concept representations were viewed as comprising a single domain. However, in reality concepts are highly distributed over a network of subnetworks, each subnetwork providing a neural representation of features of a concept that fall within a particular domain. Thus, the concept of dog corresponds to a pattern of neural activity in visual association cortices corresponding to visual attributes of dogs, a pattern in somatosensory association cortices corresponding to tactile aspects of dogs, a pattern in olfactory association cortex, a pattern in auditory association cortex, a pattern in limbic cortex (corresponding to emotional feelings regarding dogs in general or a particular dog), and a pattern in frontal cortex corresponding to predicative aspects of dogs (what they are likely to do). The fact that there is variability in the contribution of different feature domains to the meaning of particular entities provides much of the basis for category-specific naming deficits (Forde & Humphreys, 1999). Thus, the dominance of the visual representation in our conceptualization of dogs or other living things leads to a susceptibility of this knowledge to focal lesions of visual association cortex. This is essentially the explanation proposed by Warrington and Shallice (1984).

Grammar

For purposes of this discussion, we break down grammatic function into syntax and grammatic morphology. Syntax is knowledge of acceptable word order and sentence structure. Grammatic morphology refers both to the modifications of words that are made in their use in sentences (bound grammatic morphology, e.g., affixes conveying case, number, or tense) and to the use of individual words that primarily serve sentence composition rather than meaning (free grammatical morphemes, e.g., articles, auxiliary verbs, conjunctions, and certain prepositions). We break down syntax into (1) *sentence organization*, which encompasses such things as the necessary relationships between verbs and nouns or noun phrases in a sentence (verb argument relationships—see later), and embedded clauses; and (2) *phrase structure rules*, which constrain word order at the local level (e.g., the rule that constrains articles to precede nouns). In Chomskian thinking, both these components of syntax are thought to arise from the operational principles of a grammar generator. In contrast, we argue that principles of sentence organization follow directly from the way the brain manipulates concept representations, and that phrase structure rules and rules of grammatic morphology are an emergent property of the pattern associator networks responsible for articulatory and inscriptional (written) output.

Syntax: Sentence Organization

It is easy to conceive of spoken concrete nouns as the product of distributed representations of concepts that are linked, through a pattern associator network, to the sequences of oropharyngeal movements that actually produce the speech sounds of the noun, as discussed in the section on phonology. The same cannot be said about other types of words, most particularly adjectives, verbs, and abstract nouns.

Adjectives represent the simplest case and therefore are a reasonable place to start. In principle, the distributed representations corresponding to noun concepts are infinitely malleable. We can easily modify the general distributed representation of dog to capture any species of dog or any particular dog we have personally known. We can easily contemplate the most complicated and arbitrary of distributed representations—for example, "the obese, pockmarked, oily-haired, slovenly, unctuous, check-shirted, plaid-jacketed man with the striped pants, food-stained paisley tie, goatee, wire-rimmed glasses, bundle of pens in his pocket, and clip board in his hand"—a sort of Uriah Heep cum used-car salesman. The process of pairing an adjective or adjectival phrase with a noun corresponds to a particular modification of the distributed representation of the noun.

Verbs are viewed as the work masters in traditional linguistic formulations because they specify the major participants in the action that is described by the verb, thereby defining sentence structure. These participants are "the arguments" of the verb. Arguments are usually noun phrases but may also be prepositional phrases, adjectival phrases, or sentential clauses. They fill argument positions (e.g., subject, object, and indirect object positions). Each argument is assigned a purpose in the sentence by the verb—its "thematic role." For example, the agent is the perpetrator of the action ("The *man* gave flowers to Mary"); the theme is the object of the verb's action (flowers in the preceding sentence); and the goal is the recipient of the action (Mary). Verbs differ with respect to the arguments they specify—some require only an agent; some an agent and a theme; others an agent, theme, and goal. They also differ with respect to the nature of the arguments they can specify (e.g., "knew" easily accommodates a sentential clause in the predicate—e.g., "He knew Mary would arrive soon"— whereas "hit" does not).

Does the argument-specification property of verbs provide direct insight into the cerebral processing of verbs? To date, no one has succeeded in answering this question using a traditional linguistic formulation. How might a verb be represented in PDP terms? First, consider what might be the distributed representation of a verb (e.g., the verb "to shoot"). What features underlie this distributed representation? A problem is immediately apparent. In fact, our conceptualization of shooting actually consists of the juxtaposition of two distributed concept representations: a person who is the shooter and a person who has been shot or is about to be shot. The sentence "the old man shot the burglar" generates two distributed-concept representations, one of an old man appropriately altered to incorporate the act of shooting, the second of a burglar, appropriately altered to incorporate the fact of having been shot. Thus, "shot" achieves its meaning not through the generation of its own distributed representation but, rather, through the elicitation of two reciprocally modified distributed representations ("old man shooter" and "shot burglar") that are in addition meaningfully linked, in effect constituting a composite, "super-distributed" representation that incorporates the entire shooting scene. The two components of this composite representation are implicitly linked by their complementarity (shooter and shot) and their simultaneity. They become explicitly linked when this particular reciprocal pair of distributed representations generates a pattern of activation in articulatory motor cortex that will produce the sound sequence of /shot/. They may also become explicitly linked when a pattern of activity in acoustic cortex, generated by the sound of /shot/ (occurring in the context of preceding and following noun-generated concepts), leads to production of the reciprocal pair of distributed representations underlying "old man shooter" and "shot burglar."

Intransitive verbs function in a fashion essentially identical to adjectives (e.g., "the soldier salutes"). A transitive verb functions as a sort of super-adjective, reciprocally modifying the distributed representations of the concepts underlying the two or three nouns phrases in the sentence and at the same time, linking them to form a new, superdistributed representation. Thus, in our new conceptualization, verbs are defined exclusively by the effect they have on the distributed representations of the nouns they constrain.

The autoassociator network representation of a concept can be translated by the lexical semantic–articulatory pattern associator network into any one of a number of different word sequences. The actual word sequence chosen depends on several factors, including (1) the modifiability of the core distributed representation of the concept; (2) whether the modification occurs nearly simultaneously with the generation of the core distributed representation or at some later time; and (3) the availability of words to be elicited by the autoassociator network representation of the concept. To provide a sense of the concept manipulation demands that are met by the normal brain, we consider each of these possibilities in some detail.

Modifiability of the Core Representation. Consider the core representation of "burglar" in our previous example. "Old man-shot burglar" is not likely to be a modification of the distributed representation of burglar that is readily available to us. Thus, we are forced to use a superdistributed representation to capture this concept—a representation that therefore engages a verb (e.g., "the burglar that had been shot by the old man"). On the other hand, consider the concept of streets wet with rain. Here, the concept of "rain-wet streets" falls well within the various modifications of street that are readily available to us. Thus, we have a choice in expressing this idea. We can employ a single distributed representation, modified by an adjective, yielding "rain-wet streets," or we can employ a superdistributed representation, thus engaging a verb (e.g., "the streets made wet by the rain").

Simultaneous versus Sequential Modification. Whether a modification of the distributed representation underlying a concept occurs as the concept is formed or sometime later is likely to influence the word sequence corresponding to that concept. Thus, someone viewing a romantic Parisian street in her mind's eye might incorporate "rain-wet" from the beginning, favoring the verbal product "rain-wet streets." On the other hand, the wetness modification might be conceptualized only after the street concept has been realized and verbalization has been initiated, hence "the car skidded on the street that was still wet from the rain," "the car skidded on the street because the street was still wet from the rain," or "The car skidded on the street. The street was still wet from the rain." The way the sequence of conceptual development happens to emerge is probably not the only factor at play here. We may have the luxury of shaping the conceptual stream according to our intent to place emphasis or imply causality. On the other hand, working-memory capacity may limit the number and complexity of modifications we can make in a distributed representation at one time, forcing us to use a narrative stream employing multiple clauses or sentences, each further modifying the original distributed-concept representation.

The Availability of Words. Word representations corresponding to certain distributed-concept representations may be completely unavailable, available but inappropriate to the context, or temporarily unavailable. Each of these circumstances would necessitate a clause construction in lieu of an adjective construction. Thus, "rain-wet" might simply not be in a person's vocabulary. Alternatively, it might be available but carry with it a sense of inappropriateness to the context (possibly a limbic component to the distributed representation generated by the word in this context). Thus, "rain-wet" is satisfactory in a novel but would sound contrived in ordinary conversation and would be inappropriate in formal discourse. Finally, the word may be transiently unavailable because of the "tip-of-the-tongue" phenomenon, necessitating a circumlocutory clause or sentence to convey the concept.

In this way, the aspect of syntax we have defined as sentence organization does not depend on the machinations of a sophisticated language processor but, rather, constitutes an emergent property of the distributed representations of concepts, the modification of concepts, the linking of concepts into super-distributed representations, and the interaction of network systems defining concepts with the pattern associator networks defining language output. Concept representations and their manipulations invoke association cortices (and subcortical structures such as the amygdala) throughout the brain. Therefore, the ways in which concepts are handled provide a window to fundamental properties of higher brain function. The pattern associators linking concept representations to language input and output systems terminate predominantly though somewhat variably in dominant perisylvian cortex.

Two aspects of a common aphasia, Broca's aphasia, are explainable on the basis of a breakdown in the processes just outlined. Broca's aphasia is commonly characterized by two grammatic attributes: simplification of syntax and a characteristic abnormality of grammatic morphology known as agrammatism—the propensity for leaving out words of primarily grammatic importance, such as articles, auxiliary verbs, conjunctions, and, to some extent, prepositions. These two aspects of Broca's aphasia may be dissociated: A number of cases of morphological agrammatism without simplification of syntax have been reported and at least two cases of simplification of syntax without morphological agrammatism have been reported (Nadeau, 1988; Nadeau & Gonzalez Rothi, 1993). As we have noted, sentence production reflects the flexible modification and manipulation of the distributed representations underlying concepts. Simplification of syntax (including a paucity of embedded clauses and inability to use strings of adjectives) can be accounted for in terms of a defect in the ability to alter the distributed representations of single or multiple concepts at will. This may be due to a general inability to maintain selective engagement of the specific neural networks incorporating the featural basis for the concepts and their intended nuances. Consistent with this interpretation is the fact that patients with Broca's aphasia exhibit limited lexical priming (Prather, Zurif, Stern, & Rosen, 1992). By *selective engagement* we mean the bringing on line of selected representations in selected neural networks, either by eliciting sustained neural activity in those networks or by altering the state of polarization of the neurons such that they are more susceptible to firing by other afferent input (Moran & Desimone, 1985). "Selective engagement" is a general term that embraces the many processes by which the brain allocates resources, and it includes processes commonly referred to as working memory—the specific type of selective engagement we refer to here—as well as attention (Nadeau & Crosson, 1997). In normal subjects engaged in a lexical decision task, preceding a lexical target with a semantically related word reduces the time needed to determine whether the target is a word or a nonword. Seeing the semantically related word has led to the selective engagement of a number of semantically related distributed-concept representations and their associated articulatory motor representations, one of which is the target. In patients with Broca's aphasia, the range and number of the distributed-concept representations selectively engaged appear to be limited, with the result that speeding of lexical decision by semantic priming is less likely to occur.

Generating verbs also normally invokes a particular form of selective engagement in order to modify two or more distributed representations in reciprocal fashion and link them to form a superdistributed representation. It thus makes special demands on selective engagement mechanisms. Patients with Broca's aphasia exhibit relatively greater difficulty accessing verbs than nouns, and their production of verbs with complex argument structures is more impaired than is production of simple verbs (e.g., intransitive verbs) (Thompson, Lange, Schneider, & Shapiro, 1997)—further evidence of impairment in ability to simultaneously manipulate multiple distributed representations. Notably, the ability of subjects with agrammatism to produce verbs in tasks of picture naming, whether naturally or as a result of treatment (in our nomenclature, to use verbs as adjectives), does not translate into ability to use verbs in sentences (i.e., to link and reciprocally modify distributed-concept representations), a far more demanding skill (Mitchum & Berndt, 2001).

One of the most widely accepted theories regarding the fundamental deficit in Broca's aphasia is the "mapping deficit hypothesis" (Saffran & Schwartz, 1988; Saffran, Schwartz, & Marin, 1980; Schwartz, Linebarger, Saffran, & Pate, 1987). This hypothesis characterizes the deficit as an inability to produce ordered sentence components (e.g., noun phrase–verb–noun phrase) that reflect the underling thematic roles (e.g., agent, theme, and goal) in order to link sentence structure to meaning. Two components are identified: (1) lexical, referring to argument information specified by verbs; and (2) procedural, referring to operations governing thematic role assignment for sentences that require interpretation of structural cues (word order, verb morphology) in order to relate noun phrases as they literally appear in the sentence to underlying sentence meaning. For example, to understand who did what to whom in the passive voice sentence "Joe was hit by John," one must cue not just on word order but on the auxiliary verb "was" and the preposition "by." These mapping capacities correspond quite directly to the capacities for distributed-concept manipulation and association discussed in the foregoing. The advantage of the sentence organization hypothesis we have introduced is that it relates these functions directly to neural network processes.

Syntax: Phrase-Structure Rules

One of the most remarkable attributes of words in spoken language is their consistent respect for phrase-structure rules (e.g., articles always precede and never follow nouns). Only in the occasional jargon aphasic does this rule seem to be broken, and even then it is far from clear whether inappropriate sequences emerge in continuous discourse or whether they result just by happenstance as a result of the juxtaposition of phrase fragments. Clearly these immutable phrase-structure rules reflect some fundamental and redundantly represented attributes of cerebral language networks that govern word sequence. To gain some insight into such network properties, we return to the pattern associator model of single-syllable word reading developed by Plaut et al. (1996) (see the subsection "A Parallel Distributed Processing Model of Language," "Phonological Processing"). Had the model been designed to accommodate multisyllabic words rather than only single-syllable words, we would have seen it acquire sequence knowledge about syllables, polysyllables, root forms, and affixes as they combine to form words, simply from its experience with English vocabulary. This sequence knowledge incorporates the sequential relationship of these various sublexical phoneme clumps to each other: the lexical equivalent of phrase-structure rules.

The inferential leap we make at this point is that sequential relationships *between words* are also represented in various neural pattern associator networks, in the same way that sequential relationships between phonemes *within* words are represented. Specifically, we need to posit that for phrase-structure rules to be represented in oral-language output, there needs to be a pattern associator network *between* the autoassociator network underlying semantics and the pattern associator network that serves as the phonological output lexicon, the two pattern associators linked to form a hierarchy (see Figure 5.2). This additional pattern associator links distributed representations of concepts underlying words, characterized by the properties of their network representation (e.g., nouns, adjectives, and verbs, as we have discussed), with distributed representations of the articulatory forms of these words in proper sequence. In effect, it is a property–sequence transducer in which the systematic relationships between concept-representation properties and articulatory sequences emerge as implicit knowledge through extended experience with heard and spoken language. At first one is inclined to protest that as the number of possible word sequences is virtually infinite, no system, even one comprised of tens of billions of units and involving combinatorial mathematics, could possibly represent all the possibilities. However, the actual amount of information relevant to word sequence that is implicit in all the allowable word sequences is actually much less than it seems and quite plausibly is incorporated within neural connectivity. This is because word-sequence information implicitly incorporates rules governing the order of *classes* of words, precisely as a multisyllabic phonemic processor would implicitly incorporate rules about the placement of suffixes and prefixes. Thus, in English, words that have the attribute of modifying the distributed representation of a concept (adjectives) uniformly precede nouns and knowledge about the proper order of adjective–noun sequences simply emerges from the network's experience with heard and written English. PDP networks can also learn specific exceptional representations as well as patterns that are common to many representations. Thus, the reading model of Plaut et al. (1996) was able to learn to read such extremely exceptional words as "aisle," "guide," and "fugue." By the same token, a word-sequence network should be able to learn certain sequences with few exemplars, such as those involving the placement of articles. In fact, because articles are among the most commonly encountered words in the language, the network would be expected to instantiate the sequential relationship between articles and nouns with particular redundancy.

How long are the word sequences that are likely to be entrained by the pattern associator network contemplated here? The answer is not known. There is some evidence that the length of commonly used sequences grows with practice through the lifespan. Elderly people are relatively more likely than younger people to develop Wernicke's aphasia and relatively less likely than younger people to develop Broca's aphasia, whether the lesion is due to stroke, neoplasm, or trauma (Basso, Bracchi, Capitani, Laiacona, & Zanobio, 1987; Brown & Grober, 1983; Kertesz & Sheppard, 1981; Miceli et al., 1981). One possible explanation for this likelihood is that elderly people are able to maintain reasonable fluency given a frontal lobe lesion because of their considerable capability for generating relatively lengthy word sequences through the posteriorly located pattern associator network we have discussed. Only when the lesion directly affects that pattern associator and/or its downstream phonological pattern associator does aphasia result, and then it is, as expected, a Wernicke's aphasia or a conduction aphasia. This hypothesis finds further support in the observation that normal elderly subjects tend to use more elaborate sentence structures than do young subjects (Obler & Albert, 1981).

Grammatic Morphology

Morphological grammar refers to the use of words (free grammatical morphemes, e.g., articles, auxiliary verbs, conjunctions, and some prepositions) and suffixes (bound grammatical morphemes, e.g., affixes specifying case, number, or tense) whose role appears to be primarily grammatical. The distinctiveness of these free grammatical morphemes and the apparently fundamental differences between them and major lexical items (nouns and main verbs) is further conveyed in the other terms by which they are known: "functors" and "closed-class words."

This way of classifying these words has a certain appeal if one posits the existence of a grammatic processor, such as that proposed by Chomsky and others. However, as we have noted, there has not been a successful effort to account for a grammatic processor in terms of known principles of neural network function. Therefore, in this section, we continue the approach taken earlier, assuming that all aspects of language can be understood in terms of (1) the properties of distributed representations; (2) the mechanisms that manipulate distributed representations; and (3) the interface of the autoassociator network supporting semantic distributed representations with pattern associator networks that translate these semantic distributed representations into alternate forms (e.g., acoustic, orthographic, articulatory, and inscriptional). The essential currency of semantic distributed representations is meaning. Constraints on sequence are primarily provided by implicit sequence rules latent in the connectivity of the acoustic–articulatory pattern associator network, but also derive from the fact that language formulation, production, and comprehension evolve over hundreds or thousands of milliseconds. In the spirit of this dialogue, we attempt to approach the problem of grammatic morphology from the perspective of meaning constrained by sequence.

Articles. We have already noted in the section on phrase-structure rules that representations of articles such as "the" are probably engaged to some degree by virtue of their incorporation in multiword sequence knowledge. In addition, although articles have minimal meaning, they cannot be characterized as having no meaning whatsoever: They do indicate definite or indefinite. However, as modifiers in noun phrases, they differ from adjectives in that their meaning is contextual, whereas the meaning of adjectives is absolute. That is, whether the article "a" or "the" is used depends on the preceding discourse; in contrast, the use of an adjective such as "big" depends only on the attributes of the noun distributed representation it is linked to. Thus, in part, the use of articles depends on the maintenance of some working memory of what has already been said (i.e., sustained selective engagement of immediately prior distributed-concept representations and their relationship to each other). To the extent that working-memory (selective engagement) mechanisms are defective, we might expect impetus to article use from this source to be reduced. In English-speaking patients with Broca's aphasia, as we have noted, there is some evidence of such a defect. As predicted by our hypothesis of defective selective engagement, these patients tend to omit articles (agrammatism). In other languages (e.g., German), articles are marked for case, gender, and number, additional meaningful information that derives from the semantic representation of the nouns with which they are associated. Apparently because of these additional contributors to engagement of article representations, German subjects with Broca's aphasia are much more likely to produce incorrect articles (paragrammatisms) than to omit articles (Bates, Friederici, & Wulfeck, 1987); these substitutions can be viewed as syllabic sequence errors.

The essential lesion for producing agrammatism in spontaneous language appears to involve dominant postcentral perisylvian cortex (Nadeau, 1988). However, if our hypothesis regarding the contextual and hence working-memory dependence of article use is correct, we should see some evidence of article omission in English-speaking patients with dominant frontal lobe convexity cortex lesions. The fact that patients with frontal lesions with sparing of postcentral perisylvian cortex are not conspicuously agrammatic may reflect two things: (1) that frontal systems engaged in working-memory processes underlying article use are highly distributed, and (2) that frontal lesions spare the neural-network representation of multiword sequence knowledge (e.g., phrase-structure rules). Thus, a modest lesion in postcentral perisylvian cortex may produce agrammatism (Kolk & Friederici, 1985) because it is at the point in which frontal projections converge on the pattern associator networks producing language output and it is the locus of relevant sequence knowledge.

Auxiliary verbs. There are four attributes of auxiliary verbs (e.g., "The boy *was* fishing") that might make them particularly prone to omission by subjects with Broca's aphasia, given the model we have been considering. First, they are linked to the main verb. We have reasoned that main verbs function by simultaneously reciprocally modifying and linking as many as three distributed representations corresponding to the verb arguments in the sentence, a process particularly demanding of selective engagement mechanisms. Main verbs are differentially affected in subjects with Broca's aphasia. Second, most often the purpose of an auxiliary verb is to convey tense. Frontal systems may provide the chief substrate for the neural instantiation of the time concept by virtue of their primary role in planning. Time tagging of memories is impaired in patients with frontal lobe lesions. Third, auxiliary verbs are often used only to reconcile the tense of the sentence with the tense of the preceding narrative (e.g., "She has a headache now. She has been having headaches for six months."). That is, the inclusion and choice of auxiliary verbs are based, like those of articles, on narrative context—hence, working memory. Finally, auxiliary verbs may be linked to main verbs within the domain of sequence knowledge. The fact that the neural mechanisms underlying all four of these are impaired in patients with Broca's aphasia may account for the tendency for these patients to omit these words.

Prepositions. Although there are many types of prepositions, here we focus only on locative prepositions (e.g., "The book is *on* the table"). These words strongly resemble main verbs in that they are the product of reciprocal alterations in the distributed representations of the concepts underlying the nouns on which they operate, coupled with linkage of these noun concepts. On this basis alone, we might expect them to be differentially affected by brain lesions that impair the selective engagement processes necessary for this to happen, as in the case of verbs.

Pronouns. Pronouns, because they derive their meaning only through reference to antecedent nouns, depend on sustained engagement (working memory) of the noun representations that have been used recently. Again, to the extent that such selective-engagement mechanisms are impaired, one would expect defective use of pronouns. This is indeed the case in subjects with Broca's aphasia. By contrast, people with aphasia due to more posterior lesions, which leave frontally mediated selective-engagement mechanisms intact, use pronouns to excess as a device to deal with their problems with lexical semantic access.

Grammar: A Synthesis

Lexical semantic function is based on three domains of knowledge: semantic, sequence, and the pattern associators linking semantic and sequence knowledge, which provide the basis for the phonological lexicons. Grammatic expression demands an elaboration of sequence knowledge to the extent that word stems may attach grammatical morphemes and multiword sequences are governed by phrase-structure rules. Grammatic expression demands an additional domain of knowledge, which may be characterized as lexical syntactic. That is, a phonological sequence may be selected not just by a concept representation but also by a configuration of concept representations. This configuration may include representations that are reciprocally related to each other, as in the case of transitive verbs and locative prepositions. Alternatively, the configuration may involve a relationship between unspoken concept representations and already spoken representations (maintained as working memory), as in the case of pronouns, articles, and many auxiliary verbs.

In this conceptualization, anomia may represent a breakdown in lexical semantic or lexical syntactic knowledge (or both). The degree to which a word is affected depends on the degree to which its phonological engagement relies on lexical semantic and lexical syntactic knowledge (which may vary from language to language), the locus of the lesion, and perhaps the degree of reliance on lexical semantic and lexical syntactic knowledge relative to sequence knowledge. Grammatic morphemes are most susceptible to deficits in lexical syntactic knowledge, whereas nouns are most susceptible to deficits in lexical semantic knowledge. Main verbs require both domains of knowledge, and the breakdown in verb use in aphasia is revealing of the underlying basis for lexical syntactic knowledge: Even when agrammatic subjects produce a relatively normal number of verbs, their verb use tends to ignore argument structure (Thompson, Lange, Schneider, & Shapiro, 1997), which is based on concept relationships.

MEMORY

Any behavioral therapy, language therapy included, involves the addition of new knowledge to the brain to replace that lost as a result of brain injury or disease. Because the properties of the neural systems that incorporate new knowledge have major implications for the therapeutic strategies employed in presenting that information, we address this topic in some detail.

Language processes explicitly involve two well-known types of memory, procedural and declarative (Squire & Knowlton, 2000), and may involve other as yet unrecognized types of memory. Each is discussed separately.

Procedural Memory

Procedural memories, often referred to as skill memories, are acquired incrementally by the neural systems representing the skills as they are practiced. For example, skill in playing tennis is enhanced gradually through extended practice as connectivity in the premotor and motor cortices, basal ganglia, cerebellum, brainstem, and spinal motor systems is incrementally modified. In language, the neural-network knowledge that enables translation of continuous incoming sound into the acoustic representation of phonemes, which are discrete, not continuous, probably represents a form of procedural knowledge. By the same token, the neural-network knowledge that enables the translation of the articulatory representation of phonemes, also discrete, into continuous programs of movement involving oropharyngeal musculature and the diaphragm also probably represents a form of procedural knowledge. It also seems likely that knowledge of the phonemic sequence repertoire of a given language is procedural, at least insofar as this knowledge is actually used in speech. The development of phonological awareness—awareness of the discrete phoneme structure of words—may correspond to the addition of a declarative form of this knowledge.

Declarative Memory

Declarative memories, or memories for discrete facts, are acquired all at once in approximately 1 second in a process that is thought to involve fast Hebbian learning within Ammon's horn (the "cornu Ammonis") of the hippocampus (McClelland et al., 1995; Rolls & Treves, 1998). This nearly instantaneous establishment of new connections between active neurons within the hippocampus serves to close long loops linking neural networks in the cerebral cortex. Cerebral association cortices project to the parahippocampal gyrus and perirhinal cortex, which in turn project to the entorhinal cortex and then to the dentate gyrus of the hippocampus. Dentate neurons project to the pyramidal neurons in the cornu Ammonis (CA3 and CA1 fields) of the hippocampus. The pyramidal neurons then project via the subiculum to the entorhinal cortex, which then projects back to cerebral association cortices. These circuitous new connections instantiate new knowledge. Initially this new knowledge constitutes episodic memory in that it is memory of a particular aspect of a particular event at a particular place and time. Eventually, to one extent or another, this new knowledge may be incorporated into neural-network connectivity in the cerebral cortex in a process referred to as consolidation. The process of declarative memory consolidation is not completely understood and is currently somewhat controversial. It appears most likely that memories are incorporated into cortical network connectivity to the extent that they share features with knowledge that is already represented in the cortex. In this process of consolidation, the hippocampus appears to serve as a teacher to the cortex, repeatedly subjecting the cortex to patterns of activation congruent with the new information the hippocampus has incorporated. There is growing evidence that this process occurs during sleep and, particularly, during dream sleep. If this theory of consolidation is correct, it follows that memories that cannot be readily incorporated into the cortex because they share few features with existent cortical knowledge will remain permanently dependent on connections within the hippocampus and its immediately adjacent neural structures. This appears to be the case: Autobiographical memories generally share few features with knowledge represented in cortex (they represent knowledge of particular places and times that are of only personal significance); autobiographical memories are highly susceptible to disruption by lesions of the hippocampus and its associated structures.

It is currently thought that the hippocampal system is required because in neural-network simulations, the sustained presentation of new information to a network results in replacement of old knowledge already represented in the network by the new knowledge; that is, there is catastrophic degradation of the old information (McClelland et al., 1995). However, if presentation of new information is interleaved with rehearsal of the old information, a network is capable of instantiating both old and new knowledge simultaneously. It is thought that the hippocampal system provides the brain with a means to circumvent this impasse: It at once serves as a repository of newly acquired declarative knowledge and a teacher to the cortex that, presumably during dream sleep, serves to interleave the new knowledge with rehearsal of old, related knowledge. The new knowledge is added to the old gradually, and because the changes in neural connections are made incrementally, and new interleaved with old, catastrophic degradation of old knowledge does not occur.

Properties of Procedural and Declarative Memory Systems Relevant to Aphasia Therapy

Both procedural and declarative memory systems have characteristic strengths and weaknesses relevant to their recruitment in aphasia therapy. One major advantage of procedural knowledge underlying language is that it generalizes widely. That is, the acquisition of skills in decoding of sound sequences into phonemic acoustic representations (rarely a source of difficulty), translating phonemic articulatory representations into motor programs, and of phonemic sequence knowledge will provide the procedural knowledge basis for decoding and producing all words in the native vocabulary. A second major advantage is that achieving an adequate foundation of procedural language skills potentially gives the patient the tools to continue growth of language capacity on his or her own in the course of routine conversation—in direct analogy to the normal process of language acquisition in early childhood.

The major disadvantage of procedural knowledge acquisition is that it is incremental. Therefore, the ultimate development of a useful level of skill will require extensive practice. In addition, successful procedural linguistic memory acquisition in the domain of phonological knowledge would only build the phonemic/articulatory foundation for acquisition of lexical semantic knowledge. The actual links between distributed-concept representations (semantic knowledge) and phonemic/articulatory sequences would still have to be established, either through further therapy or by the patient in the course of daily use of language. Our major hypothesis (yet to be proven) motivating phonological therapy (training of phonologic sequences, among other things) for naming disorders in aphasic patients is that once a solid phonemic/articulatory sequence foundation is built, lexical semantic knowledge will be established relatively easily, perhaps even without further therapy.

The advantage of declarative knowledge underlying language is that it can potentially be acquired all at once (assuming that declarative memory acquisition is 100% efficient despite damage to cerebral cortex—clearly an over-optimistic assumption). The major disadvantage of declarative knowledge acquisition with respect to language therapy is that it generalizes only minimally because there is little relationship between the meaning of a word and its sound. Thus, for any therapeutic strategy that depends on declarative knowledge acquisition to achieve practical value for a patient, the learning process must be extended to incorporate a full useful working vocabulary for the patient. The number of words that would be necessary for this, the demographic and cultural modifications in this vocabulary that would be needed, and the practical means for training patients in this extended vocabulary are unknown.

Lexical Semantic Memory

In our discussion thus far, we have suggested that knowledge underlying translation of sound sequences into phonemic acoustic representations, knowledge underlying translation of phonemic articulatory representations into motor sequences, and phonemic sequence knowledge may all constitute varieties of procedural memory. In contrast, knowledge of concepts, by virtue of being discrete and consciously accessible, is prototypical declarative knowledge. What about knowledge linking distributed-concept representations to phonemic sequence or articulatory or acoustic representations? This, the basis for lexical semantic knowledge, spans the declarative–procedural divide. In the immediately foregoing discussion, we blithely assumed that this knowledge has declarative properties. However, this information is not known, and this type of "bridging knowledge" may have unique properties of its own. Certainly the neural-network simulations that demonstrated the phenomenon of catastrophic degradation did not use networks incorporating a declarative–procedural interface. If this interface has unique properties, can they be used to advantage in treatment of aphasia? What are their limitations with respect to treatment of aphasia?

To our knowledge, the linguistic declarative–procedural interface has not been the explicit subject of any research, even though the problem lies at the heart of language acquisition and has profound implications for the operational domain of hippocampal function. However, we briefly discuss two lines of evidence that bear on this issue.

In an already famous paper, Vargha-Khadem et al. (1997) reported three subjects who early in life had experienced severe bilateral damage to the hippocampus as a result of anoxic insults. During subsequent intensive neuropsychological testing, these subjects demonstrated expected severe deficits in episodic memory acquisition. However, all three had acquired language function that appeared to be nearly normal. There had been similar reports of this phenomenon in prior case studies, but none nearly as compelling as the Vargha-Khadem paper. The nearly normal language function and the remarkably good general knowledge acquisition of these subjects, in conjunction with the results of studies in nonhuman primates, suggested to the authors that there are two separate declarative memory acquisition systems, one resident in the hippocampus that is essential to acquisition of episodic memories and one in entorhinal/perirhinal cortex (spared in the three subjects reported) that suffices for declarative semantic memory acquisition. This hypothesis remains to be fully tested. Against it is the evidence that the hippocampus and adjacent cortices are anatomically and functionally organized as a cascade system, not a binary system, and that the most essential property conferred by the unique architecture of the dentate–hippocampal apparatus is the capacity for almost instantaneous learning without catastrophic degradation (McClelland et al., 1995; Rolls & Treves, 1998). We propose an alternative explanation.

The alternative explanation lies in the possibility that the declarative–procedural interface posed by language cortex has unique properties and affords some unique opportunities. The data to be presented come from a study of the potential impact of repetitive transcranial magnetic stimulation on a variety of learning processes (Roth, Triggs, & Nadeau, unpublished observations). In one test, a typical test of verbal declarative memory acquisition, 20 normal subjects (college students) were on one single occasion verbally presented a list of 20 word pairs and then asked to produce the second word of each pair given the first. They were then re-presented the entire list of 20 pairs and the test process repeated. In the second iteration of the test, subjects correctly produced 17.35 ± 3.87 words. In a second test, a test of memory acquisition involving the semantic–phonological sequence interface, subjects were twice verbally presented a list of 10 word–nonword pairs and then asked to produce the corresponding nonword when given each word. They were then twice presented a list of 16 word–nonword pairs that included the original 10, and the testing process repeated. In the testing of the 16 word–nonword pairs, subjects correctly produced 11.40 ± 3.73 nonwords. The most interesting outcome of this experiment was that the correlation between word–word and word–nonword performance was only .60. Although highly statistically significant ($p = .0053$), this means that only 36% of the variance in word–nonword performance was accounted for by word–word performance. In other words, there is evidence in normal subjects of a dissociation between verbal declarative memory acquisition and memory acquisition involving links between semantic representations and phonemic and/or articulatory sequences. It is possible that this dissociation reflects differences between subjects in the extent to which they rely on phonemic sequence knowledge in language production (e.g., some subjects may rely primarily on the "whole word" naming route) (Nadeau, 2001; Plaut et al., 1996). However, it is also possible that subjects rely on a memory-acquisition process that does not involve the hippocampus for the word–nonword pair task (which after all emulates normal language acquisition in early childhood), and that the efficiency of this process correlates only roughly with the efficiency of the hippocampal system in these subjects. It is possible that this process depends on nonhippocampal mesial temporal structures as Vargha-Khadem et al. suggest, but it is also possible that it occurs in certain cortical systems (e.g., at declarative–procedural interfaces). Because word meaning and sound bear little relationship to each other, we would not expect much generalization of knowledge in this system (as discussed previously in the section "Properties of Procedural and Declarative Memory Systems Relevant to Aphasia Therapy"). However, if this separate nonhippocampal memory-acquisition system does exist, it suggests that naming therapy may be feasible even in aphasic patients with severe impairment of dominant hippocampal function (e.g., due to traumatic brain injury).

SUMMARY: NEURAL PROCESSES UNDERLYING LANGUAGE FUNCTION AND IMPLICATIONS FOR DEFICIT-SPECIFIC REHABILITATIVE STRATEGIES

This has been an extremely brief and, in the case of grammar, a substantially speculative review of neural mechanisms of language. Nevertheless, our review provides a basis for a tentative list of the underlying neural processes, processes that are the logical targets of therapy in patients with impaired language function. This dissection of these processes, together with some consideration of the nature of the memory-acquisition processes likely to be involved in them, provides a basis for some hypotheses about therapeutic strategies.

Phonological and Lexical Semantic Impairment

Our model of phonological processes defines three domains of knowledge: sequence (latent in the acoustic–articulatory motor pathway), semantic (latent in concept representations), and lexical semantic (latent in the pattern associator networks linking concept representations to the acoustic–articulatory motor pathway). Impairment of lexical access (manifested as anomia and word-finding difficulty), whether in internally generated language or in naming to confrontation, is by far the most common and the most debilitating component of aphasia. Traditional approaches have confronted the problem of anomia head-on, through naming therapy (reteaching of the names of things). However, our delineation of the knowledge domains involved in phonological processing indicates that two additional approaches may be of value in selected patients. If naming is failing because of damage to unimodal, polymodal, and supramodal association cortices supporting distributed-concept representations, it might be improved by redeveloping the knowledge underlying these representations (i.e., semantic therapy) (see below). If naming is failing because of impaired lexical semantic function, the presence of two pathways linking distributed-concept representations with phonological representations suggests two potential treatment strategies. The traditional naming-therapy approach might logically be directed to patients in whom the target is the direct-concept-representations–articulatory-motor-representations pathway (pathway 1-2 in Figure 5.2). This target would be most logical in patients with essentially no evidence of phonological function (poor repetition, reduced auditory verbal short-term memory, no phonemic paraphasias in spontaneous language or repetition, and no improvement in naming with phonemic cues) (e.g., deep dysphasia or repetition conduction aphasia). On the other hand, if patients have some evidence of phonological function, albeit impaired, the presence of an in-direct-concept-representations–acoustic/articulatory-motor pathway suggests that phonological therapy might improve naming. The presence of phonemic paraphasias in naming or repetition (especially nonword repetition) or evidence of improved naming with phonemic cueing would constitute evidence of some residual phonological sequence knowledge and partial integrity of the acoustic–articulatory motor pathway. To what extent training of phonological sequence knowledge will facilitate subsequent acquisition of lexical semantic knowledge (and in particular whether this will occur spontaneously in subsequent routine language use or require further speech therapy) remains to be established. Phonological sequence knowledge appears to represent procedural knowledge. For example, patients with amnesia due to mesial temporal lobe lesions are not impaired in learning artificial "grammars" characterized by rule-bound letter strings (Squire & Knowlton, 2000). Therefore, speech therapy will necessarily involve intensive practice within a relatively limited domain and the results can be expected to generalize widely to the native vocabulary. On the other hand, although lexical semantic knowledge apparently spans the declarative–procedural divide, and may depend at least in part on a unique memory-acquisition system, the fact that there is little resemblance between word meaning and word sound means that there is relatively little basis for generalization, and that practical and relatively inexpensive techniques will have to be developed to extend training to encompass useful working vocabularies. Just how many words comprise a useful working vocabulary would need to be determined. Age, gender, and culture specific vocabularies would need to be developed. An individualized, ongoing dynamic vocabulary list development project involving both patient and caregivers may be the best way to define such personal vocabularies. Once a target vocabulary starts to emerge, a training algorithm that does not require a therapist would then need to be developed, almost certainly involving caregivers, possibly using computers. This algorithm would then need to be executed over many months, perhaps indefinitely, to enable maintenance and expansion of the vocabulary over time.

In this discussion, access to articulatory motor representations during internally generated language and during naming to confrontation have been treated as if they were supported by identical neural structure. This assumption provided the basis for the implicit conclusion that if patients are adequately trained in naming to confrontation, this capacity will generalize to spontaneous language. This is not necessarily so. There appear to be two pathways by which we name to confrontation. In the best known (the "semantic route"), the object is seen, a concept representation is formed, and then an articulatory motor representation is elicited in one of the ways described in the foregoing. The second pathway (the "direct route") provides the basis for directly associating an object representation in visual association cortex with an articulatory motor representation—that is, without recourse to an intervening concept or any associated meaning. For example, if you are told that the symbol ❏ is a framezoid, if later shown this symbol, you will be able to provide the correct name despite the complete absence of any meaning beyond the visual configuration. Two clinical syndromes, reflecting a double dissociation, provide support for this two-pathway confrontation naming hypothesis. Severe damage to the direct route and partial damage to the indirect route presumably provide the basis for optic aphasia; patients with this disorder exhibit some knowledge of the object they are looking at but cannot name it. Typically they can name the object given a definition and they have relatively preserved lexical access during internally generated language (Bauer & Demery, 2003). Severe damage to the semantic route with relative preservation of the direct route presumably provides the basis for nonoptic aphasia (Shuren & Heilman, 1993). Patients with this disorder may have difficulty describing attributes or functions of objects they see but can name them with relative facility; they typically exhibit impaired lexical access during internally generated language, presumably because of associated damage to the neural basis for concept representations. Thus, we see the risk latent in naming therapy: It might train the direct route without affecting the semantic route, the route invoking concept representations, which a patient must employ in internally generated language. To what extent this occurs is unknown; it might depend in part on the degree of semantic impairment that is present. To the extent that it does occur, it might be necessary to complement confrontation naming therapy with naming to definition therapy or sufficient semantic therapy to ensure that the patient adopts a semantic set (see the next section). Training of naming in narrative context might also help to address this problem.

Semantic Impairment

In a PDP conceptualization, anomia, to the extent that it is due to semantic impairment, reflects insufficient engagement of representations of the critical features that distinguish concepts from each other (see Raymer & Rothi, 2000) for detection and quantitation of semantic impairment). The goal of therapy is to alter network connectivity such that these distinguishing features are more reliably engaged at the same time that features shared with other items are relatively disengaged. A variety of approaches invoking this general theme have been employed with some success (Raymer & Rothi, 2000). These have included (1) word–picture matching tasks using semantically related foils; (2) answering yes–no questions about semantic features of pictured objects; (3) semantic sorting of objects; (4) variously cued matching of semantic associates as the number and relatedness of semantic foils is increased; (5) correction of naming errors by provision of additional semantic information that distinguishes the erroneous response from the correct response; and (6) systematic training in the semantic features of objects. Unlike naming therapy directed to lexical semantic deficits, therapy directed to more purely semantic deficits might be expected to generalize substantially as refining featural relationships of trained items (the regularities in the knowledge implicit in the network) will benefit naming of untrained items to the extent that they share some of these featural relationships (Plaut, 1996). Counterintuitively, training on a spectrum of unusual exemplars of a category might be more effective in inducing generalization than training on typical exemplars (Plaut, 1996). This is because unusual exemplars convey information about both the core regularities defining the category (which help to distinguish it from other categories) and the greater range of regularities that are crucial in distinguishing all the different within-category exemplars from each other. Recent clinical work has confirmed this concept (Kiran & Thompson, 2003).

Even a damaged network still contains a great deal of information, so that the task of therapy is to refine network knowledge rather than to reestablish it. The distributed nature of semantics may provide some rationale for the targeting of semantic therapy at particular representational domains (e.g., representations with a substantial visual component in patients with selective deficits in naming living things). Individualization of vocabulary development, as in therapy for lexical semantic impairment (see the preceding section), would also be needed.

Grammatic Impairment

For patients who have good lexical semantic function, impairment in grammatic function may represent but a modest handicap and therefore provides relatively less motivation for language therapy than do lexical semantic deficits. Assuming that therapy of grammatic impairment is desired, we have identified a number of facilities underlying grammatic function that may be logical targets of therapy:

- Capacity for arbitrary modification of single-noun-concept representations.
- Capacity for simultaneous endogenous generation of multiple-noun-concept representations.
- Capacity for maintenance of memory of the immediately preceding discourse.
- Capacity for manipulation of multiple related, modified noun-concept representations to fit the particular situation.
- Multiword sequence knowledge (underlying grammatic morphology and phrase-structure rules).

The essential neural processes underlying these capacities have not yet been well defined. We suggest at least three: (1) working memory (engagement of one or more concept representations and recall of immediately preceding linguistic history); (2) concept manipulation (modification of individual concepts, adaptation of temporal order and content relationships of multiple concept representations to meet the situation at hand); and (3) sequence knowledge. These are discussed in some detail in the following sections.

Working Memory

Working memory is an intrinsic brain function that appears to be particularly dependent on frontal lobe systems, and thus it is no accident that grammatic impairment is seen predominantly in patients with major dominant frontal lesions. It is possible that treatment of working-memory impairment relevant to language will have to be specific to particular language constructs. However, it may be that generic improvement in working-memory capacity will enable improvement in grammatic function. We suggest two possible strategies, one pharmacological and one behavioral. The pharmacological therapy, involving either methylphenidate or d-amphetamine, is motivated by experience with subjects with attention-deficit/hyperactivity disorder (ADHD) (Heilman, Voeller, & Nadeau, 1991). These subjects appear to have a disorder involving the selection of plans for action. Plans for action may be formulated (often on the basis of memory or reflex) in more or less automatic response to environmental stimuli, a process that might be termed "reactive intention." Reactive intention is primarily driven by temporoparietal and brainstem systems. Plans for action may alternatively be formulated deliberately as part of an ongoing problem-solving strategy, a process that might be termed "intentional intention." Intentional intention is primarily driven by frontal systems. In this view, subjects with ADHD have a relative imbalance between reactive and intentional plan formulation such that their behavior is dominated by reactive planning. Treating these subjects with methylphenidate appears to redress this imbalance, enabling these subjects to achieve more balanced plan formulation and, most particularly, to sustain the intentional intention that is necessary to successfully complete tasks. We propose methylphenidate treatment of patients with grammatic dysfunction, most particularly those with simplification of syntax and difficulty articulating complex concepts that might be related in part to working-memory deficits. Because these patients are likely to have multicomponent deficits, methylphenidate treatment might have to be accompanied by behavioral treatment of associated deficits (see the next section) to demonstrate efficacy.

Our proposal for behavioral treatment of working-memory deficits contributing to syntactic dysfunction is also predicated on the concept that there is something approaching a generic working-memory capacity for language and that training of this capacity in one domain will generalize to other domains. Two tests commonly used to probe working memory, the Brown–Peterson paradigm (Peterson & Peterson, 1959) and the Paced Auditory Serial Addition Test (PASAT) (Gronwall, 1977), lend themselves to adaptation as training devices to enhance working-memory capacity (the main problem being to reduce task difficulty such that aphasic subjects can make some correct responses). Both tasks require the maintenance of two working-memory compartments: one to support recall of a prior stimulus and one to support a computation (in direct analogy to the working-memory demands of language). As we cautioned in the testing of methylphenidate effects, it may be necessary to couple working-memory training with other behavioral training in patients with syntactic dysfunction before the benefit of working-memory training becomes evident. The study of Stablum, Umiltà, Mogentale, Carlan, and Guerrini (2000) suggests that facility with operating two working-memory compartments can be trained but provides no insight into how this might affect language. They trained patients with closed head injury and patients who had experienced an anterior communicating artery aneurysm rupture on a dual-task paradigm in which the stimuli consisted of two letters, one above the other, placed to the right or left of the center of a display screen. Subjects had to indicate, first, the side of the stimulus (manual reaction-time paradigm) and second, whether the letters were the same or different (verbal report). The chief dependent measure was the reaction-time cost of introducing the second task. With the training on this task, subjects showed significant improvement that was sustained over time (to the extent that they became indistinguishable from controls), together with comparable improvement in PASAT performance, which was highly correlated with dual-task cost. The effect on PASAT performance suggests generalization of the trained dual-task skill to other content domains.

Concept Manipulation

Concept manipulation may have declarative components that render it domain specific, but we suspect that it predominantly represents a set of skills (i.e., nondeclarative memories akin to procedural memory). This means that effective training will require extensive practice and that there should be good generalization of skills across exemplars of particular manipulations. However, one would not necessarily expect generalization from one type of concept manipulation to another, any more than one would expect much generalization from training on serves in tennis to backhand skills. Thus, the extensive practice will need to involve a variety of constructions no less than phonological therapy must involve a substantial portion of the repertoire of native phonemic sequences to be successful. Thompson (2001) has shown explicitly that patients can be trained in specific distributed-concept manipulation skills and show generalization to different applications of these skills but not a generic improvement in concept manipulation capacity. Patients with agrammatism trained to produce "who" questions showed generalization to the production of "what" questions (both involve a verb that requires an agent and a theme) but not to production of "when" or "where" questions (in which the verb does not take a theme but may take an adjunctive phrase, e.g., "He is sleeping in the bedroom" → "Where is he sleeping?"). Patients trained to produce "when" questions showed generalization to "where" questions (which also involve verbs that take adjunctive phrases) but not to "who" or "what" questions. None of these patients showed generalization to passive voice sentence production. Notably, patients trained on more complex variants of a particular distributed-concept manipulation (e.g., cleft object constructions) show generalization to simpler variants of the same manipulation (e.g., "who" questions) but not vice versa (Thompson, Shapiro, Kiran, & Sobecks, 2003). This suggests that training on more complex variants may constitute a more efficient therapeutic approach. What constitutes a useful repertoire of syntactic skills has not been defined, much less the extended line of therapies that would be needed to train enough of these skills to make a clinically significant difference.

Word-Sequence Knowledge

To the extent that multiword sequence knowledge is like phonological sequence knowledge, it is procedural in nature and will require extensive practice. At first glance, it might seem that this training process would require repeated exposure to an almost infinite number of word sequences. However, as discussed earlier, this may not be so because the essential memories that are being acquired are between word classes (agent, theme, verb, adjective, etc.) rather than between word exemplars. To the extent that word-class knowledge is incorporated in distributed-concept representations and their modifications (which are relatively less susceptible to the effects of discrete lesions), the size of the training task will be reduced.

IMPLICATIONS FOR PRAGMATIC THERAPY

Up to this point, we have discussed language rehabilitation strategies that are linked precisely to specific deficits. They are predicated on careful evaluation of the various components of the patient's aphasia, identification of the salient neural system deficits, and design of a specific treatment that takes into account the underlying mechanisms. The achievement of success with such therapies would not only be clinically important, but it would yield scientific information about the neural basis of language processes (e.g., Thompson, 2001). These therapies face challenges from two directions. First, as we have noted, much work is required before the scientific principles we have elaborated can be accepted. Second, even if these therapies are proven in principle, much further work will be in order to translate them into approaches that substantially improve the communicative lives of patients.

The question arises as to whether therapies can be developed that still respect the underlying scientific principles but, by taking a more pragmatic approach, can achieve important clinical gains more quickly, at less cost, and with better subject acceptance, than the head-on deficit-specific approaches we have discussed. The prototype pragmatic therapy is constraint-induced language therapy (CILT) (Maher et al., 2003; Pulvermüller et al., 2001). CILT seeks to engage patients in intensive language production by limiting their opportunities for communication to spoken language and by placing them in situations—for example, partially scripted scenarios, games, or problem-solving—tasks that absolutely require verbally mediated collaboration with others, thus placing considerable pressure on patients to speak at length. By thus maximizing language production, and by concentrating therapy into long sessions over a relatively brief period, the technique potentially achieves the extensive practice requirements of procedural memory acquisition—thereby addressing the needs of patients with phonological sequence deficits, speech apraxia (disruption of the motor programs supporting speech articulation), and grammatic impairment. Extended practice involving naming also addresses the problem that declarative memory acquisition may be much less than 100% efficient. Although CILT can be consistent with principles of knowledge acquisition in various domains of language function, the challenges in developing this therapy lie not in teasing apart neural mechanisms and directly engaging them. Rather, the goals of CILT development are how to most effectively and efficiently achieve the most practice; how to achieve the most useful practice content; how, in a pragmatic therapy setting, to enhance the learning of individual words, phonological sequences, or syntactic structures in patients with differential impairment in these domains; how to best entrain patient motivation to drive some of these strategies; and what role the therapist should take in such therapy (see the next section "Errorful and Errorless Learning"). CILT is a very new therapy, and we do not yet have the answers to these questions.

Errorful and Errorless Learning

Space does not allow an extended discussion of the therapist–patient interaction during delivery of therapy. However, one aspect of that interaction, the therapist's best response to errors, does bear discussion because it relates directly to both the principles of knowledge acquisition in various language domains and the practicalities of therapist intervention in pragmatic therapies.

The efficacy of errorless learning was first demonstrated in studies of pigeons; later studies of human subjects with severe learning disabilities provided some further support for the concept (Jones & Eayrs, 1992). In 1994,

Baddeley and Wilson applied it for the first time to subjects with acquired brain damage—subjects with severe anterograde amnesia (see Glisky, Chapter 4, this volume). The experimental paradigm was somewhat contrived: subjects were presented with the first two letters of a five-letter word. In the errorful condition, they had to make three guesses regarding the word before being told the correct answer, which they were instructed to write down. In the errorless condition, they were immediately told the correct answer. Subjects trained in the errorless condition showed better retention of word knowledge given the two letter cues. Baddeley and Wilson interpreted this as supporting their hypothesis that these patients, with their severe impairment in explicit memory function, were relying substantially on implicit memory function for performance of the task. Their results have since been replicated many times over, but the implicit memory hypothesis has been successfully challenged (Hunkin, Squires, Parkin, & Tidy, 1998). Errorless learning techniques have since been tried in amnesic populations in a variety of tasks, including associating names with photos of unfamiliar people (with or without cuing with the first letter of the names), learning routes around a room defined in relationship to objects in the room, learning a route through an array of patterned stepping-stones, and programming an electronic organizer (Evans et al., 2000). While errorless learning techniques facilitated cued learning of names of unfamiliar people, it either provided no clinically important advantage or actually conduced to worse performance on these other tasks.

The errorless-learning literature does not provide an adequate basis for drawing conclusions about the mechanisms by which errorless learning might or might not provide benefit, nor about the deficit domains in which it might be effective. Most important, it does not provide information on the potential benefit of errorless learning for patients with intact memory function who already have partial knowledge of the correct answer—simply not enough to reliably produce the correct response. This is the situation in patients with aphasia. Nevertheless, errorless-learning techniques have recently gained some popularity in aphasia treatment, at least in part on the presumption that errorless learning obeys Hebbian principles (i.e., that to the extent that two connected neurons are coactive, the strength of the synaptic connection between them will increase). For example, in naming therapy, it is posited that if the subject is asked to name an object and is left to his or her own devices, if the subject arrives at the wrong answer, there is an opportunity for strengthening of connections between that particular concept representation and the articulatory motor representation of that wrong answer. There are two immediate problems with this conceptualization. First, Hebbian learning (and the related synaptic process, long-term potentiation) is a complex and incompletely understood process that requires, among other things, a burst of acetylcholine delivered to the cortex by the nucleus basalis or to the hippocampus by the medial septal nuclei that signals to the neurons in question that the activity in which they are engaged is important (Kilgard & Merzenich, 1998). This will occur only if the behavior is rewarded, which a wrong answer would not be. Second, in naming therapy, this conceptualization will apply only to the extent that auditory input delivered by the therapist elicits the correct articulatory motor representation. If the patient has no phonological function (e.g., he or she has deep dysphasia or repetition conduction aphasia), simultaneous auditory presentation of the object name will not be of value, because auditory input will not elicit an articulatory representation except via the concept representation. If repetition is commonly associated with production of phonemic paraphasias, then simultaneous auditory presentation might actually be dysfunctional as it will lead to production of incorrect patterns of activity in cortex supporting articulatory motor representations.

Under what circumstances might an errorless learning paradigm be beneficial or harmful? Because of the limitations of the literature, we can only offer some tentative hypotheses. Errorless learning might be beneficial in naming therapy (with the caveats noted in the foregoing) not so much because of its impact on Hebbian learning but rather because it can markedly speed therapy and cut through perseverative responses, thereby vastly increasing the number of stimuli presented and reducing patient frustration. In naming therapy directed at lexical semantic deficits, there is only one correct answer and there is no evident reason why permitting the patient to struggle might be beneficial. The same may be true for phonological therapy directed at disorders of phonemic sequencing. However, for other therapies (e.g., for speech apraxia and semantic deficits), the therapeutic goal is for the patient to redifferentiate functions that have become dedifferentiated because of injury. In apraxia of speech, a reduced number of crude motor responses must be differentiated into a larger number of more refined and specific responses. With semantic deficits, the various exemplars of semantic categories must be redifferentiated from the central tendency of those categories—for example, from the general concept of "dogness" must be differentiated specific breeds of dogs and particular individual dogs, as well as wolves, coyotes, foxes, hyenas, and dingoes. In the realm of syntax, there are typically many different syntactic approaches (multiple concept manipulations) to any particular communicative problem. In patients with syntactic impairment, as in patents with semantic impairment or apraxia of speech, there may be value in allowing the patient to produce responses with successive corrections by the therapist. Thus, we may tentatively posit that errorless learning should be of value when only one response is correct, as in treatment of lexical semantic deficits, but that it may be less effective or deleterious when redifferentiation of procedural or semantic representations is needed. These hypotheses (yet unproven) are broadly congruent with the conclusions drawn by Jones and Eayrs (1992) in their critique of errorless learning. They are summarized, together with our prior conclusions regarding deficit-specific therapy, in Table 5.1.

TABLE 5.1. Summary of Neurally Motivated Treatments of Aphasia

Circumstance	Nature of knowledge	Therapy	Therapeutic goal	Potential for generalization	Error management
Phonological sequence and articulatory motor function					
Speech apraxia	Procedural	Phonological	Redifferentiation	High	Allow and correct
Impaired phonological sequence knowledge	? Procedural or specialized	Phonological	? Redifferentiation versus learning of single correct target	High to all words containing the trained sequences	? Errorless versus allow and correct
Lexical semantic					
Present but impaired phonological function	? Procedural versus specialized	Phonological	? Redifferentiation versus learning of single correct target	High to all words containing the trained sequences; may require subsequent naming therapy	? Errorless versus allow and correct
Normal or absent phonological function	Declarative	Naming to confrontation Naming to definition or in semantic context	Learning of single correct target	None	Errorless
Impaired semantics	Declarative	Semantic	Redifferentiation	High to semantically related items	Allow and correct errors
Syntax					
Impaired concept manipulation abilities	Procedural	Syntactic	Redifferentiation	High to sentences employing trained grammatic structures	Allow and correct errors
Impaired working memory	Procedural	Behavioral/ pharmacological	NA	High	NA

These ideas may have implications for CILT. It should not be too difficult or intrusive for a therapist to quickly provide names as soon as a patient exhibits word-finding difficulty. Because anomia is the most common disabling deficit seen in aphasia, this means that CILT should have fairly broad applicability. However, it is not so clear how a therapist can promote redifferentiation in the context of CILT. Therefore, this may not be the best approach to patients whose aphasia is primarily characterized by dedifferentiation.

Finally, studies of neural-network reorganization in somatosensory cortex (Buonomano & Merzenich, 1998) suggest that for change to occur in response to somatosensory stimuli, those stimuli must be attended. If this is true throughout the brain, including the association cortices supporting language function, it suggests that in errorless learning paradigms the target of the subject's attention must be adequately constrained. This should pose no major difficulty at the single word level (barring subject fatigue and given a task paradigm that sustains subject interest, attention, and effort), but it may be a problem at the sentence level. If whole sentences are provided by the therapist in pursuit of errorless syntactic therapy, it is quite possible that the subject will attend to the phonological sequence (i.e., performing repetition) rather than to the syntactic structure.

CONCLUSION

In this review, we have introduced a general neural-network conceptualization of spoken language processes, attempting to be as specific as possible about the nature of the knowledge represented in the various domains and the neural principles underlying modification of that knowledge. A substantial body of evidence supports certain aspects of this conceptualization (particularly phonology) while other aspects are fairly speculative (e.g., grammar). Nevertheless, all aspects of our model represent merely hypotheses. The particular value of these hypotheses is that experiments testing them will challenge not just a conceptualization of language function but also a conceptualization of the neural-network organization of the brain. This is because we have avidly sought to make these hypotheses neurally plausible (O'Reilly, 1998). As tentative as these hypotheses are, they make many specific predictions regarding approaches to be taken in language therapy, as discussed throughout this chapter. The success or failure of implementation of these therapeutic strategies will further test these underlying hypotheses and will add specificity to their predictions (e.g., the work of Thompson, 2001). In the final sections of this chapter, we briefly considered pragmatic therapies (e.g., CILT). We strove to show that even though the primary goal of these therapies is to achieve greater clinical gains at less cost, they can be related in logical fashion to our understanding of neural-network function as it bears on language processes; furthermore, there are specific constraints deriving from neural-network principles that probably need to be respected in the implementation of these therapies.

NOTES

1. A variety of phonemic errors may be observed in slips of the tongue by normal subjects and in paraphasic errors by aphasic subjects (Blumstein, 1973; Shattuck-Hufnagel, 1979):

> Substitution: /timz/ "teams" → /kimz/
> Simplification: /prIti/ "pretty" → /pIti/
> Addition: /papa/ "papa" → /papra/
> Environmental:
>> Assimilation within a word: "Crete" → /trit/
>> Assimilation across word boundaries: "roast beef" → /rof bif/
>> Shifts: "in a black box" → "In a b_ack blox"
>> Metathesis (exchange): "degrees" → /gedriz/
>> "sphinx in the moonlight" → "minx in the spoonlight"

Exchanges may also involve affixes:

> "When Monday isn't sunny" → "When Monny isn't Sunday"

word roots:

> "wearing a name tag" → "naming a wear tag"

or words:

> "I used to sit in her room and read." → "I used to sit in her read and room."

2. Examples of chaotic order include the ornate structure of a flower and the marvelous computational machine that is the human brain; they reflect the order that emerges from the precise behavior of individual cells interacting with each other. Deterministic order is exemplified by the movement of planets in the solar system (and the satellites we send to them), which can be explained entirely by equations that characterize the force of gravity and its effect on mass.

3. The only major departure of neural-network theory from PDP theory is that the former seeks to apply exclusively local learning processes, whereas PDP simulations employ predominantly heuristic learning devices that are for the most part not local. The prototypical example of a local learning process is Hebbian learning, named after Donald Hebb, who first elucidated the concept (Hebb, 1949). Hebb postulated that to the extent that two connected neurons are simultaneously active, the strength of the synaptic connection between them will increase. This concept has since been validated in extensive research on long-term potentiation (Buonomano &

Merzenich, 1998). This work has also revealed evidence of a reciprocal process, long-term depression, which occurs to the extent that the activity of connected neurons is discrepant. Hebbian learning is intrinsically local and therefore eminently plausible neuroscientifically. It requires only a peculiar neurotransmitter receptor such as the NMDA-glutamate receptor, which functions as a detector of the coincidence of high activity of the postsynaptic neurons (reflected in a depression in membrane voltage) and high activity of the presynaptic neuron (reflected in large amounts of glutamate released from the presynaptic axon terminal). In contrast, the most common learning algorithm employed in PDP simulations is back propagation (see text), which requires a change in the strength of interunit connections based upon events occurring at the output end of the network, which could be many synapses away. This intrinsically nonlocal learning algorithm is biologically implausible but it remains possible that some nonlocal learning processes are instantiated in the brain (O'Reilly, 1996). Although subsequent discussion in this chapter focus exclusively on PDP approaches, there do not appear to be any fundamental scientific impediments to the realization of the language model we develop incorporating a local learning process.

4. A unit is the smallest functional entity within a connectionist model. It has a level of activation that is defined as a nonlinear mathematical function of its combined inputs at any one time (in many models a sigmoid curve that asymptotically approaches a minimum value of 0 or a maximum value of 1). It has an output that is a nonlinear mathematical function of its level of activation, often incorporating a threshold such that for activation levels below that threshold, there is no output. Each unit is connected to a large number of other units. The patterns of connectivity within a network define its functional capacity. The precise neural counterpart of a unit is uncertain and may vary from region to region. Thus, it is not implausible that single neurons function as units in the superior colliculus, whereas in the cortex, it is possible that a cortical column comes closer to meeting our definition of a unit. The neurobiology of cortical neural network function is currently understood at only the most rudimentary level.

GLOSSARY

Grammar: The principles governing the organization of words and major components of words within a sentence. The major domains of grammar are syntax and grammatic morphology.

Lexicon: The inventory of words available to a person. Implicit in the concept is that these words have both meaning and representational forms (e.g. articulatory, acoustic, orthographic, inscriptional, or, in the blind, tactile).

Morphology: The subfield of linguistics involving the internal structure of words and some interrelationships between words. The domain of morphology includes grammatic morphology and derivational morphology. Grammatic morphology involves (1) the modifications of words that are made in the service of incorporating them into sentences (bound grammatic morphology, e.g., affixes conveying case, number, or tense) and (2) the use of individual words that primarily serve sentence composition rather than meaning (free grammatical morphemes, e.g., articles, auxiliary verbs, conjunctions, and certain prepositions). Derivational morphology involves the combination of affixes with words or word stems to create new words or stems (e.g., govern, government, or governable, but not governing, wherein "ing" is a bound grammatical morpheme).

Phoneme: The smallest discrete units of spoken language. They can be conveniently represented by letters or letter pairs, e.g., /b/, /t/, and /sh/. This method of notation indicates that an articulated sound (e.g., "b-"), and not a letter sound (e.g., "bee"), is intended. Any phoneme in any language reflects a combination of several of a total of 18 distinctive features—attributes of the oropharyngeal apparatus as it produces that phoneme. Thus, /b/ has distinctive features including labial occlusion (the lips momentarily brought together to stop the airflow) and vocalization; /p/ is similar but lacks vocalization. In a PDP model, distinctive features would be discrete—they would be present or absent; it is not so clear how they are represented in the brain.

Phonetics: The study of speech sounds. When phonemes are actually produced in spoken language, their corresponding articulatory motor programs of muscle contractions are modified in graded fashion according to the phonemic environment. For example, the "i" of "fit" and "fish" is the same phoneme but the sound is more prolonged in "fish." This is phonetic modification.

Phonology: The subfield of linguistics that involves the structure and systematic patterning of sounds in human language. The major focus of this field is the phoneme.

Semantics: The meaning of words.

Syntax: The domain of grammar having to do with knowledge of acceptable word order and sentence structure.

REFERENCES

Baddeley, A. D., & Wilson, B. A. (1994). When implicit learning fails: Amnesia and the problem of error elimination. *Neuropsychologia, 32,* 53–68.

Basso, A., Bracchi, M., Capitani, E., Laiacona, M., & Zanobio, M. E. (1987). Age and evolution of language area functions. A study of adult stroke patients. *Cortex, 23,* 475–483.

Bates, E., Friederici, A., & Wulfeck, B. (1987). Grammatical morphology in aphasia: Evidence from three languages. *Cortex, 23,* 545–574.

Bauer, R. M., & Demery, J. A. (2003). Agnosia. In K. M. Heilman & E. Valenstein (Eds.), *Clinical neuropsychology* (4th ed., pp. 236–295). New York: Oxford University Press.

Blumstein, S. (1973). *A phonological investigation of aphasic speech.* The Hague: Mouton.

Brown, J. W., & Grober, E. (1983). Age, sex, and aphasia type. Evidence for a regional cerebral growth process underlying lateralization. *Journal of Nervous and Mental Disease, 171,* 431–434.

Buonomano, D. V., & Merzenich, M. M. (1998). Cortical plasticity: From synapses to maps. *Annual Review of Neuroscience, 21,* 149–186.

Chapey, R. (Ed.). (2001). *Language intervention strategies in aphasia and related neurogenic communication disorders.* Philadelphia: Lippincott Williams & Wilkins.

Cheung, S. W., Bedenbaugh, P. H., Nagarajan, S. S., & Schreiner, C. E. (2001). Functional organization of squirrel monkey primary auditory cortex: Responses to pure tones. *Journal of Neurophysiology, 85,* 1732–1749.

Dell, G. S. (1986). A spreading-activation theory of retrieval in sentence production. *Psychological Review, 93,* 283–321.

Dell, G. S., & Reich, P. A. (1981). Stages in sentence production: An analysis of speech error data. *Journal of Verbal Learning and Verbal Behavior, 20,* 611–629.

Dell, G. S., Schwartz, M. F., Martin, N., Saffran, E. M., & Gagnon, D. A. (1997). Lexical access in normal and aphasic speakers. *Psychological Review, 104,* 801–838.

Evans, J. J., Wilson, B. A., Schuri, U., Andrade, J., Baddeley, A. D., Bruna, O., et al. (2000). A comparison of "errorless" and "trial-and-error" learning methods for teaching individuals with acquired memory deficits. *Neuropsychological Rehabilitation, 10,* 67–101.

Forde, E. M. E., & Humphreys, G. W. (1999). Category specific recognition impairments: A review of important case studies and influential theories. *Aphasiology, 13,* 169–193.

Gleick, J. (1987). *Chaos: Making a new science.* New York: Viking.

Goldman-Rakic, P. S. (1990). Cellular and circuit basis of working memory in prefrontal cortex of nonhuman primates. *Progress in Brain Research, 85,* 325–336.

Gronwall, D. M. A. (1977). Paced Auditory Serial Addition Test: A measure of recovery from concussion. *Perceptual Motor Skills, 44,* 367–373.

Harley, T. A. (1984). A critique of top-down independent levels models of speech production: Evidence from non-plan-internal speech errors. *Cognitive Science, 8,* 191–219.

Hebb, D. O. (1949). *The organization of behavior.* New York: Wiley.

Heilman, K. M., Voeller, K. S., & Nadeau, S. E. (1991). A possible pathophysiological substrate of attention-deficit-hyperactivity disorder. *Journal of Child Neurology, 6*(Suppl.), S76–S78.

Hunkin, N. M., Squires, E. J., Parkin, A. J., & Tidy, J. A. (1998). Are the benefits of errorless learning dependent on implicit memory? *Neuropsychologia, 36,* 25–36.

Jones, R. S., & Eayrs, C. B. (1992). The use of errorless learning procedures in teaching people with a learning disability: A critical review. *Mental Handicap Research, 5,* 204–212.

Kertesz, A., & Sheppard, A. (1981). The epidemiology of aphasic and cognitive impairment in stroke. Age, sex, aphasia type, and laterality differences. *Brain, 104,* 117–128.

Kilgard, M. P., & Merzenich, M. M. (1998). Cortical map reorganization enabled by nucleus basalis activity. *Science, 279,* 1714–1718.

Kiran, S., & Thompson, C. K. (2003). The role of semantic complexity in treatment of naming deficits: Training semantic categories in fluent aphasia by controlling exemplar typicality. *Journal of Speech, Language and Hearing Research, 46,* 608–622.

Kolk, H. H. J., & Friederici, A. D. (1985). Strategy and impairment in sentence understanding by Broca's and Wernicke's aphasics. *Cortex, 21,* 47–67.

Lichtheim, L. (1885). On aphasia. *Brain, 7,* 433–484.

Maher, L. M., Kendall, D., Swearengin, J. A., Pingel, K., Holland, A., & Roth, L. J. G. (2003). Constraint induced language therapy for chronic aphasia: Preliminary findings. *Journal of the International Neuropsychological Society, 9,* 192.

McClelland, J. L., McNaughton, B. L., & O'Reilly, R. C. (1995). Why there are complementary learning systems in the hippocampus and neocortex: Insights from the successes and failures of connectionist models of learning and memory. *Psychological Review, 102,* 419–457.

McClelland, J. L., & Rumelhart, D. E. (1981). An interactive activation model of context effects in letter perception: Part 1. An account of basic findings. *Psychological Review, 88,* 375–407.

Miceli, G., Caltagirone, C., Gainotti, G., Masullo, C., Silveri, M. C., & Villa, G. (1981). Influence of age, sex, literacy and pathologic lesion on incidence, severity and type of aphasia. *Acta Neurologica Scandinavica, 64,* 370–382.

Mitchum, C. C., & Berndt, R. S. (2001). Cognitive neuropsychological approaches to diagnosing and treating language disorders. In R. Chapey (Ed.), *Language intervention strategies in aphasia and related neurogenic communication disorders* (pp. 551–571). Philadelphia: Lippincott Williams & Wilkins.

Moran, J., & Desimone, R. (1985). Selective attention gates visual processing in extrastriate cortex. *Science, 229,* 782–784.

Nadeau, S. E. (1988). Impaired grammar with normal fluency and phonology. Implications for Broca's aphasia. *Brain, 111,* 1111–1137.

Nadeau, S. E. (2000). Connectionist models and language. In S. E. Nadeau, L. J. Gonzalez Rothi, & B. A. Crosson (Eds.), *Aphasia and language: Theory to practice* (pp. 299–347). New York: Guilford Press.

Nadeau, S. E. (2001). Phonology: A review and proposals from a connectionist perspective. *Brain and Language, 79,* 511–579.

Nadeau, S. E., & Crosson, B. (1997). Subcortical aphasia. *Brain and Language, 58,* 355–402, 436–458.

Nadeau, S. E., & Gonzalez Rothi, L. J. (1993). Morphologic agrammatism following a right hemisphere stroke in a dextral patient. *Brain and Language, 43,* 642–667.

Nadeau, S. E., Gonzalez Rothi, L. J., & Crosson, B. (Eds.). (2000). *Aphasia and language: Theory to practice.* New York: Guilford Press.

Obler, L. K., & Albert, M. L. (1981). Language and aging: A neurobehavioral analysis. In D. S. Beasley & G. A. Davis (Eds.), *Aging: Communication processes and disorders* (pp. 107–121). New York: Grune & Stratton.

O'Reilly, R. C. (1996). Biologically plausible error-driven learning using local activation differences: The generalized recirculation algorithm. *Neural Computing, 8,* 895–938.

O'Reilly, R. C. (1998). Six principles for biologically based computational models of cortical cognition. *Trends in Cognitive Sciences, 2,* 455–462.

Peterson, L. R., & Peterson, M. J. (1959). Short-term retention of individual verbal items. *Journal of Experimental Psychology, 58,* 193–198.

Plaut, D. C. (1996). Relearning after damage in connectionist networks: Toward a theory of rehabilitation. *Brain and Language, 52,* 25–82.

Plaut, D. C., McClelland, J. L., Seidenberg, M. S., & Patterson, K. (1996). Understanding normal and impaired word reading: Computational principles in quasi-regular domains. *Psychological Review, 103,* 56–115.

Prather, P., Zurif, E., Stern, C., & Rosen, T. J. (1992). Slowed lexical access in nonfluent aphasia: A case study. *Brain and Language, 43,* 336–348.

Pulvermüller, F., Neininger, B., Elbert, T., Mohr, B., Rockstroh, B., Koebbel, P., et al. (2001). Constraint-induced therapy of chronic aphasia after stroke. *Stroke, 32,* 1621–1626.

Raymer, A. M., & Rothi, L. J. G. (2000). The semantic system. In S. E. Nadeau, L. J. Gonzalez Rothi, & B. A. Crosson (Eds.), *Aphasia and language: Theory to practice* (pp. 108–132). New York: Guilford Press.

Rolls, E. T., & Deco, G. (2002). *Computational neuroscience of vision.* Oxford, UK: Oxford University Press.

Rolls, E. T., & Treves, A. (1998). *Neural networks and brain function.* New York: Oxford University Press.

Rumelhart, D. E., & McClelland, J. L. (1982). An interactive activation model of context effects in letter perception: Part 2. The contextual enhancement effect and some tests and extensions of the model. *Psychological Review, 89,* 60–94.

Rumelhart, D. E., Smolensky, P., McClelland, J. L., & Hinton, G. E. (1986). Schemata and sequential thought processes in PDP models. In J. L. McClelland, D. E. Rumelhart, & PDP Research Group (Eds.), *Parallel distributed processing* (Vol. 2, pp. 7–57). Cambridge, MA: MIT Press.

Saffran, E. M., & Schwartz, M. F. (1988). "Agrammatic" comprehension it's not: Alternatives and implications. *Aphasiology, 2,* 389–394.

Saffran, E. M., Schwartz, M. F., & Marin, O. (1980). The word order problem in agrammatism: Production. *Brain and Language, 10,* 263–280.

Schwartz, M. F., Linebarger, M. C., Saffran, E. M., & Pate, D. S. (1987). Syntactic transparency and sentence interpretation in aphasia. *Language and Cognitive Processes, 2,* 85–113.

Seidenberg, M. S., & McClelland, J. L. (1989). A distributed, developmental model of word recognition and naming. *Psychological Review, 96,* 523–568.

Shattuck-Hufnagel, S. (1979). Speech errors as evidence for a serial-ordering mechanism in sentence production. In W. E. Cooper & E. C. T. Walker (Eds.), *Sentence processing: Psycholinguistic studies* (pp. 295–341). Hillsdale, NJ: Erlbaum.

Shuren, J., & Heilman, K. M. (1993). Non-optic aphasia. *Neurology, 43,* 1900–1907.

Squire, L. R., & Knowlton, B. J. (2000). The medial temporal lobe, the hippocampus and the memory systems of the brain. In M. S. Gazzaniga (Ed.), *The new cognitive neurosciences* (pp. 765–779). Cambridge, MA: MIT Press.

Stablum, F., Umiltà, C., Mogentale, C., Carlan, M., & Guerrini, C. (2000). Rehabilitation of executive deficits in closed head injury and anterior communicating artery aneurysm patients. *Psychological Research, 63,* 265–278.

Stemberger, J. P. (1985). An interactive activation model of language production. In A. W. Ellis (Ed.), *Progress in the psychology of language* (Vol. 1, pp. 143–186). Hillsdale, NJ: Erlbaum.

Thompson, C. K. (2001). Treatment of underlying forms: A linguistic specific approach to sentence production deficits in agrammatic aphasia. In R. Chapey (Ed.), *Language intervention strategies in aphasia and related neurogenic communication disorders* (4th ed., pp. 605–625). Philadelphia: Lippincott Williams & Wilkins.

Thompson, C. K., Lange, K. L., Schneider, S. L., & Shapiro, L. P. (1997). Agrammatic and non-brain damaged subjects' verb and verb argument structure production. *Aphasiology, 11,* 473–490.

Thompson, C. K., Shapiro, L. P., Kiran, S., & Sobecks, J. (2003). The role of syntactic complexity in treatment of sentence deficits in agrammatic aphasia: The complexity account of treatment efficacy (CATE). *Journal of Speech, Language, and Hearing Research, 46,* 591–607.

Vargha-Khadem, F., Gadian, D. G., Watkins, K. E., Connelly, A., Van Paesschen, W., & Mishkin, M. (1997). Differential effects of early hippocampal pathology on episodic and semantic memory. *Science, 277,* 376–380.

Vitevitch, M. S. (1997). The neighborhood characteristics of malapropisms. *Language and Speech, 40,* 211–228.

Warrington, E. K., & Shallice, T. (1984). Category specific semantic impairments. *Brain, 107,* 829–854.

6

Disorders of Spatial Orientation and Awareness

UNILATERAL NEGLECT

Anne Aimola Davies

THEORETICAL MODELS OF SPATIAL ORIENTATION AND AWARENESS, SPECIFICALLY UNILATERAL NEGLECT

Introduction to Unilateral Neglect

In the acute or transitory phase immediately following a cerebrovascular accident (CVA), the classical signs of severe unilateral neglect (UN) can be easily recognized. The individual with UN has an obvious deviation of eyes, head, and trunk away from the contralesional hemispace (i.e., the side of space opposite to his or her cerebral lesion), as if captivated by the ipsilesional side (i.e., the same side as his or her lesion). These extreme neglect behaviors seen in the acute phase may improve for most individuals with UN, but there is a subgroup who have persisting or chronic symptoms of neglect that continue for many months or years post-CVA.

The everyday activities of individuals with UN are marked by a "magnetic attraction" toward ipsilesional space that results in difficulties specific to the contralesional side of their world. For example, these individuals may collide with objects on the contralesional side; fail to eat food on the contralesional side of the plate; ignore someone attempting to engage them in conversation from the contralesional side; or fail to negotiate the entrance to a doorway that requires a contralesional turn. Dramatic demonstrations are also illustrated by individuals with UN who are diagnosed as having personal neglect, which is manifested by attention that is directed exclusively to the ipsilesional side of their body when grooming. For example, these individuals with UN will dress, shave, or apply lipstick only to the ipsilesional side. Clinical dissociations demonstrate that individuals with UN may have neglect that is limited to personal space (directed toward the body), peripersonal space (within arm's reach), or extrapersonal space (beyond arm's reach) (Bisiach, Perani, Vallar, & Berti, 1986; Cowey, Small, & Ellis, 1994; Halligan & Marshall, 1991a).[1]

Unilateral neglect is most commonly assessed with paper-and-pencil drawings, in which the individual will make a fairly accurate and detailed reproduction of the ipsilesional side of a drawing but omit details on the contralesional side. To the interested observer (such as family members and rehabilitation staff), one surprising aspect of UN is that these individuals are physically capable of exploring and reporting contralesional information, especially if they are specifically requested to attend contralesionally (Riddoch & Humphreys, 1983) or to ignore ipsilesional events (Karnath, 1988). These findings imply that the failure to orient attention toward the contralesional hemispace can be counteracted to some degree by voluntary control (Làdavas, 1987). It is also well known that individuals with UN do not always acknowledge contralesional information even when cued, and that in more extreme examples, these individuals with UN will either deny the existence of contralesional information or will give an elaborate and often nonsensical explanation for their behavior. For example, Bisiach described a patient, P. R., who "obstinately refused" to acknowledge that his left (contralesional) arm belonged to him. On one occasion when the examiner placed P. R.'s left hand on the bedclothes between his own two hands, P. R. maintained that the third hand belonged to the examiner, even when questioned as to the logic of a three-handed man (Bisiach & Geminiani, 1991).

Individuals with UN have also been known to become distressed at what they reasonably argue is a false accusation. After all, how can they be accused of neglecting something that is outside their awareness? The puzzle is further complicated by results from neurological and neuropsychological testing that demonstrate that the individual with UN generating these explanations may have neither a visual impairment nor an impairment of cognitive functioning. The difficulties experienced by individuals with UN may thus best be captured in Mesulam's (1981) description, "the deficit therefore is not one of seeing, hearing, feeling, or moving but one of looking, listening, touching, and exploring" (p. 318).

Most descriptions of UN have a common theme that assumes an asymmetrical spatially selective disorder that biases attention away from the side opposite to the brain lesion (and toward the ipsilesional side). But many different explanatory accounts have been offered for the numerous dissociations within the constellation of UN symptoms that have been described in the literature (Mesulam, 1981; Milner & Goodale, 1997; Posner & Petersen, 1990; Rizzolatti & Gallese, 1988). In addition to explaining these numerous dissociations, theories of UN also attempt to explain the fairly consistent finding that although UN can be found after right- and left-hemisphere damage (Ogden, 1985a), it is most often found following right-hemisphere damage (Albert, 1973; Gainotti, Messerli, & Tissot, 1972). While there are many different theories, this chapter is not intended as an exhaustive review of the numerous articles and books devoted to the study of UN and its rehabilitation.[2] Instead, the focus will be on theoretical accounts that summarize our current understanding of UN and its rehabilitation, without contradicting empirical evidence that UN is not a unitary disorder and that a single explanation cannot encompass all symptoms and types. These theoretical accounts provide explanations for (1) the gradient of attention in UN, and (2) the role of the right hemisphere for (a) alerting and vigilance and (b) guiding global processing.

A Gradient of Attention in Unilateral Neglect

Kinsbourne (1987, 1993, 1994) contends that it is not adequate to conceive of UN as a hemispace phenomenon. He believes that it is misleading to describe UN as bisecting perception and performance at the vertical meridian. Instead, he proposes that UN is a directional phenomenon caused by a breakdown in the balance of reciprocally inhibitory opponent processors that control and direct lateral attention on the left/right axis (Kinsbourne, 1993). Leftward movements are under right-hemisphere influence and rightward movements are under left-hemisphere influence. But following brain damage, the nonlesioned hemisphere is believed to generate an unopposed orienting response to the ipsilesional side of space, and this biases attention to the ipsilesional side.

Most important to Kinsbourne's theory is the claim that the imbalance that occurs between the opponent processing systems not only biases attention to the ipsilesional hemispace but also biases attention to the ipsilesional region within both hemispaces. The expectation is that a monotonic gradient of attention along the left/right axis will be created, so that the area most activated (ipsilesional to the lesion) will be best represented, and the area least activated (contralesional to the lesion) will not be experienced. Another important claim is that the particular subtype of UN demonstrated is determined by which of the many uniquely localized lateral opponent processors are damaged, and to what degree they are damaged (Kinsbourne, 1994). This claim has allowed

Kinsbourne's theory to withstand the onslaught of growing evidence for dissociations within UN. By specifying that there are many opponent processors
vulnerable to damage, Kinsbourne's theory can also encompass forms of UN
that are "display-centered, not space-centered" (Kinsbourne, 1993). In such
forms, the neglect can affect the contralesional half of the display even if the
display is presented in the ipsilesional half of space. More generally, for a right-
hemisphere-damaged patient, the neglected stimuli may be those to the left in
a viewer-centered, in an environment-centered, or in an object-centered frame
of reference.

Kinsbourne's proposed gradient of attention is not demonstrated in most
studies because the experimental set-up places one stimulus on the left and one
on the right of the midline, so that there is no way to test the difference between the relative-left and relative-right locations within a single hemisphere.
This problem is easily overcome by having two stimulus positions in each of
the two hemispaces and measuring the responses to targets presented in the
relative-left and relative-right positions in each hemispace. With this improved
experimental set-up, the main distinction between the hemispace and directional theories of UN is based on the predictions of best performance. The
hemispace (or step-function) theory predicts normal performance in the ipsilesional hemispace and impaired performance in the contralesional hemispace.
In contrast, the directional (or gradient of attention) theory predicts that superior performance will be found in the extreme lateral position within the
ipsilesional hemispace, that a gradual decline in performance will be evident as
early as the more central (compared with the more lateral) region within the
ipsilesional hemispace, and that this performance will deteriorate further as it
moves toward the central and lateral regions of the contralesional hemispace.
Visual attention studies that have adopted this experimental set-up are reviewed in the following section.

Three Cognitive Operations for Shifting Attention

Ládavas and colleagues used Kinsbourne's suggested experimental set-up of
two stimulus positions (left or right) within each hemispace to demonstrate that
UN patients with a right-parietal-lobe lesion had the longest reaction times to
targets at the relative-left position of both the right visual field and the left visual field (Làdavas, 1987), and patients with a left-parietal-lobe lesion had
the longest reaction times at the relative-right position of each visual field
(Làdavas, Del Pesce, & Provinciali, 1989). In a second experiment, a similar
set-up was used with two stimulus positions in the right visual field only, to
demonstrate that UN patients with right-parietal-lobe lesions not only responded faster to the stimuli in the relative-right position (compared to the left)
but also responded faster in that position than the control patients, who had a
CVA of the right hemisphere and did not have extrapersonal neglect (Làdavas,

Petronio, & Umilta, 1990). The authors interpreted these results as supporting Kinsbourne's proposal that there is a pattern of attentional benefits for stimuli in a relative-right position and costs for stimuli in a relative-left position within a hemispace.

In most studies with neurological patients, the task is simply to make a key press in response to the appearance of a target, which is a bright visual signal presented either to the right or to the left of fixation. The efficiency of target detection is measured by the reaction time to the target. Posner and colleagues (Posner, Walker, Friedrich, & Rafal, 1984) were able to make visual field distinctions, in addition to those described by Ládavas and colleagues, because they used a location-precueing paradigm to examine the effects of a parietal-lobe lesion on shifting attention. In the location-precueing paradigm, the presentation of the target is preceded by a cue that directs attention either to the correct target location (valid-cue condition) or to an incorrect target location (invalid-cue condition). By this method, the participant's reaction times when responding to validly-cued targets can be contrasted with their reaction times to invalidly-cued targets. An invalid cue requires the participant to disengage attention from the cued location before shifting attention to the unexpected target location.

The findings from Posner and colleagues demonstrated, first, that although shifting attention contralesionally was a major difficulty following a parietal-lobe lesion, the patients' contralesional shifts in the contralesional hemispace were more costly than the same operation performed in the ipsilesional hemispace, and second, that ipsilesional shifts of attention had an advantage over contralesional shifts of attention, irrespective of the visual field of presentation (Posner, Walker, Friedrich, & Rafal, 1987). In addition, their findings demonstrated that individuals with a left-parietal-lobe lesion generally had faster reaction times than individuals with a right-parietal-lobe lesion, even though both groups showed similar trends.

As a result of these findings, Posner and colleagues proposed that the posterior-parietal attentional system is designed to disengage attention from its current focus in preparation for movement to a new target. Following damage to this area, the ability to disengage attention for a contralesional shift is disadvantaged in comparison to disengaging for an ipsilesional shift. In fact, Posner and his colleagues were the first to propose that covert orienting of attention[3] to a target involved the following three separate cognitive operations, each of which could be disrupted as a result of damage to specific anatomic structures within the posterior brain system: (1) the operation of disengaging attention from the current attentional focus to direct attention to a contralesional target, which is affected by damage to the posterior parietal lobe; (2) the operation of moving attention to a new focus, which is affected by damage to the superior colliculus (and surrounding midbrain areas); and (3) the operation of fully engaging selective attention at a new target location in such a way as to avoid any distracting events, which is affected by damage to the lateral pulvinar nucleus of the thalamus (Posner, 1995; Posner, Inhoff, Friedrich, & Cohen, 1987; Posner & Petersen, 1990).

The Role of the Rostral Inferior Parietal Lobe in Maintaining Attention

The final study to be presented used a variation of the Posner location-precueing paradigm (Posner et al., 1984), as designed by Egly, Rafal, Driver, and Starrveveld (1994),[4] to study five patients with UN persisting at least 3 months post-CVA (one with a left CVA and four with a right CVA), and 17 neurologically intact control participants. Aimola (1999) chose this experimental paradigm because its set-up included two rectangles on each side of fixation, which was ideal for investigating Kinsbourne's gradient of attention theory of UN, and for directly contrasting the directional, hemispace, and disengage theories of UN.

The *valid-cue* condition of the location-precueing paradigm demonstrated that a monotonic increase in reaction time consistent with Kinsbourne's proposed gradient of attention was revealed only in the patients with a rostral-inferior-parietal-lobe lesion of the right hemisphere. These patients demonstrated a clear left-side neglect, with a monotonic increase in reaction time as the stimuli were presented further into their left visual field. In contrast, the two patients without a parietal-lobe lesion (one left CVA and one right CVA) did not demonstrate the monotonic gradient of attention in the valid-cue condition. They had significantly longer reaction times (compared with the control participants) across all positions in both the right and left visual fields. But they did not demonstrate specific costs for the right or left hemispace or for the lateral positions within the two hemispaces.

The *invalid-cue* condition of the location-precueing paradigm demonstrated that all five patients with UN had problems with disengaging attention when making a contralesional shift of attention. Aimola (1999) concluded that the role of the rostral inferior parietal lobe was to maintain attention, as demonstrated in the valid-cue condition, as opposed to Posner's proposal that the role of the posterior parietal lobe was to disengage attention. The argument was not that the patients with UN did not have problems with disengaging attention, as this difficulty was demonstrated by all, once attention was captured ipsilesionally, but that assigning this role to the parietal lobe may be inaccurate given that two patients (one with a right-hemisphere lesion and the other with a left-hemisphere lesion) had difficulties with disengaging attention but did not have parietal-lobe involvement. Interestingly, the invalid-cue condition also demonstrated that three patients clearly had difficulties with contralesional shifts that occurred irrespective of the visual field of presentation, in support of Kinsbourne's directional theory of attention, and two had difficulties that were specific to contralesional shifts of attention in the contralesional visual field only, as might be more consistent with Heilman's hemispace theory.

In summary, these findings, from the studies of Ládavas and colleagues, Posner and colleagues, and Aimola, which utilize the suggested experimental set-up of two stimulus positions within each hemispace, are broadly consistent with Kinsbourne's monotonic gradient of attention theory of UN. But it is important to note that different theories of attention and UN come into play as we consider different task requirements and individuals with UN who have different lesion locations.

Hemispheric Asymmetries in Unilateral Neglect

This discussion of the hemispheric asymmetries found in UN begins with a brief review of two theories that dominated this literature in the early stages of research on UN. It then turns to a fuller consideration of the two current attentional theories, that is, the alerting/vigilance systems theory and the global/local processing theory. The first of the early theories was an adjunct to Kinsbourne's gradient of attention theory mentioned previously. Kinsbourne further proposed that the right- and left-hemisphere opponent processors that direct attention laterally are not equal in power. Most importantly, he proposed that the left-hemisphere activation is the more powerful in neurologically intact individuals, especially in conditions of orienting conflict such as location uncertainty or competing stimulation (Kinsbourne, 1987; Reuter-Lorenz, Kinsbourne, & Moscovitch, 1990). In these conditions, the right hemisphere's leftward directional orienting is believed to be weak and barely able to maintain control of the left hemisphere's rightward directional orienting. Therefore, UN is believed more likely to occur following right- than left-hemisphere damage because the more powerful rightward directional orienting of the left hemisphere takes over and dramatically shifts attention rightward.

The second of the early theories postulates that the right hemisphere is dominant for spatial attention because it has neural mechanisms for attending to both hemispaces, whereas the left hemisphere attends only to the right hemispace (Heilman & Valenstein, 1979; Mesulam, 1981; Weintraub & Mesulam, 1987). This theory predicts that UN is less severe following a left-hemisphere lesion because the right hemisphere can continue to direct attention to both the left and the right hemispace. There is more severe UN following a right-hemisphere lesion because attention is limited to the contralesional hemispace. Positron emission tomographic (PET) studies with neurologically intact individuals have supported this hypothesis, by demonstrating that although there is left- and right-superior-parietal-cortex activation for spatial shifts of attention, the right-superior-parietal-cortex activation occurs following attention shifts in both visual fields, whereas the left-superior-parietal-cortex activation occurs following shifts of attention in the right visual field only (Corbetta, Miezin, Shulman, & Petersen, 1993; Petersen, Corbetta, Miezin, & Shulman, 1994).

The two current attentional theories that support our understanding of hemispheric asymmetries in UN, the alerting/vigilance systems theory and the global/local processing theory are reviewed next. Examples of the rehabilitation implications are reviewed later in this chapter.

The Alerting/Vigilance Systems Theory

Posner and Petersen (1990) proposed that the attention system is divided into the following three subsystems that perform different but interrelated functions: (1) the anterior attentional system, which is believed responsible for target detection, that is, selection and focal awareness of a relevant target; (2) the posterior attentional system, which has directional components that control orienting of attention; and (3) the nondirectional attentional system, which has components that function to alert or sustain attention. Disruption of the directional components that orient attention toward a contralesional target is believed to cause left or right neglect because those components are located in the posterior attentional system of both hemispheres. In contrast, the nondirectional components for generalized attention are located principally in the right hemisphere, so that the right hemisphere is dominant for maintaining a state of alertness or sustained attention. Thus, a right-hemisphere lesion may cause more severe and persisting neglect because both the directional and nondirectional components of attention are affected.

Evidence for the dominant role of the right hemisphere in maintaining alertness has come from different types of investigations in humans and animals. For example, animal studies with rats have demonstrated that depletion of norepinephrine that is specific to lesions of the right hemisphere leads to changes in vigilance (Robinson, 1985). And Ládavas and colleagues discuss a simple reaction-time measure that can differentiate patients with right- and left-hemisphere damage, with the finding that those patients with right-hemisphere lesions have significantly longer overall reaction times that are independent of the spatial location of the visual stimuli (Ládavas et al., 1989). It has also been shown that omitting a warning or alerting signal before the presentation of targets greatly affects patients with right (but not left) parietal-lobe lesions (Posner, Inhoff, et al., 1987). Finally, in a unique approach to the study of the role of sustained attention in UN patients with a right-hemisphere lesion, Robertson and colleagues demonstrated that a nonlateralized, nonspatial rehabilitation strategy, which increased alertness with a warning sound or a verbal self-alerting technique, significantly decreased UN (Robertson, Mattingley, Rorden, & Driver, 1998; Robertson, Tegnér, Tham, Lo, & Nimmo-Smith, 1995).

These results are consistent with Posner and Petersen's (1990) hypothesis that the alerting system has a direct impact on the posterior attention system responsible for directing attention in space. A PET study with 23 neurologically intact individuals has specifically implicated the prefrontal and superior parietal cortex of the right hemisphere in mediating sustained attention to sensory input (Pardo, Fox, & Raichle, 1991). An important point from this study is that the laterality of brain activation was found to be independent of the laterality of sensory input.

Posner and Petersen (1990) consider that a distinction between neural mechanisms for alerting and for target detection—between systems (3) and (1) above—is vital because the alert state is a disengaged state. In the alert state, action is suspended while the subject waits for low probability or unpredictable signals. This is in contrast to the engaged state of target detection, which involves action on the part of the subject. A more recent study with neurologically intact individuals has provided further evidence for the distinction between the alerting and orienting mechanisms—between systems (3) and (2) above. For example, Posner and colleagues demonstrated that presenting alerting cues at four locations simultaneously (to prevent orienting) resulted in a global mode of alertness, which facilitated responding when compared to a no-cue situation (Fernandez-Duque & Posner, 1997). More important, they demonstrated that these alerting cues were equally facilitative for all target responses, which could be presented in a position that was either near or far from one of the four cues.

The Global/Local Processing Theory

The global/local processing theory provides an alternative explanation for the fact that right-hemisphere damage is more likely to lead to severe and persisting UN than left-hemisphere damage (Halligan & Marshall, 1994b). According to this theory, a right CVA may result in damage to the global guidance system of the right hemisphere that is believed to be responsible for directing focal attention to the spatial locations that require further analysis. A right-hemisphere lesion thus leaves the individual with UN with a left-hemisphere processing system that amplifies local-level information. Marshall and Halligan (1994a) suggest that even in severe UN, the issue is not that the individual cannot redirect focal attention leftward but that this act is not done voluntarily or without prompting. They argue that the overall global representation, which may be available at the preattentive stage of processing, is lost (or unable to be sustained) once local-level attention is engaged.

This global/local hypothesis complements Kinsbourne's theory of mutual inhibitory interaction between the hemispheres, and indicates that a right-hemisphere lesion leads to ipsilesional capture and the ultimate failure to redirect attention leftward because of the unopposed influence from the nonlesioned left hemisphere (Kinsbourne, 1987, 1993, 1994). Halligan and Marshall (1991b, 1994a, 1994b) propose that attention is not only shifted rightward by this unopposed left hemisphere influence but that local-level ipsilesional information is amplified at the cost of global-level information. Together, these two theories predict that the damaged right hemisphere (with a predilection for global processing and leftward attention shifts) is pitted against the undamaged left hemisphere (with a predilection for focal processing and rightward attention shifts), and this competition is resolved by an attention shift to a local-level rightward feature, followed by ipsilesional capture and the ultimate failure to redirect attention leftward. These authors further believe that ipsilesional capture could be the key to understanding UN, and that the difficulties that individuals with UN have with contralesional shifts of attention are a consequence of this process rather than the main component (Halligan, Marshall, & Wade, 1989).

Evidence supporting the global/local processing hypothesis comes from neuropsychological tests that have long been known to demonstrate that right- and left-hemisphere brain damage results in very different visuospatial deficits. One of the classic examples of this distinction, historically referred to as part/whole processing, can be seen in the drawings of individuals following brain injury. For example, when an individual with a right-hemisphere lesion copies the Rey Complex Figure (a standard neuropsychological test) there is a loss of the rectangular global whole but the separate local units remain intact. In contrast, when an individual with a left-hemisphere lesion copies it, the problems are specific to the separate local units within the rectangular global whole (Robertson & Lamb, 1991). These findings are important for understanding the role of global/local level processing in the severity of UN because visual stimuli are organized, not only next to one another in space but also in a spatial hierarchy with global-level objects made up of a number of local-level objects. Other examples of neuropsychological tests used to investigate global/local level processing include scene tests (a scene made up of trees, a house, and a fence, which are in turn made up of their respective individual parts) (Gainotti et al., 1972; Ogden, 1987), and composite figures. Examples of composite figures include the Navon Figure (a hierarchical figure consisting of a large global-level letter—S, made up of numerous smaller local-level letters that can be either congruent—small Ss—or incongruent—small Js) (Navon, 1977) and Halligan and Marshall's (1993) flowers (one is a drawing of two flowers converging on a single stem protruding from a single pot and the other is a drawing of two flowers in a similar position but without the common stem or pot).

When Halligan and Marshall (1993) presented P. B., a right-CVA patient, with these two drawings of the flowers to copy, they found that UN was directly influenced by whether the stimuli were presented as parts of the same object (a single potted plant with two flowers) or as two separate objects (two flowers). P. B. neglected the entire flower on the left in the first instance, and the left half of each of the two flowers in the second. Halligan and Marshall explained these results by proposing a hierarchy of attentional control, from global-level to local-level analyses of the stimulus configuration. They believe that the global-level aspects of the stimulus are perceived, and what follows is the assignment of a principal axis of elongation or symmetry (Driver & Halligan, 1991; Marr,

1982). The omission of local-level components is thus determined in relation to these global properties, and it is specifically at this stage that global-level processes are unable to guide focal attention leftward in individuals with UN following right-hemisphere damage.

One advantage of composite figures is that they avoid some the ambiguities of scene tests, in which the component elements may be perceived as a series of individual objects rather than as making up an integrated scene. But Navon Figures have an additional advantage when testing the global/local processing hypothesis because these figures have been used both as paper-and-pencil measures (Delis, Kiefner, & Fridlund, 1988) and in detailed reaction-time studies, in which the motor output requirements of the task can separated from the perceptual input components (Robertson, Lamb, & Knight, 1988). Research with the paper-and-pencil version of the Navon Figures has demonstrated that individuals with left-hemisphere lesions maintain the global configuration but miss the local components of the letters, whereas individuals with right-hemisphere lesions reproduce the local letters but miss the global organization.

The findings across numerous reaction-time studies with brain-injured individuals have further demonstrated that the temporoparietal junction is the area that is critical for hemispheric asymmetries that affect differential efficiency, speed of responding, and priority given to a stimulus. Lateralized presentations of the Navon Figures demonstrate that individuals with left-temporoparietal-lobe damage have a global-level advantage and individuals with right-temporoparietal-lobe damage have a local-level advantage (regardless of field of presentation), when compared with neurologically intact individuals. In other words, damage to the temporoparietal region results in an advantage to the nonpreferred level of responding (e.g., right-temporoparietal-lobe damage results in a local-level advantage) (Ivry & Robertson, 1998).

These results from reaction-time studies are broadly consistent with the findings from the drawings of individuals following a left- or right-hemisphere lesion, which emphasize one level at the expense of the other. But we need to explain why, in the *drawings* of the Navon figures, the disadvantaged level of processing is hardly manifested at all whereas, in the reaction-time studies, the disadvantaged level of processing is still manifested, but with slower responses. The results from the drawings of the Navon figures do not obviously conform to our current understanding of hemispheric asymmetry for global/local analysis. For neither hemisphere is believed to be solely responsible for global-level or local-level processing. So, following damage to the left hemisphere, the right hemisphere should still be able to perform local-level processing, although less efficiently; similarly, following damage to the right hemisphere, the left hemisphere should still be able to perform global-level processing. This is the pattern that we find in the reaction-time studies. But while the intact hemisphere can perform processing at either level, the advantaged level of processing completely dominates when the task demands processing at both levels simultaneously, as in drawing the Navon figures. (This explanation presupposes that the reaction-time tasks do not demand simultaneous processing at both levels.)

In addition to these findings of level-dependent advantages associated with the temporoparietal junction, there are additional anatomical findings that demonstrate interesting dissociations between this area and the inferior parietal lobe.[5] The research in this area has been extensively reviewed (Ivry & Robertson, 1998; Rafal & Robertson, 1995; Robertson, Lamb, & Knight, 1991), and it is noteworthy that these findings indicate that the inferior parietal lobe may have a dual spatial attentional function: (1) a regional attentional function, which guides attention to spatial locations; and (2) a categorical attentional function, which guides attention to the spatial resolution or spatial frequency of relevant or expected stimuli (Robertson, 1996; Robertson, Egly, Lamb, & Kerth, 1993). In support of these findings, a recent PET study used a divided-attention task with global/local figures to demonstrate that, for neurologically intact individuals, increases in the relative regional cerebral blood flow (rCBF) in the supplementary motor area and the medial parietal cortex (or rostral inferior parietal cortex) were significantly correlated with increasing numbers of target switches from the global level to the local level (Fink et al., 1997).

In summary, the evidence reviewed for both the alerting/vigilance systems theory and the global/local processing theory demonstrates that there are at least these two reasons why there should be more severe symptoms in individuals with UN following right-hemisphere damage. Taken together with the findings from the previous section, the results indicate that individuals with UN may have problems in at least two distinct areas that require consideration in rehabilitation planning: (1) problems in the directional attentional system that manifest as difficulties with disengaging, reorienting and maintaining attention; and (2) problems in the nondirectional attentional system that, following a right CVA, manifest as difficulties with (a) alerting and vigilance and (b) preferential processing of local-level information at the expense of global-level information.

NEUROANATOMICAL AND NEUROPHYSIOLOGICAL BASIS OF DISORDERS OF SPATIAL ORIENTATION AND AWARENESS, SPECIFICALLY UNILATERAL NEGLECT AND EXTINCTION

Evidence of a Time Course That Distinguishes Acute from Persisting Neglect

Many studies of UN are conducted within the first few weeks post-CVA, when the incidence of UN is high. Research findings have demonstrated that half of all individuals with a right CVA experience UN immediately following their stroke (Gainotti, 1968). In one study a "visual neglect recovery index," based on a battery of six neglect tests from the Behavioural Inattention Test (BIT), was used to test 171 consecutive patients admitted with an acute first CVA (Stone, Patel, Greenwood, & Halligan, 1992). Three time intervals were chosen for testing (3 days, 3 months, and 6 months). The findings demonstrated that patients with UN recover most quickly in the first 10 days post-CVA. Of the original 171 patients tested at 2–3 days post-CVA, 68 patients demonstrated UN, and, more important, of these 68, only 7 demonstrated residual UN at 3 months.

Time post-CVA is seldom considered as a variable in the study of UN. But from behavioral studies, as well as studies of lesion location and metabolic dysfunction, evidence is mounting that *persisting* neglect may be a different phenomenon from transitory neglect (i.e., neglect that resolves within the first few days or weeks post-CVA). Some of the findings from lesion studies comparing persisting and transitory neglect symptoms are now discussed.

Lesion Location in Unilateral Neglect

The inferior parietal lobe (Vallar, 1993; Vallar & Perani, 1986, 1987) and/or the temporoparietal junction of the right hemisphere (Bisiach, Capitani, Luzzatti, & Perani, 1981) are the areas most often implicated in UN. However, UN has also been demonstrated as a result of damage to the left hemisphere (Ogden, 1985b, 1987) and to the frontal lobe (Heilman & Valenstein, 1972; Husain & Kennard, 1996; Vallar & Perani, 1986), the thalamus (Colombo, De Renzi, & Gentilini, 1982; Motomura et al., 1986), and the basal ganglia (Damasio, Damasio, & Chang Chui, 1980; Egelko et al., 1988; Ferro, Kertesz, & Black, 1987).

Some studies that have failed to support a dominant role for the parietal lobe in UN have suggested that this is because the interval between onset of disease and testing was longer than is commonly used in such studies—longer than 4 weeks (Egelko et al., 1988). For example, over a 3-year period in a rehabilitation unit in New York, Egelko and colleagues recruited 57 right-hemisphere stroke patients with visuospatial neglect, who were at a minimum of 4 weeks post-CVA (median = 7 weeks; range = 4–120 weeks). A combination of computerized tomography (CT) scans, neurological examination, and psychometric measures revealed a surprising lack of lesion specificity in relation to the tests of visuospatial attention used. Most important, the patients' visuospatial attention was not found to be specifically related to parietal damage. Damage involved the frontal (72% of patients), basal ganglia (77% of patients), temporal (70% of patients), parietal (81% of patients), and occipital (16% of patients) regions. Amongst only six patients who demonstrated damage confined to a single region, five showed lesions confined to the basal ganglia. These findings raise the interesting possibility that the structural and neurological correlates of UN may be different in the minority of patients whose neglect persists into the post-acute stage.

Two recent studies have addressed this question (Maguire & Ogden, 2002; Samuelsson, Jensen, Ekholm, Naver, & Blomstrand, 1997). Samuelsson and colleagues tested 181 consecutive admissions to a stroke unit in Sweden over 2 years and found that 53 patients met the criteria for the study. At 1–4 weeks post-CVA, only 18 of these 53 patients demonstrated UN on seven modified tests from the BIT (Wilson, Cockburn, & Halligan, 1987). At follow-up 6 months later, only six patients continued to demonstrate UN (nine did not demonstrate UN and three were lost to follow-up). These results indicate that persisting neglect is a relatively rare phenomenon. Once again, these findings did not support the hypothesis put forward for an exclusive role of the parietal lobe for individuals with UN. Instead, the results implicate the posterior middle temporal gyrus and the (deep) temporoparietal paraventricular white matter in transitory neglect at the acute stage, and the central white matter below the collateral trigone of the temporal lobe (deep white matter of the temporal lobe) in persisting neglect at the post-acute stage (Samuelsson et al., 1997).

In the most recent of these two studies, Maguire tested all right- and left-CVA patients admitted to two stroke-rehabilitation units in Auckland, New Zealand, over an 18-month period, and identified nine patients who met the criteria for study inclusion (Maguire & Ogden, 2002). The patients were tested for UN at 4–6 weeks post-CVA using the six conventional sub-tests of the BIT and were tested again at a minimum of 3 months post-CVA (range 3–22 months) using a full neuropsychological test battery, which included tests of visual neglect, personal neglect, extinction (visual, auditory, and tactile), and anosognosia (literally, unawareness of or failure to acknowledge one's hemiplegia or other disability). The study also included magnetic resonance imaging (MRI), which was conducted specifically to look for lesions in the neuroanatomical areas hypothesized to be associated with UN. These MRI findings demonstrated that the lesions in patients with persisting neglect were large (14–111 cm^3) and affected three or more cortical or subcortical structures of the brain. Most notable was the finding that parietal (or temporoparietal junction) lesions are common but not essential for persisting neglect. Although seven patients did demonstrate parietal involvement, specifically the rostral inferior parietal lobe and the parietofrontal junction, there were two patients (one right-hemisphere CVA and one left-hemisphere CVA) who did not demonstrate parietal (or temporoparietal junction) involvement. The MRI investigation also demonstrated that all the patients had some degree of basal-ganglia involvement, and with one exception they all demonstrated involvement of the temporal lobe and the frontal lobe, including the frontal eye fields (within Brodmann area 8). Only two patients had any thalamic involvement.

In summary, these findings indicate that persisting neglect is a rare phenomenon (Maguire & Ogden, 2002; Samuelsson et al., 1997), and that it may involve extensive lesions (Egelko et al., 1988; Heir, Mondlock, & Caplan, 1983; Maguire & Ogden, 2002). Neglect—either acute or persisting—has been described following lesions to the right or left, anterior or posterior, and cortical or subcortical regions of the brain and is most often associated with damage to the right inferior parietal lobe or the temporoparietal junction of the right hemisphere. But the time post-CVA is an important factor for identifying the dominant lesion location. Lesion location studies in the post-acute stage have either failed to find a unique role for the parietal lobe in UN persisting at least 4 weeks post-CVA (Egelko et al., 1988; Maguire & Ogden, 2002; Samuelsson et al., 1997), or have implicated other regions, such as the basal ganglia (Egelko et al., 1988; Maguire & Ogden, 2002) or the deep white matter below the collateral trigone of the temporal lobe (Samuelsson et al., 1997). The findings also indicate that the many reported associations and dissociations in UN are unlikely to be symptoms of a unitary, coherent syndrome.

Metabolic Dysfunction Following a Cerebral Vascular Accident

Further evidence that patients with UN tested in the acute stage may represent a different population from patients with persisting neglect comes from research findings in humans and macaque monkeys, which have demonstrated widespread metabolic dysfunction during the early weeks post-CVA. The extent of this dysfunction has been demonstrated clearly in a study of 13 macaque monkeys with neglect induced by lesions to the right frontal polysensory cortex (Deuel & Collins, 1983). During the acute stages the monkey was likely to demonstrate spontaneous circling to the side of the lesion, disuse of the contralesional extremities, and failure to orient to contralesional stimuli. At this time, a decrement was found in unilateral local glucose utilization in unlesioned areas (e.g., the striatum and motor nuclei of the thalamus, the nucleus medialis dorsalis, and the deep layers of the superior colliculus). Spontaneous recovery was completed by 10 weeks post-injury and resulted not only in a return of normal behavioral responses (including orienting that was indistinguishable from normal monkeys) but also in a return of normal local glucose utilization in the outflow pathway from the frontal polysensory cortex to efferent motor structures. These results demonstrate that acute behavioral symptoms are based on widespread depression of neuronal activity in uninjured regions of the brain quite distant from the lesion site but with synaptic relations to damaged cortex. The authors hypothesize that recovery of neuronal activity in the undamaged cortical regions must reach sufficient capacity to activate the striatum, which in these cases allows for the restitution of behavioral function.

In 1914, following observations of the recovery process in humans suffering from a CVA, von Monakow proposed the term "diaschisis" to describe the phenomenon of reduction of cerebral profusion or metabolism in undamaged cerebral regions that are distant from the structural lesions. This interest has recently been renewed in the study of humans because of the availability of functional imaging methods to measure regional cerebral blood flow and functional metabolic recovery. For example, spontaneous recovery from UN (as measured by a battery of UN tests) was found to parallel the reduction of hypoperfusion, as measured by single photon emission computed tomography (SPECT), in undamaged cortical regions far removed from the subcortical right-hemisphere lesions of two patients with UN who were at 1 month and 6 months post-CVA (Vallar et al., 1988). Further, it has been demonstrated that the presence of a remote decrease in cortical cerebral blood flow (as measured by SPECT at 41 days post-CVA) in the right-temporoparietal region can distinguish UN patients with subcortical right-hemisphere lesions that spare the cortex (as measured by CT or MRI at 17 days post-CVA) from patients with the same lesion sites but without UN (Demeurisse, Hublet, Paternot, Colson, & Serniclaes, 1997).

The implications of these results can be extended by reviewing PET data, which demonstrates that restoration of metabolism in undamaged regions of the right hemisphere contributes to recovery from UN, but in addition that restoration can also occur in the left hemisphere (Perani, Vallar, Paulesu, Alberoni, & Fazio, 1993). Two patients were tested. The first patient had a right-basal-ganglia lesion (but no cortical damage as evidenced by CT scan), and demonstrated UN and a severe reduction of metabolism in both hemispheres on PET when tested in the acute stages (3 days post-CVA). For this patient, substantial recovery from UN was paralleled by a complete reduction of hypometabolism in the left hemisphere, and an almost complete recovery in the right hemisphere when tested at follow-up 8 months later. The right frontoparietal lobe and thalamic regions continued to demonstrate a persistent hypometabolism, which was hypothesized to be related to the persisting mild neglect. The second patient had extensive cortical and subcortical damage resulting from an infarct of the right middle and posterior cerebral artery, which spared the anterior cerebral artery territory. This patient had both severe neurological deficits and UN. A single PET study, conducted at 4 months post-CVA, demonstrated widespread metabolic reduction in unaffected areas of the left hemisphere and frontal lobe areas of the right hemisphere. In the first patient the time factor for recovery was clearly evident. For the second patient it is unknown how widespread the hypometabolism was in the acute stages, but in the post-acute stage he continued to demonstrate severe metabolic depression believed to result from the extremely large areas of the brain originally damaged.

In summary, these findings of complex underlying neurophysiological disturbances, which are most severe and widespread in the acute stage following CVA, make it vitally important that stage of recovery post-CVA (acute or post-acute) should be reported in research results for individuals with UN. CT or structural MRI scans in the *acute* stage post-CVA are informative, but they may not fully indicate the extent of lesion involvement, because metabolic dysfunction (and even consequential structural damage) has been demonstrated up to 6 months following CVA in areas of the brain that are quite distant from the original lesion site (Perani et al., 1993). Neglect may resolve when the recovery of neuronal activity in the *undamaged* cortical regions reaches sufficient capacity and allows for the restitution of behavioral function.

Distinguishing Neglect from Extinction and from a Primary Sensory or Motor Deficit

The distinction between UN and extinction is known but not always explicitly reported. This is probably because, even in the recent past, extinction has been considered a less severe form of UN that persists after recovery from the more severe form. The existence of extinction without UN is widely acknowledged. But behavioral and neuroanatomical evidence clearly demonstrates a double dissociation between UN and extinction (Findlay & Walker, 1996; Goodrich & Ward, 1997; Vallar, Rusconi, Bignamini, Geminiani, & Perani, 1994). In a particularly striking single-case study, a patient, V. H., had a left visuospatial neglect following a right-parietal infarct and demonstrated *better* detection and identification of contralesional targets when they appeared simultaneously with an ipsilesional target than when they appeared alone: that is, V. H. not only had UN in the absence of extinction but actually demonstrated "anti-extinction" (Goodrich & Ward, 1997).

Most studies of UN and extinction make reference to which disorder they are studying. But few clearly report clinical findings for tests of both UN and extinction. Distinguishing UN from extinction and distinguishing both disorders from a visual field (or somatosensory or motor) deficit is important, not only because of the double dissociation between UN and extinction, but also because the clinical evidence demonstrates that there are serious difficulties when making a differential diagnosis between primary sensory or motor deficits and UN (Vallar, 1993, 1998). Selective findings from neuroanatomical studies that take into account the distinctions between lesion location in UN and extinction are now discussed, in relation to the problems with making a differential diagnosis between a primary sensory or motor deficit and UN.

Lesion Location in Extinction

Extinction is usually defined as the inability to report a contralesional stimulus (visual, tactile, auditory) if, and only if, it is presented at the same time as a symmetrically located ipsilesional stimulus. Extinction is assessed using the confrontation method. This tests for visual extinction by having patients with UN fix their gaze on the examiner's nose and report if they see the examiner's forefingers (presented on the left only, right only, or both sides) extending from closed fists held at eye level from outstretched arms. Patients are diagnosed as having a visual extinction if they report single contralesional (80% or more) and ipsilesional (100%) stimuli but fail to report contralesional stimuli (30% or fewer) in the double-stimulation condition (Vallar et al., 1994).[6] The ability to detect a single contralesional stimulus is taken as evidence that sensory function is intact, and that the difficulties with double stimulus presentations are more likely to be caused by attentional competition between the two stimuli than by sensory processing.

Vallar and colleagues (Vallar et al., 1994) completed the first large systematic anatomical–clinical CT study of extinction (both visual and tactile), which included 159 continuous admissions of patients with a right CVA. The patients were assessed within 30 days of stroke using an extrapersonal neglect test that required them to cross out 13 circles printed on paper; tests for tactile and visual extinction; a standard clinical neurological examination; and a CT scan. The results demonstrated that UN and extinction do not necessarily co-occur and that the two disorders probably have different underlying neural bases.

The findings from their investigation of the co-occurrence of UN and extinction indicated that 46 patients (29%) showed visual or tactile extinction (22 tactile, 14 visual, 10 tactile and visual) but only 13 of these patients also showed UN; 58 patients (36.5%) showed UN but only 13 of these patients also showed either tactile or visual extinction; and none of the patients showed difficulties in all three areas (UN, visual extinction, and tactile extinction). In addition, there were dissociations demonstrated within extinction, that is, tactile and visual extinction did not always co-occur as only 10 of the 46 patients with extinction had both visual and tactile extinction. Although all these patients were tested at the acute stage post-CVA, similar dissociations between UN and extinction and within the disorder of extinction (visual, auditory, and tactile) have been demonstrated in persisting neglect (Maguire & Ogden, 2002).

There is evidence that extinction occurs following left- and right-hemisphere lesions in both cortical and subcortical regions of the brain, and, as with UN, the region most often implicated is the right inferior parietal lobe (Vallar & Perani, 1987). But the results of Vallar and colleagues (Vallar et al., 1994) show that lesions confined to subcortical structures were more often found in patients with extinction in the absence of UN than in patients with UN in the absence of extinction (50% of patients with subcortical damage had only extinction, whereas only 25% of patients with subcortical damage had only UN). Of the 46 patients studied with extinction, 24 patients had lesions confined to deep structures (and the basal ganglia was the most commonly damaged structure). Of the 22 patients with cortical/subcortical lesions, the right inferior parietal lobe was *not* the most commonly damaged structure, unless the patient demonstrated both extinction and UN.

In summary, these findings reveal the importance of testing for both UN and extinction because the behavioral and neuroanatomical evidence demonstrates that although UN (acute and persisting) and extinction may co-occur, they are distinct disorders. The findings also indicate that extinction should be tested across modalities because extinction has been found to dissociate by modality of testing (e.g., visual, auditory, and tactile).[7]

Differential Diagnosis

In spite of the many studies that have demonstrated a double dissociation between primary sensory or motor deficits and extinction, the confidence in the assertion that either an homonymous hemianopia (HH) or a somatosensory deficit can be distinguished from UN at assessment remains controversial, mainly due to the difficulties with differential diagnosis (Vallar, 1998). For example, it has recently been proposed that apparent contralesional somatosensory and motor deficits associated with right-hemisphere lesions may not result from a primary sensory or motor disorder, and, in fact, may be a manifestation of UN (Sterzi et al., 1993; Vallar, 1993).

Similar issues arise with the assessment of visual field deficits resulting from damage to the primary visual striate cortex of the occipital lobe. Tests that are used to assess visual field deficits are based on the belief that patients with a visual field deficit will not respond to stimulus presentations in the contralesional blind field during either single presentations (presentation to one visual field at a time) or double presentations (presentation of one stimulus to each visual field simultaneously). Using the confrontation method, the patient is diagnosed as having a visual field deficit if they fail to report contralesional stimuli while reporting ipsilesional stimuli (Vallar et al., 1994).

Distinguishing an HH from extinction using confrontation methods is relatively easy as patients with extinction will report visual information presented in isolation in the contralesional visual field but fail to report this information on double simultaneous stimulation (i.e., when contralesional sensory stimuli are simultaneously competing with ipsilesional stimuli). But distinguishing an HH from UN is more difficult as UN, like a contralesional blind region, is characterised by the failure to report a single stimulus presentation in the contralesional visual field. The patient with UN may fail to make a response in these testing situations even though their primary visual cortex is intact, whereas the patient with an HH fails to respond due to a blind region in the visual field (Heilman, Bowers, Valenstein, & Watson, 1987). Walker and colleagues have demonstrated difficulties with misdiagnosis of HH (in the presence of UN) not only with confrontation testing but also with perimetric visual field plotting, which is another standard measure for assessing the visual fields of individuals with UN (Walker, Findlay, Young, & Welch, 1991).

In summary, it is well accepted that the disorders of UN and extinction cannot be attributed to the patients' difficulties with primary sensory or motor deficits (somatosensory, motor, or visual field deficits), because they can occur in the absence of these deficits (Halligan, Burn, Marshall, & Wade, 1990). But the assessment issues discussed demonstrate that it remains essential to assess fully (and to report) the patients' primary sensory and motor deficits and to distinguish these deficits clearly from UN. These issues of differential diagnosis are not always considered in research on lesion location in patients with UN but clinical evidence indicates that primary sensory or motor deficits are likely to be amplified by the presence of UN (Bisiach, Vallar, Perani, Papagno, & Berti, 1986; Vallar, Bottini, Rusconi, & Sterzi, 1993). Studies of UN that include patients with symptoms of HH, for instance, are in fact including a confounding variable that may lead to possible misrepresentation of primary lesion location sites in UN. For example, the results of a recent lesion-location study have been used directly to challenge earlier findings that the inferior parietal lobe and/or the temporoparietal junction of the right hemisphere are the areas most often implicated in UN (Karnath, Ferber, & Himmelbach, 2001; Karnath & Himmelbach, 2002; Karnath, Himmelbach, & Rorden, 2002). Instead the authors implicate the right superior temporal cortex (in a cortical/subcortical anatomical network which includes the subcortical structures of the right putamen, caudate nucleus, and pulvinar) in spatial neglect in humans. Importantly, their challenge is not made on the grounds discussed in the section on metabolic dysfunction following a CVA. That is, it is not made on the grounds that information about the stage of recovery post-CVA (acute or post-acute) is crucial for interpreting scans identifying lesion location. Instead, they argue that the inclusion of patients with visual field deficits can bias the region of cortical lesion overlap to the inferior parietal lobe and/or the temporoparietal junction of the right hemisphere, which they claim are the brain areas most likely to mortify following the occurrence of an HH.

REVIEW OF THEORETICALLY BASED APPROACHES TO THE REHABILITATION OF UNILATERAL NEGLECT

A comprehensive discussion of the rehabilitation of attentional deficits in UN requires consideration of the role of damage to both the directional (or spatial) and the nondirectional (or nonspatial) attentional systems. As reviewed at the end of the first section of this chapter, damage to the directional attentional system may lead to difficulties that are specific to disengaging, reorienting and maintaining attention. Damage to the nondirectional attentional system may lead to difficulties with alerting and vigilance and with global-level processing. Both these difficulties with the nondirectional system of attention are appealed to in explanations of the finding that there is right-hemisphere involvement in the majority of individuals with persisting neglect. As we consider these two kinds of damage, it is helpful to keep in mind that there are reported findings of a facilitating relationship between the directional and the nondirectional attentional systems, namely, facilitation of the posterior-spatial-orientation system by the alerting/vigilance system (Posner & Petersen, 1990; Robertson, Mattingley, et al., 1998; Robertson et al., 1995). In addition, any discussion of the rehabilitation of UN requires some consideration of the literature reviewed in the second section of this chapter, which indicates that there are neuroanatomical, neurophysiological, and functional differences between acute and persisting neglect.

This section begins with a review of the attempts that have been made to address the directional (or spatial) attentional problems in UN. As the early studies in this area have had variable success, the first question addressed will be, "Is it profitable to continue to use standard visual-scanning training methods in the rehabilitation of individuals with UN?" At this point the discussion turns to more recent studies that have successfully used limb activation and prism adaptation to redirect the attention of individuals with UN. Following this, the discussion focuses on the following two clinical questions that are raised by considerations specifically related to the nondirectional attentional system, "When is it best to begin the implementation of rehabilitation strategies for a disorder that demonstrates much spontaneous recovery?" and "What role is there for developing effective rehabilitation strategies that increase motivation in those patients who experience problems in addition to the UN, for example, problems with either anosognosia or with alerting and vigilance, both of which are likely to make the UN persist?" Following a discussion of the rehabilitation strategies for anosognosia and for alerting and vigilance, the final question addressed is, "Which rehabilitation strategies are most likely to overcome the effects of preferential processing of local-level information at the expense of global-level information following right-hemisphere damage?"

Directional (or Spatial) Attentional Systems in Unilateral Neglect

Rehabilitation Strategies for the Redirection of Attention: Visual Scanning

The earliest attempts at the rehabilitation of UN focused on training individuals with UN to make habitual use of the voluntary orienting of attention system (believed to be undamaged in individuals with UN), as opposed to attempting to restore function in the automatic orienting of attention system (believed to be disrupted in individuals with UN). These rehabilitation strategies involved teaching individuals with UN to look to the left and have included methods such as visuoperceptual anchoring (i.e., reporting a visual cue, such as a letter or brightly colored marking, in the contralesional hemispace) (Ferro et al., 1987; Heilman & Valenstein, 1979; Riddoch & Humphreys, 1983) and visual scanning (i.e., scanning a board with a movable peripheral light target) (Diller & Riley, 1993; Weinberg et al., 1977).

These behavioral cueing methods, using progressively fading cues to teach individuals with UN to orient attention leftward voluntarily, have produced variable results. The reported outcomes range from no success (Heilman & Valenstein, 1979) to excellent success (Antonucci et al., 1995; Paolucci et al., 1996; Pizzamiglio et al., 1992; Zoccolotti et al., 1992). But importantly, there is a general finding that this form of rehabilitation is time-consuming, the effects are transitory, and there is often poor generalization from treatment conditions to untrained task conditions or to everyday functioning. However, there have been *some* successful results in this area of rehabilitation, especially in skills useful for reading and cancellation tasks (Brunila, Lincoln, Lindell, Tenovuo, & Hamalainen, 2002; Weinberg et al., 1977). And some studies have also reported generalization of the effects from training to untrained tasks and to everyday functioning in individuals with persisting neglect (Antonucci et al., 1995; Paolucci et al., 1996). In at least one study using a within-subjects design, these successes were maintained at a 5-month follow-up (Pizzamiglio et al., 1992). It is noted that generalization in the studies demonstrating success has been attributed to treatment duration, which included systematic, progressive training over 40 sessions (each lasting longer than 1 hour).

In response to the first question posed earlier, "Is it profitable to continue to use standard visual-scanning training methods in the rehabilitation of individuals with UN?" one needs to consider not only the resource and time demands involved in the successful use of these strategies but also whether the strategies generalize from the tasks used during training to everyday tasks. And, from a theoretical perspective, it is important to consider whether the difficulties with generalization can be explained by some of the findings from the research studies reported in the first section of this chapter.

These studies clearly demonstrated that individuals with UN have at least three kinds of directional attentional problems, that is, with disengaging attention, reorienting attention, and maintaining attention. But the visual-scanning training strategies have focused on the rehabilitation of, at most, only the first two of these kinds of problems. In developing theoretically viable rehabilitation strategies, one must consider not only the findings that demonstrate that individuals with UN fail to disengage and reorient their attention contralesionally but also the findings that, on demand, some individuals with UN can redirect their attention contralesionally but then fail to maintain their attention at the new location. For example, the research reported in the first section of this chapter provides findings that support Kinsbourne's (1987, 1993, 1994) gradient of attention theory for UN. In the valid-cue condition of the location-precueing paradigm, individuals with UN following a right-hemisphere lesion did respond to targets in the contralesional hemispace. These responses take significantly longer and are affected not only by the side of space but also by the relative-left location in both sides of space. The reported findings further indicate that the reason that some individuals with UN fail to maintain attention in the valid-cue condition, even though they can make contralesional shifts of attention on demand, may be explained by lesion location, in particular, by a rostral-inferior-parietal-lobe lesion of the right hemisphere (Aimola, 1999). Thus, when considering the issue of generalization in the rehabilitation of the directional (or spatial) aspects of attention, one needs to assess the specific individual difficulties experienced, as these are likely to include more than one kind of difficulty with redirecting attention.

Most commonly used behavioral cueing techniques have not proven to be especially effective rehabilitation strategies. But it was through these original training procedures for redirecting attention leftward that more successful strategies, such as limb-activation treatment, were discovered. This process of discovery is reviewed, along with possible theoretical reasons for the success.

Rehabilitation Strategies for the Redirection of Attention: Limb Activation

The discovery that contralesional limb activation could prove to be an effective rehabilitation strategy is based on research findings from two studies, which demonstrated that overall UN could be reduced by having the individual with UN use the contralesional hand to perform a task (Halligan & Marshall, 1989; Joanette, Brouchon, Gauthier, & Samson, 1986). Although these early studies attributed their findings of reduced UN (following the use of a contralesional limb) to an effect of ipsilesional hemisphere arousal, careful investigations of hand-start positions in a later line-bisection study led to the questioning of this hypothesis in favor of a spatio-motor cueing hypothesis (Halligan, Manning, & Marshall, 1991). Halligan and colleagues demonstrated that using the contralesional hand in contralesional space effectively reduced UN because the contralesional hand served as a contralesional stimulus cue, as was demonstrated in previously reported behavioral cueing studies (e.g., visuoperceptual anchoring and visual scanning studies). Importantly, they also demonstrated that using the contralesional hand but starting in the ipsilesional hemispace resulted in worse performance on line bisection than the more common ipsilesional-start position of the ipsilesional hand.

These findings have led to an active research program looking specifically at the role of visuoperceptual cueing in the effectiveness of limb activation as a rehabilitation strategy for individuals with UN, and to the related research question of whether it is *active*, as compared with *passive*, contralesional limb use that leads to the most significant reductions in UN (see Robertson & Hawkins, 1999). Passive-limb activation involves one of two conditions:

(1) teaching the individual with UN to place and hold their contralesional limb on the contralesional side of the proposed task set-up, and visually locating this contralesional limb before commencing the task (Robertson, North, & Geggie, 1992); or (2) activation of the contralesional limb by the experimenter/clinician (Robertson & North, 1993). The active-limb condition involves self-movement (even if only minimally) of the contralesional limb (be it the arm, leg, or sometimes the shoulder). If self-movement is not made spontaneously, this condition can also involve prompting by one of two methods: (1) the experimenter/clinician makes a single knock on the desk and instructs the individual with UN to make a movement by saying the single word "Now" at intervals of 8–10 seconds; or (2) the individual with UN is instructed to make a contralesional-limb movement that consists of pressing a cable-activated switch attached to a neglect alerting device (NAD)[8] and, if there is no movement, the NAD makes a buzzing tone at variable intervals (approximately every 8 seconds) to remind the individual with UN to make a movement. This is a promising area of rehabilitation research, as pointed out by Robertson and colleagues, because the use of the contralesional limb has the added advantage that it is a stimulus cue that is reliably present in all situations (Robertson, Halligan, & Marshall, 1993).

In response to the research question concerning passive and active contralesional-limb activation, the overall findings demonstrate that active contralesional-limb use in the contralesional hemispace is what is most effective as a rehabilitation strategy for reducing UN on the letter cancellation subtest of the BIT (Wilson et al., 1987), even when the contralesional limb is hidden from view. Active contralesional-limb activation (with the limb hidden from view) was also found to reduce left-sided visual extinction with a paradigm requiring the individual to fixate centrally, thus controlling for the possible confounding effects of eye movements (Mattingley, Robertson, & Driver, 1998). A noted exception to these findings was presented by Ládavas and colleagues, who demonstrated the reduction of UN symptoms with passive-contralesional limb use (albeit with an object-search paradigm which was considered to be a perceptual task that had a much reduced verbal/linguistic load from that used by Robertson and colleagues) (Làdavas, Berti, Ruozzi, & Barboni, 1997). Importantly, the findings from Robertson and colleagues (Robertson & North, 1992) demonstrate that the element of visuoperceptual anchoring (i.e., using one's own hand as a visual cue in the contralesional hemispace) may be an irrelevant aspect of the overall success of this strategy. For *ipsilesional*-limb use in the contralesional hemispace did not significantly reduce UN (but see Brown, Walker, Gray, & Findlay, 1999; Mattingley et al., 1998; Robertson & North, 1994).

Robertson and colleagues have proposed an alternative hypothesis to explain these findings, as well as the unexpected finding that the effectiveness of contralesional-limb movements in the contralesional hemispace is abolished if these movements are accompanied by simultaneous active ipsilesional-hand movements in either hemispace (Robertson & North, 1994). They suggest that the explanation that encompasses all the findings reported above is based on the work of Rizzolatti and colleagues (Rizzolatti & Berti, 1993; Rizzolatti & Camarda, 1987; Rizzolatti & Gallese, 1988). These authors argue, first, that spatial attention is not a supramodal function controlling the whole brain, but that it is distributed in several independent circuits, so that multiple but dissociable representations of space interact to form a coherent spatial reference system that can be selectively impaired. And second, they argue that spatial attention is a consequence of the activation of premotor neurons that facilitate functionally related sensory cells. The selection of a motor plan for action is believed to automatically shift attention toward the spatial sector where the action will be executed, because spatial attention is a correlate of the collaboration and organization for a motor act. Rizzolatti and colleagues have offered three suggestions about the potential consequences for spatial attention of selective impairment to sensorimotor circuits: (1) simultaneous activiation in several circuits is required for stimulus awareness in any one spatial location, so that disruption to any one circuit leads to insufficient overall activation; (2) the circuits that control any one sector of space are interconnected, so that a breakdown in any one of these circuits leads to hypoactivity in the connected circuits; and (3) attentional movements are controlled by a dynamic balance between various sensorimotor circuits, so that a lesion in any one circuit leads to an imbalance because of hyperactivity in other circuits (Rizzolatti & Gallese, 1988).

It will be recalled, from the first section of this chapter, that Rizzolatti and colleagues' third explanation for the mechanisms underlying the breakdown of spatial awareness was also put forward by Kinsbourne (1987, 1993, 1994). Kinsbourne proposed that UN results from a breakdown in the balance of reciprocally inhibitory opponent processors that control and direct lateral attention on the left/right axis (leftward movements are under right-hemisphere influence and rightward movements are under left-hemisphere influence). Robertson and colleagues argue that even minimal movements of the contralesional limb in the contralesional hemispace may cause sufficient activation to lead to a reduction in inhibitory competition from the nonlesioned hemisphere (Robertson, Hogg, & McMillan, 1998). This explanation of the competition for attention, of course, also explains the unexpected finding that active simultaneous limb movements abolish the effectiveness of single contralesional-limb movements (Robertson & North, 1994). To explain the findings that the contralesional limb in the ipsilesional space does not reduce UN, Robertson and colleagues have argued in favor of Rizzolatti and colleagues' second explanation for the mechanisms underlying spatial awareness. That is, activation of more than one corresponding spatial sector of closely linked neuronal maps is required to overcome the deficit in representing the contralesional side of space, so that cueing the personal system alone or the reaching system alone is not enough. Only when at least two systems are activated simultaneously is there an improvement in the spatial representation of contralesional space.

One caveat concerning this proposed explanation must be entered, given the findings from Ládavas and colleagues for the reduction of UN symptoms with passive contralesional-limb use (Làdavas et al., 1997). These findings do not detract from the general hypothesis put forward. But they do introduce the possibility that proprioceptive input may also lead to sufficient activation and to a reduction in inhibitory competition from the nonlesioned hemisphere. It may be that either proprioceptive input or motor intention can lead to this activation. But, once again, spatial awareness of contralesional space requires the activation of at least two systems. Thus, passive-limb activation may, like active-limb activation, lead to spatial awareness following the activation of both the personal sector of space (related in some way to somatosensory representations of the body) and the peripersonal or reaching sectors of space.

Finally, it is important to discuss generalization issues and the long-term benefits of contralesional-limb-activation treatment, as these formed the major criticisms against the behavioral cueing studies previously reviewed. Most recently, a randomized-control study (with two treatment conditions, either perceptual training only or perceptual training plus limb-activation treatment using a limb activation device[9]) has demonstrated significant improvements in motor function of the left arm or leg (Robertson, McMillan, MacLeod, Edgeworth, & Brock, 2002). But the findings did not extend to evidence of significant differences in the two treatment conditions at 6-month follow-up on tests measuring UN, for example, the BIT (Wilson et al., 1987), the Comb and Razor test of personal neglect (Beschin & Robertson, 1997), or an adapted version of the Landmark test. Nonetheless, the results did demonstrate that eleven individuals with UN with as few as 8–9 hours of contralesional-limb-activation treatment were able to improve their contralesional-limb movements significantly, and to maintain these improvements at an 18–24 month follow-up.[10]

Rehabilitation Strategies for the Redirection of Attention: Prism Adaptation

Prism adaptation is the final rehabilitation strategy to be discussed in connection with the directional (or spatial) attentional system in UN. The use of this strategy for redirecting attention contralesionally in individuals with UN is based on findings from neurologically intact individuals. These findings demonstrate that wearing optical prisms while repeatedly pointing to visual targets leads to visuomotor adaptation[11] (for a review, see Mattingley, 2002). The proposal that adaptation to optical prisms may be a useful strategy in the rehabilitation of UN is suggested by the fact that, after adaptation to prisms creating an optical shift of 10 degrees to the right, there is a temporary *after-effect*. For example, after removal of the prisms at the end of the adaptation phase, a neurologically intact individual asked to point straight ahead in the dark—and so reliant on proprioceptive rather than visual feedback—will point somewhat to the left of straight ahead. Without prism adaptation, an individual with UN who is asked to point straight ahead will typically point somewhat to the ipsilesional side; that is, toward the right for patients following a right CVA. Thus if the prism-adaptation after-effect (a leftward shift in pointing) were to be induced in an individual with UN it would result in more accurate straight-ahead pointing behavior.

The results from a group study of individuals with UN (between 3 weeks and 14 months following a right CVA) indicate post-adaptation leftward shifts in pointing following a brief period of adaptation to prisms that created an optical shift of 10 degrees to the right[12] (Rossetti et al., 1998). During the adaptation phase, subjects made 50 pointing responses to visual targets over a period of 2–5 minutes. Following removal of the goggles at the end of the adaptation, the individuals with UN showed much reduced errors in pointing straight ahead, and, importantly, they also showed improvements on a battery of standard tests for UN. Indeed, improvements lasting for at least 2 hours were demonstrated for line bisection (Schenkenberg, Bradford, & Ajax, 1980), line cancellation (Albert, 1973), copying (Cainotti et al., 1972), drawing a daisy from memory, and reading a simple text. The authors suggest that these improvements show that the effects of the prism adaptation go beyond the establishment of new correspondences between vision, proprioception, and motor control of the pointing movement and may lead to changes in the representation of space at higher cognitive levels. They offer two possible mechanisms to explain these improvements in performance. One is the stimulation of the plasticity of the neural functions of cross-modal integration and sensorimotor co-ordination. The other is the error signal that indicates a mismatch between intended arm position and visually observed arm position during the adaptation phase (Rossetti et al., 1998).

In a subsequent group study, Frassinetti, Angeli, Meneghello, Avanzi, and Làdavas (2002) demonstrated that 20 sessions of prism-adaptation treatment (two 20-minute treatment sessions daily over 2 weeks) could lead to significant improvements for individuals with persisting neglect (between 3 and 27 months following a right CVA). The improvements in this study lasted at least 5 weeks (with some preliminary data indicating that improvements lasted 17 weeks after treatment) and extended beyond the standard battery of UN tests (which tested for both near and far space) to tests reflecting improvements in everyday activities. Like Rossetti and colleagues, these authors argue that prism adaptation has its effects not only on the recalibration of visuomotor co-ordination but also on the organisation at higher levels of visuospatial representation. If the improvement in UN symptoms were to be explained only in terms of the leftward shift in pointing with the right hand—the after-effect of the adaptation—then we would expect that improvement would be shown only on tasks performed with that hand, and only while the after-effect lasted. However, improvement extended to a wider range of tasks, including visuoverbal tasks such as room description, and lasted much longer than the after-effect. While the after-effect decayed over 12 hours or so, the improved performance on UN tasks was maintained over several weeks. It is important to note that this improvement in UN was not found in the one patient, R. D., who did not demonstrate prism adaptation and did not have a stable after-effect.

One further single-case study of C. S., an individual with persisting neglect (between 39 and 42 weeks following a right CVA), provides additional support for the claim that improvements in UN may last for at least a week following a single period of prism adaptation (3–5 minutes of prism exposure), as well as some indication that improvements may generalize to everyday activities (McIntosh, Rossetti, & Milner, 2002).

If prism adaptation can reduce the severity of some symptoms in individuals with UN, then we might expect that adaptation to prisms that create a leftward optical shift might produce, not only a rightward pointing after-effect, but also neglect-like symptoms, in neurologically intact individuals. Michel and colleagues (Michel et al., 2003) tested neurologically intact individuals on line-bisection tasks, both manual and perceptual, following adaptation to leftward distorting prisms. The results simulated many aspects of line-bisection in individuals with UN. These results, like the earlier findings, were proposed by the authors to show that plastic changes in cross-modal or sensorimotor processes can affect higher-level cognitive representations of space. In conclusion, the authors suggest that "some of the lateralized symptoms observed in [unilateral neglect] originate from secondary maladaptive responses such as those following uninhibited adaptation between intact left hemisphere and cerebellum" (Michel et al., 2003, p. 38).[13]

In summary, this review of the directional rehabilitation strategies for reducing UN indicates, first, that prism-adaptation treatment is the most promising of the therapeutic strategies that have been considered. This conclusion is based on findings that prism adaptation is an effective rehabilitation strategy, as it provides both generalization to everyday activities and long-term effects (Frassinetti et al., 2002). In addition, it does not make heavy demands on either resources or time. By comparison, treatment methods that have focused specifically on teaching individuals with UN voluntarily to redirect their attention contralesionally have demonstrated serious difficulties both with generalization to everyday activities and with long-term benefits. The exception is the rehabilitation programs that have included intensive treatment sessions over a long duration. One reason given for these variable findings is that this latter form of intervention is aimed at improvements to the systems for disengaging and/or reorienting attention but it fails to incorporate findings demonstrating that individuals with UN have an additional directional problem with maintaining attention contralesionally. Second, this review of the directional rehabilitation strategies for individuals with UN also indicates support for the use of limb-activation treatment, especially given the findings that only 8 or 9 hours of treatment can lead to significant improvements in left-sided motor functions that continue to be evident at an 18–24 month follow-up (Robertson et al., 2002).

Nondirectional Attentional Systems in Unilateral Neglect

In regard to the second of the four questions posed earlier, as to when to begin the implementation of rehabilitation strategies, Làdavas, Carletti, and Gori (1994) have recommended that rehabilitation should begin 6 months post-CVA and that there should be a UN assessment on two separate occasions (separated by at least a month) to ensure that the phase of spontaneous recovery has ended. Although valid in regard to issues of spontaneous recovery of function, such a recommendation does not accord with current knowledge which indicates that rehabilitation should begin as soon as possible following neurological insult (Kolb, Chapter 2, this volume). This is especially the case for those patients with (1) smaller lesions or (2) a sufficient number of unimpaired cells and neural connections, as is sometimes demonstrated by residual function, for example, residual function in the hemiplegic limb (Robertson, 1999).

Two bodies of literature are relevant to this second question, the anosognosia literature and the alerting/vigilance literature. This literature demonstrates that some individuals with UN may fail to make spontaneous recovery (from UN and from hemiplegia) or to develop compensatory strategies (such as voluntary leftward eye movements) due to problems with anosognosia or with alerting and vigilance, problems considered additional to the spatial problems involved in the UN disorder itself. In fact, it is believed that these additional problems may not only impair recovery but also mask existing residual function.

Thus, the additional problems of anosognosia or of alerting and vigilance at the acute stage following a neurological insult may be the determining factors for when to begin UN rehabilitation. For either problem is likely to prevent spontaneous recovery, so that waiting up to 6 months in anticipation of spontaneous recovery would be futile. For example, it has been demonstrated that the presence of anosognosia in the first few days post-CVA is a good predictor of UN severity (Stone et al., 1992). Similarly, it has been shown that functional recovery post-CVA can be predicted by the individual's capacity to sustain attention. Specifically, sustained attention, as measured by the Elevator Counting, Telephone Search, and Lottery subtests of the Test of Everyday Attention (TEA) (Robertson, Ward, Ridgeway, & Nimmo-Smith, 1994) at 2 months following a right CVA predicts motor recovery over a 2-year period (Robertson, Ridgeway, Greenfield, & Parr, 1997).

Robertson and Murre (1999) have argued for a similar recommendation as to when rehabilitation should begin. Their emphasis has been on the relevant research findings specifying that Hebbian-learning-based self-repair processes (i.e., synaptic reconnections) require not only that behavioral stimulation be directed to the affected areas in the early stages following neurological insult but also that this stimulation be both specific and repetitive (to avoid or minimize the possibility of fostering faulty neural reconnections). Their most emphatic contribution to rehabilitation practice concerns the importance of adequate attention, specifically adequate sustained attention, to the success of learning-based recovery of function. Robertson and colleagues have not only demonstrated that sustained attention measures predict recovery but also shown that there is a significant difference between right- and left-hemisphere stroke patients in their ability to sustain attention at 2 years post-CVA, even if this difference was not initially apparent at the 2-month assessment (Robertson et al., 1997). These sustained attention differences were apparent in an auditory sustained-attention task that had no spatial component and a minimal perceptual load. The authors illustrated that these differences were mainly attributable to improvements in sustained attention for the left-hemisphere patients over the 2-year period post-CVA. In comparison, the right-hemisphere patients failed to demonstrate improvements.

These findings demonstrate that if learning is the key to recovery of function, and attention to the specified rehabilitation activity is required for learning, spontaneous recovery or compensatory strategies are unlikely to occur if the individual with UN has alerting and vigilance deficits. Similarly, if learning does not take place without attention, then learning will not occur for individuals with UN and anosognosia for the UN, mainly because these individuals will not attend to rehabilitation strategies for deficits of which they are unaware. Thus, it has been suggested that treatment focusing on problems that the individual with UN can recognize are more likely to lead to successful rehabilitation outcomes (Robertson et al., 1997).

The third question posed earlier concerns the role of rehabilitation strategies that are aimed at increasing motivation for rehabilitation in patients who experience problems with either anosognosia for their deficits or alerting and vigilance. Here it is suggested that either of these two problems may prevent the individual with UN from taking advantage of rehabilitation strategies. It is thus important to assess these additional problems at an early stage post-CVA, and to commence treatment to prevent the *persisting* neglect syndrome from developing.

Rehabilitation Strategies for Anosognosia

As discussed earlier in this chapter, there are serious difficulties in making a differential diagnosis between primary sensory or motor deficits and UN. Apparent sensory and motor deficits associated with right-hemisphere lesions have in some cases been shown to be manifestations of the UN rather than the results of primary sensory and motor disorders (Sterzi et al., 1993; Vallar, 1993, 1998). Further evidence can be found in the following research findings from rehabilitation interventions which use sensory manipulations to induce a reorientation of spatial attention to the contralesional side: (1) contralesional posterior neck muscle vibration (Karnath, Christ, & Hartje, 1993; Schindler, Kerkhoff, Karnath, Keller, & Goldenberg, 2002) (or, similarly, the repositioning of the trunk 15 degrees leftward from that of the orientation of the eyes) (Karnath, Schenkel, & Fischer, 1991); (2) optokinetic (or visual vestibular) stimulation (i.e., visual presentation of tasks against a large, leftward moving background) (Pizzamiglio, Frasca, Guariglia, Incoccia, & Antonucci, 1990); and (3) caloric vestibular stimulation (i.e., irrigation of the contralesional ear canal with 20 ml of iced water for 1 minute) (Cappa, Sterzi, Vallar, & Bisiach, 1987; Rubens, 1985; Vallar et al., 1993).

These interventions lead to short-term improvements in contralesional shifting of attention, though the effects usually last only for a few minutes.[14] Importantly, the results of these interventions provide both the clinician and the individual with UN with more accurate information about the nature of the patient's disorder (Vallar et al., 1993; Vallar, Sterzi, Bottini, Cappa, & Rusconi, 1990). In particular, patients are provided with the opportunity to recognize both that they do have sensory or motor abilities where previously they may have maintained that they were incapacitated, and that they have a genuine problem of UN, which they may have previously denied (Cappa et al., 1987; Pizzamiglio et al., 1990). As long as this more accurate estimate of the situation is maintained, the individual with UN is better placed to respond appropriately to rehabilitation strategies.

Because a combination of UN and anosognosia is believed to be especially detrimental to the prospects of recovery, it is worth noting that there have been reports of a virtuous cycle when using the rehabilitation techniques developed by Pizzamiglio and colleagues (1992). These researchers have found that initial unawareness of deficit in individuals with UN can in itself be ameliorated by the attention provided during rehabilitation programs that include leftward scanning techniques, and sometimes also optokinetic stimulation (Pizzamiglio et al., 1990; but see Zoccolotti et al., 1992). As leftward attention improves through training so does the individuals' awareness of the nature of his or her own deficits. This in turn leads to more active participation in the rehabilitation training and, in the most promising cases, to the emergence of self-initiated compensatory strategies.

The symptoms of UN themselves make it difficult for the patient to gather accurate information about the nature of the disorder. Individuals with UN who do not respond to visual stimuli presented in the left side of extrapersonal space will not learn that they have failed to comb the left side of their hair by looking in a mirror. Söderback and colleagues reasoned that instead of mirrors, which are commonly used in the treatment of UN and anosognosia, video would be a more effective medium, because, of course, when individuals with UN watch video playback, the left side of their bodies appears in the right side of visual space (Söderback, Bengtsson, Ginsburg, & Ekholm, 1992). These authors videotaped four individuals with UN while they performed three household tasks (finding pastry in the refrigerator, cutting the pastry, and arranging the cakes on an oven tray) and Albert's Line Crossing test (Albert, 1973). The authors did not provide intervention during the video sessions, but they replayed the videos of the household tasks to the individuals with UN, both to demonstrate their experienced difficulties and to provide new strategies for performing the tasks. A single-case experimental design was used and the results demonstrated improvements in UN behavior by most patients on some tasks. Importantly, the improvements were maintained at follow-up 53 days following the intervention.

Although it is widely recognized that UN is a disruptive factor impeding both functional recovery and improvement in activities for independent living following a neurological insult (Denes, Semenza, Stoppa, & Lis, 1982), a closer look at this literature reveals that it is the symptom complex comprising extrapersonal neglect and anosognosia for hemiplegia that is the worst prognostic factor for functional recovery (Aimola Davies & Ogden, 2003; Gialanella & Mattioli, 1992). For example, Gialanella and Mattioli's results demonstrate that it is not the presence of extrapersonal neglect *per se* 1 month post-CVA, but the combination of extrapersonal neglect and anosognosia for motor deficits at 1 month that is associated with the poorest recovery from hemiplegia at 5 months post-CVA. Prompted by these findings, Aimola Davies and Ogden also examined whether recovery from hemiplegia (in nine patients who were from 3–22 months post-CVA) was associated with different severities of the disorders of extrapersonal neglect, personal neglect, extinction, and anosognosia for visuospatial neglect, for personal neglect, and for a motor deficit. The results from eight of the nine patients were broadly consistent with the hypothesis that the combination of *extrapersonal neglect and anosognosia for motor deficits* predicts a poor recovery from hemiplegia, and that the combination of personal neglect and anosognosia for motor deficits was a less good predictor of poor recovery from hemiplegia, and importantly, that neither extrapersonal neglect nor personal neglect is, by itself, a good predictor of recovery from hemiplegia.

Rehabilitation Strategies for the Alerting/Vigilance System

Two points were noted earlier in this chapter. First, the alerting/vigilance system is reported to have a facilitatory effect on the posterior-spatial-orientation system. This relationship explains research findings that rehabilitation treatment strategies aimed at increasing alerting and vigilance also demonstrate improvements to perceptual visuospatial neglect (Robertson, Mattingley, et al.,

1998; Robertson et al., 1995). Second, the functional recovery of an individual with UN following a CVA can be predicted by the capacity to sustain attention (Robertson et al., 1997; Robertson et al., 1995). Thus it appears that improving the performance of the alerting/vigilance system may lead to *two* important outcomes: recovery from UN and recovery from motor deficits.

The rehabilitation strategies used for increasing alerting and vigilance include (1) nonlateralized, nonspatial auditory alerting stimuli (Robertson, Mattingley, et al., 1998) and (2) self-alerting procedures (Robertson et al., 1995). The NAD and LAD (Robertson, Hogg, et al., 1998; Robertson & North, 1992; Robertson et al., 1992) should also be included in this list, as the third rehabilitation strategy for increasing alerting and vigilance, although they have not been directly discussed in the literature as such. References to the NAD and LAD in the research literature have been specifically concerned with the implementation of these devices in conjunction with limb-activation treatment. But it is apparent from the compact construction, and the built-in alerting structure, that in addition to serving as a reminder to the individual with UN to make a contralesional-limb movement, these devices could serve to increase alertness in a manner similar to nonlateralized, nonspatial auditory alerting stimuli (Manly, Hawkins, Evans, Woldt, & Robertson, 2002; Robertson & Cashman, 1991).

The success of using a nonlateralized, nonspatial auditory alerting stimulus immediately preceding a target stimulus has been argued to depend on the preserved functioning of the *phasic* alerting system (the ascending subcortical thalamic mesencephalic projections that subserve responses to novel or salient exogenous events) of the individual with UN, in comparison to their damaged *tonic* alerting system (the cortical, right-frontoparietal circuits that maintain *endogenous* self-alerting over prolonged periods without external stimulation) (Robertson, Mattingley, et al., 1998; Robertson et al., 1995; but see Sturm, Willmes, Orgass, & Hartje, 1997). In one example of the successful application of this form of intervention, Robertson and colleagues tested individuals with UN on a comparison task (i.e., comparing relative reporting speed between left and right visual events). In a previous experiment, this task demonstrated that individuals with UN become aware of right visual events, on average, approximately half a second before left visual events (Rorden, Mattingley, Karnath, & Driver, 1997). But by preceding this comparison task with a nonspatial and nonpredictive warning sound, the *prior entry* of right visual events (compared with left visual events) was abolished (Robertson, Mattingley, et al., 1998). Robertson and colleagues argued that preceding a stimulus requiring a response with a nonspatial warning sound (presented in only 25% of trials) functions to increase phasic alertness, and that this increase in phasic alertness has an impact on the tonic alertness system, which leads to an increase in awareness of contralesional stimuli. These findings are impressive if one considers the ease of implementing an auditory cue as a rehabilitation strategy.

Robertson and colleagues used these principles for increasing phasic alertness in a rehabilitation program that also included Meichenbaum's technique of self-instructional training (Meichenbaum & Goodman, 1971). They taught individuals with UN to verbally self-regulate their levels of alertness (Robertson et al., 1995). Eight patients with persisting neglect were trained to progress gradually from learning to attend to a particular task as a result of maximal experimenter/clinician intervention (i.e., the experimenter knocks loudly on the desk every 20–40 seconds, and loudly says the word "attend"), to learning to attend as a result of minimal experimenter/clinician intervention (i.e., the experimenter knocks loudly and the individual with UN says the word "attend" aloud) to the next to final stage, learning to attend with no experimenter/clinician intervention (i.e., the individual with UN takes on the task of knocking on the desk, and at first says the word "attend" aloud, and later learns to say the word "attend" subvocally). In the final stage of training, the individual with UN merely signals to the experimenter/clinician that he or she is mentally knocking on the table and saying "pay attention." By using a multiple-baseline-by-function design along with a multiple-baseline-by-subject design, Robertson and colleagues were able to show that, following only 5 hours of self-instructional training on one series of tasks, there was significant improvement demonstrated on an independent series of tests that were reported to last from 24 hours to 14 days. Individuals with UN demonstrated significant improvements in *sustained attention* on a Vertical Letter Cancellation test and an adapted version of the Elevator Counting subtest of the TEA (Robertson et al., 1994). They also demonstrated significant improvements on tests of *visuospatial neglect*, for example, Letter Cancellation (Weintraub & Mesulam, 1987) and the Baking Tray test (see Robertson et al., 1995). But importantly, the findings demonstrated that there was no improvement on tests that were not expected to be affected by rehabilitation.

Rehabilitation Strategies for the Global-Processing System

We now turn to the final question posed earlier, "Which rehabilitation strategies are most likely to overcome the effects of preferential processing of local-level information at the expense of global-level information following right-hemisphere damage?" Halligan and Marshall have proposed that the global/local processing theory may explain the finding that damage to the global-processing system in the right hemisphere results in preferential processing of local-level information (Halligan & Marshall, 1994b; Marshall & Halligan, 1994a). They have also proposed that tasks that naturally impose the requirement of global processing may be more successfully used to reduce UN than tasks that cue the contralesional hemispace (Halligan & Marshall, 1991a, 1994a).

It is important for this present discussion to be reminded of one relevant outcome from all the previously reported studies that have used either the location-precueing paradigm or behavioral cueing techniques to direct attention to the neglected hemispace. These studies have clearly demonstrated that although individuals with UN do not *automatically* orient or make contralesional shifts of attention, they are, in fact, physically capable of making these shifts under *explicit* cueing instructions, especially if *specifically instructed* to report the contralesional cue (Posner et al., 1984; Posner, Walker, et al., 1987; Riddoch & Humphreys, 1983; Weinberg et al., 1977). It is suggested, therefore, that tasks with cues in the ipsilesional hemispace that induce global processing have the potential to resolve an ongoing debate in the UN literature about the role of attentional capture. This debate attempts to distinguish difficulties with disengaging attention to make a contralesional shift of attention (once attention has been captured ipsilesionally) from the failure of contralesional stimuli fully to capture attention.

Whatever the reason why individuals with UN do not automatically make contralesional shifts of attention, there is evidence indicating that under some circumstances they are influenced by contralesional information, even when they are unaware of this influence. Some of this evidence has been gathered in experiments using the indirect questioning method. These experiments have shown that although direct questioning may result in individuals with UN failing to respond to contralesional information, switching to indirect questioning results in responding that is accurate enough to indicate that contralesional information has been processed implicitly (Karnath & Hartje, 1987; Marshall & Halligan, 1988; Volpe, Ledoux, & Gazzaniga, 1979), at least to a level that allows for lexical/semantic analysis (Làdavas, Paladini, & Cubelli, 1993; McGlinchey-Berroth et al., 1996; but see Farah, Monheit, & Wallace, 1991). There is also evidence that individuals with UN demonstrate some degree of contralesional attraction when tested with experimental paradigms that tap preattentive processing, such as in figure/ground segmentation experiments (Doricchi, Incoccia, & Galati, 1997; Driver, Baylis, & Rafal, 1992; Marshall & Halligan, 1994b) and visual search experiments (Aglioti, Smania, Barbieri, & Corbetta, 1997; Grabowecky, Robertson, & Treisman, 1993; Riddoch & Humphreys, 1987).

Of more direct relevance to Halligan and Marshall's proposals are the experimental findings demonstrating that global properties of the stimulus configuration can help to reduce UN. For example, findings from a single-case study of an individual with UN (with a right frontotemporal meningioma) have demonstrated that UN can be present for stimuli that are discontinuous or meaningless (e.g., line bisection) while being absent, or significantly reduced, when the stimulus arrays are spatially continuous or meaningfully integrated (e.g., interactive pictures) (Kartsounis & Warrington, 1989). Two final studies with similar experimental findings are now discussed in greater detail. They provide some support for Halligan and Marshall's hypothesis that a significant factor in generating symptoms of UN is the ipsilesional capture of attention by local-level information. If this hypothesis is correct, it suggests that UN symptoms may be reduced by rehabilitation strategies that prioritize global-level information.

In the first study, Seron, Coyette, and Bruyer (1989) tested six individuals with UN following a right CVA, all of whom demonstrated unilateral posterior lesions that included the parietal region. These individuals were asked to identify drawings from different categories of informational meaningfulness.[15] The results demonstrated that the responses were influenced by contralesional information only if the ipsilesional side of a drawing did not provide enough information for identification (e.g., identification-left category: a toothbrush with the handle on the right side and the bristles on the left). In fact, the responses were as accurate for this category as they were for a second category requiring only ipsilesional information for correct identification (e.g., symmetrical-left category: an audiocassette tape). These results were contrasted with performance on a third category (e.g., unexpected-left category: a house with flames on the left side only), which required processing of the more contralesional segments of the drawing for correct identification. For this category, the individuals with UN produced incorrect identifications (e.g., a house) based on the limited information from the rightmost few segments of the drawing. The authors proposed that the *interpretation* process for individuals with UN self-terminates prematurely if the ipsilesional information in a drawing is sufficient for identification (whether correct or incorrect). Self-termination leads to correct responses for drawings in the symmetrical-left category because the contralesional information in the drawing is redundant, but it leads to incorrect responses in the unexpected-left category because the contralesional information is essential for correct identification. The findings of most relevance for the rehabilitation of UN are those related to the identification-left category, which also required processing of contralesional information for correct responding. The individuals with UN were able to integrate global-level and local-level information into an organized whole which led to correct responses for this category with the least amount of useful ipsilesional information.

In the second study, Maguire (2000) tested seven individuals with UN following a right-CVA, all of whom demonstrated unilateral lesions that included the parietal lobe in six of the seven patients. These individuals were asked both to *copy* and to *identify* 21 black-and-white line drawings selected from those used by Seron and colleagues. The findings from Seron and colleagues were replicated in the identify condition, but the critical comparison was between the identify and copy conditions as the drawings were expected to provide explicit evidence of how contralesional information is represented when the ipsilesional information in a drawing is informative enough to lead to premature self-termination. As predicted, the symmetrical-left category (e.g., audiocassette tape) resulted in 100% accuracy in the identify condition, but UN was demonstrated in the copy condition (68% accuracy). The evidence suggests that these correct identifications were based solely on the ipsilesional side of the drawing. And, as expected, a comparison of the identify condition for the identification-left (e.g., toothbrush) and unexpected-left (e.g., burning house) categories demonstrated greater percent accuracy for the identification-left category, the drawings with the least amount of useful ipsilesional information (identification-left category = 82% accuracy; unexpected-left category = 69% accuracy). The critical finding was that the copy condition also revealed a consistently better performance for the category with the least amount of useful ipsilesional information. The effect was particularly striking for a subgroup of individuals with UN who achieved 91% accuracy for the identification-left category compared with 60% accuracy for the unexpected-left category.

Overall, these findings demonstrate that the typical symptoms of UN on copying a drawing were present in both the symmetrical-left and unexpected-left categories. Indeed, the percent accuracy scores of all individuals with UN in the copy conditions for the symmetrical-left category (68% accuracy) were quite similar to those for the unexpected-left category (62% accuracy). However, the symptoms of UN were strikingly reduced in the identification-left category. It is proposed that for all three categories, individuals with UN use some global-level information to make an identification, whether correct or incorrect. For the symmetrical-left and unexpected-left categories, there is considerable local-level detail on the ipsilesional side, and individuals with UN do not attend to local-level information on the contralesional side of the drawing. For the identification-left category, in contrast, there is little local-level detail on the ipsilesional side and individuals with UN reproduce contralesional local-level information in their drawings.

In summary, this review of the nondirectional rehabilitation strategies for individuals with UN indicates, first, that there are therapeutic benefits to be gained by including treatment strategies that target problems additional to the spatial problems involved in the UN disorder itself (i.e., problems with anosognosia or with alerting and vigilance). It was proposed that these additional problems affect the decision of when to begin UN rehabilitation, because these problems may not only prevent spontaneous recovery but also mask existing residual function. As was discussed, the results clearly indicate that it is the presence of extrapersonal neglect and anosognosia for motor deficits that predicts a poor recovery from hemiplegia (Aimola Davies & Ogden, 2003; Gialanella & Mattioli, 1992). The experimental findings from studies treating individuals with UN for alerting and vigilance deficits similarly indicate benefits in addition to the immediate impact on this system itself, as a facilitatory effect on the posterior-spatial-orientation system leading to improvements in perceptual visuospatial neglect has been demonstrated (Robertson, Mattingley, et al., 1998; Robertson et al., 1995). Second, this review of the nondirectional rehabilitation strategies for individuals with UN indicates support for the hypothesis that damage to the global-processing system is a significant factor in generating symptoms of UN following a right CVA. This damage leads to preferential processing of local-level ipsilesional information at the expense of global-level information (Halligan & Marshall, 1991a, 1994a). The two studies presented indicate that UN symptoms may be reduced by including rehabilitation strategies that prioritize global-level information and thus lead to the reintegration of global- and local-level information into an organized whole (Maguire, 2000; Seron et al., 1989).

CONCLUSION

This chapter has provided an overview of some of the theoretically based approaches to the rehabilitation of UN and an evaluation of the effectiveness of treatment strategies in regard to generalization and long-term benefits. It has also provided an evaluation of the effectiveness of strategies that target problems that co-exist with UN, such as anosognosia, alerting and vigilance deficits, and global-processing deficits. The rehabilitation strategies discussed in the last section of the chapter were linked to the theories of UN presented in the first section and to the neuroanatomical and neurophysiological issues in the second section. These findings indicate that UN is not a unitary phenomenon and that it results in both directional and nondirectional attentional problems. The findings also suggest that persisting neglect may be a different phenomenon from transitory or acute neglect and that there is a need to specify the recovery stage under consideration in the development of theory-driven rehabilitation strategies. Although we are far from having a full understanding of UN, the problems that we know to exist need to be identified and specifically targeted when creating individualized treatment programs. The rehabilitation literature clearly shows that treatment effectiveness is dependent on choosing rehabilitation strategies that are theory-driven and thus directly related to the specific problems demonstrated by the individual with UN (Robertson et al., 1993). For example, Sturm and colleagues (1997) have shown that specific attention deficits need specific training if improvement is to be realized. These various problems, which may be caused by lesions in different locations, are likely to be revealed by different task requirements. Specifying these problems requires a full rehabilitation-oriented neuropsychological and neurological assessment of the individual's strengths, deficits, and residual functions (Robertson & Murre, 1999), in addition to monitored observations of the individual with UN during everyday activities.

NOTES

1. Although Halligan and Marshall (1991a) have made a valid distinction between peripersonal and extrapersonal neglect, in this chapter "extrapersonal neglect" includes the neglect of stimuli within arm's reach, which is the more commonly accepted usage of this term in the UN literature.

2. The reader is referred to the recent articles by Vallar (1998) and Manly (2002).

3. The visual attention studies that have used Kinsbourne's suggested experimental set-up are most often studies of covert orienting of attention, that is, studies conducted under conditions of restricted eye movements that allow for measurements specifically of the allocation of attention to a point in space independent of the eye movements to that point in space.

4. This paradigm presents four rectangles (two each side of the fixation point), and the participant's task is to press a button as quickly as possible in response to the target, which is a salient luminance increment. On 75% of trials (not including catch trials) the cue is a valid indicator of the target location, but for the other 25% of trials the target could appear in one of two unqued locations within the same visual field. The stimuli for each trial are restricted to one visual field, and the cue-to-target movements are always horizontal or vertical rather than diagonal.

5. As discussed later in this chapter, UN has been described following lesions to the right or left, anterior or posterior, and cortical or subcortical regions of the brain, but it is most often associated with damage to the right inferior parietal lobe or the temporoparietal junction of the right hemisphere.

6. Note that both the definition of extinction and the confrontation method for assessing it are subject to problems. Problems for the confrontation method include (unintentional) variability of stimulus intensity and floor/ceiling effects (Rorden, Mattingley, Karnath, & Driver, 1997).

7. It is important to note that different studies use different tests of UN and of extinction. Patient V. H. was tested for UN on line bisection, reading, and line cancellation, and was tested for extinction (and "anti-extinction") by single and double presentations of stimuli on a computer screen (Goodrich & Ward, 1997). Vallar and colleagues used a cancellation task to assess UN and the confrontation method to assess extinction (Vallar et al., 1994).

8. The NAD is a small metal box (12 cm × 8 cm × 2 cm) with an on/off cable-activated switch. The device is set to buzz if not turned off within a predetermined, and variable, time interval. A red light remains on if the buzzer is not activated (Robertson, Hogg, & McMillan, 1998; Robertson & North, 1992; Robertson et al., 1992). In addition, the device can be used differently; that is, rather than have the individual with UN make a contralesional-limb movement to turn off the device, so as to avoid the buzzer sounding, the individual with UN can be required to turn off the device when the buzzer sounds (Robertson et al., 1992).

9. The limb activation device (LAD) is a new version of the previously described NAD and consists of two components. The first is attached to the left wrist, leg, or shoulder of the individual with UN, and the second component is a small plastic control box attached to a trouser belt. As with the NAD, the LAD emits an auditory tone if there is no movement from the individual with UN within a specified time, and

continues to emit this tone until a movement is made (Robertson, McMillan, MacLeod, Edgeworth, & Brock, 2002).

10. Note that there are research findings that have demonstrated improvements following contralesional-limb activation in some but not all individuals with UN (Brunila et al., 2002; Cubelli, Nichelli, Bonito, De Tanti, & Inzaghi, 1991), and in some (e.g., a significant reduction in left-side word omissions) but not all task conditions (Brown et al., 1999).

11. Visuomotor coordination involves being able to point or reach toward visually presented objects. If visual space is distorted by wearing optical prisms, so that objects are seen 10 degrees to the right of where they really are then, initially, pointing errors occur. Pointing to where an object looks to be is pointing 10 degrees to the right of where the object is really located. During the adaptation phase, the neurologically intact individual initiates pointing toward visually presented objects. At the completion of the pointing movement, the subject is presented with visual feedback that shows the finger as being further to the right than expected, and further to the right than the target object. Gradually, with repeated pointing, the pointing error is reduced until pointing is once again aligned with the real location of objects. This is the direct-effect of the adaptation. At this stage, the proprioceptive feedback from the pointing movement and the visual presentation of the object are in correspondence again, and this is achieved by a kind of compromise between vision and proprioception, so that a pointing movement toward an object that is really straight ahead is experienced as being somewhat to the right. This adaptation is believed to demonstrate the plasticity of the spatial transformations that the brain uses to integrate information from different sensory modalities and to integrate sensory information with motor instructions.

12. It is worth noting that individuals with UN responded differently from the control group (inpatients without a neurological history) in two ways. First, their leftward shifts in pointing were more pronounced. Second, the effect was not symmetrical. Unlike control participants, the individuals with UN did not show a corresponding post-adaptation rightward shift in pointing after using goggles that produced a 10-degree leftward optical shift.

13. Harvey, Hood, North, and Robertson (2003) provide data for another effective rehabilitation method that makes use of visuomotor-feedback training: grasping and lifting rods centrally while allowing for unlimited readjustment in locating a central grip. At 1-month follow-up, 14 patients with persisting neglect (between 5 and 25 months post-CVA) demonstrated significant improvements on the conventional subtests of the BIT and on the landmark test, but these improvements did not generalize to everyday activities. The authors explain these findings according to the Milner and Goodale (1995) theory of neglect, which indicates that preserved visuomotor (dorsal) control systems are possibly mediated by the undamaged superior parietal cortex in individuals with UN.

14. Longer-term benefits have been demonstrated at a 2–3 month follow-up when standard treatments (such as visual scanning procedures) have been combined with either neck muscle vibration (Schindler et al., 2002) or optokinetic stimulation (Zoccolotti et al., 1992).

15. These categories had been developed by first presenting the drawings to neurologically intact individuals, dividing each drawing into 12 one-centimetre segments,

and presenting each segment from right-to-left for identification. This procedure allowed the experimenters to determine the segment boundary (from 1 to 12) at which neurologically intact individuals could correctly name a particular drawing. For the purpose of comparison between the two studies to be presented, the categories have been renamed in this discussion: identification-left, unexpected-left, and symmetrical-left.

REFERENCES

Aglioti, S., Smania, N., Barbieri, C., & Corbetta, M. (1997). Influence of stimulus salience and attentional demands on visual search patterns in hemispatial neglect. *Brain and Cognition, 34*, 388–403.

Aimola, A. M. (1999). *Dark side of the moon: Studies in unilateral neglect.* Unpublished doctoral dissertation, University of Auckland, Auckland, New Zealand.

Aimola Davies, A. M., & Ogden, J. A. (2003). Anosognosia for extrapersonal neglect, personal neglect, and hemiplegia: A study of nine patients with persisting unilateral neglect. Manuscript submitted for publication.

Albert, M. L. (1973). A simple test of visual neglect. *Neurology, 23*, 658–664.

Antonucci, G., Guariglia, C., Judica, A., Magnotti, L., Paolucci, S., Pizzamiglio, L., & Zoccolotti, P. (1995). Effectiveness of neglect rehabilitation in a randomized group study. *Journal of Clinical and Experimental Neuropsychology, 17*, 383–389.

Beschin, N., & Robertson, I. H. (1997). Personal versus extrapersonal neglect: A group study of their dissociation using a reliable clinical test. *Cortex, 33*, 379–384.

Bisiach, E., Capitani, E., Luzzatti, C., & Perani, D. (1981). Brain and conscious representation of outside reality. *Neuropsychologia, 19*, 543–551.

Bisiach, E., & Geminiani, G. (1991). Anosognosia related to hemiplegia and hemianopia. In G. P. Prigatano & D. L. Schacter (Eds.), *Awareness of deficit after brain injury: Clinical and theoretical issues.* Oxford: Oxford University Press

Bisiach, E., Perani, D., Vallar, G., & Berti, A. (1986). Unilateral neglect: Personal and extra-personal. *Neuropsychologia, 24*, 759–767.

Bisiach, E., Vallar, G., Perani, D., Papagno, C., & Berti, A. (1986). Unawareness of disease following lesions of the right hemisphere: Anosognosia for hemiplegia and anosognosia for hemianopia. *Neuropsychologia, 24*, 471–482.

Brown, V., Walker, R., Gray, C., & Findlay, J. M. (1999). Limb activation and the rehabilitation of unilateral neglect: Evidence of task specific effects. *Neurocase, 5*, 129–142.

Brunila, T., Lincoln, N., Lindell, A., Tenovuo, O., & Hamalainen, H. (2002). Experiences of combined visual training and arm activation in the rehabilitation of unilateral visual neglect: A clinical study. *Neuropsychological Rehabilitation, 12*, 27–40.

Cappa, S., Sterzi, R., Vallar, G., & Bisiach, E. (1987). Remission of hemineglect and anosognosia during vestibular stimulation. *Neuropsychologia, 25*, 775–782.

Colombo, A., De Renzi, E., & Gentilini, M. (1982). The time course of visual hemi-inattention. *Archiv für Psychiatrie und Nervenkrankheiten, 29*, 644–653.

Corbetta, M., Miezin, F. M., Shulman, G. L., & Petersen, S. E. (1993). A PET study of visuospatial attention. *Journal of Neuroscience, 13*, 1202–1226.

Cowey, A., Small, M., & Ellis, S. (1994). Left visuo-spatial neglect can be worse in far than in near space. *Neuropsychologia, 32*, 1059–1066.

Cubelli, R., Nichelli, P., Bonito, V., De Tanti, A., & Inzaghi, M. G. (1991). Different patterns of dissociation in unilateral spatial neglect. *Brain and Cognition, 15,* 139–159.

Damasio, A. R., Damasio, H., & Chang Chui, H. (1980). Neglect following damage to frontal lobe and basal ganglia. *Neuropsychologia, 18,* 123–132.

Delis, D. C., Kiefner, M., & Fridlund, A. J. (1988). Visuospatial dysfunctions following unilateral brain damage: Dissociations in hierarchical and hemispatial analysis. *Journal of Clinical and Experimental Neuropsychology, 10,* 421–431.

Demeurisse, G., Hublet, C., Paternot, J., Colson, C., & Serniclaes, W. (1997). Pathogenesis of subcortical visuo-spatial neglect: A HMPAO SPECT study. *Neuropsychologia, 35,* 731–735.

Denes, G., Semenza, C., Stoppa, E., & Lis, A. (1982). Unilateral spatial neglect and recovery from hemiplegia. *Brain, 105,* 543–552.

Deuel, R. K., & Collins, R. C. (1983). Recovery from unilateral neglect. *Experimental Neurology, 81,* 733–748.

Diller, L., & Riley, E. (1993). The behavioural management of neglect. In I. H. Robertson & J. C. Marshall (Eds.), *Unilateral neglect: Clinical and experimental studies.* Hove, UK: Erlbaum.

Doricchi, F., Incoccia, C., & Galati, G. (1997). Influence of figure-ground contrast on the implicit and explicit processing of line drawings in patients with left unilateral neglect. *Cognitive Neuropsychology, 14,* 573–594.

Driver, J., Baylis, G. C., & Rafal, R. (1992). Preserved figure-ground segregation and symmetry perception in visual neglect. *Nature, 360,* 73–75.

Driver, J., & Halligan, P. W. (1991). Can visual neglect operate in object-centered co-ordinates? an affirmative single-case study. *Cognitive Neuropsychology, 8,* 475–496.

Egelko, S., Gordon, W. A., Hibbard, M. R., Diller, L., Lieberman, A., Holliday, R., et al. (1988). Relationship among CT scans, neurological exam, and neuropsychological test performance in right brain damaged stroke patients. *Journal of Clinical and Experimental Neuropsychology, 10,* 539–564.

Egly, R., Rafal, R., Driver, J., & Starrveveld, Y. (1994). Covert orienting in the split brain reveals hemispheric specialization for object-based attention. *Psychological Science, 5,* 380–383.

Farah, M. J., Monheit, M. A., & Wallace, M. A. (1991). Unconscious perception of "extinguished" visual stimuli: Reassessing the evidence. *Neuropsychologia, 29,* 949–958.

Fernandez-Duque, D., & Posner, M. I. (1997). Relating the mechanism of orienting and alerting. *Neuropsychologia, 35,* 477–486.

Ferro, J. M., Kertesz, A., & Black, S. E. (1987). Subcortical neglect: Quantitation, anatomy, and recovery. *Neurology, 37,* 1487–1492.

Findlay, J. M., & Walker, R. (1996). Visual attention and saccadic eye movements in normal human subjects and in patients with unilateral neglect. In H. S. Stiehl, W. H. Zangemeister, & C. Freska (Eds.), *Visual attention and cognition.* Amsterdam: Elsevier Science.

Fink, G. R., Halligan, P. W., Marshall, J. C., Frith, C. D., Frackowiak, S. J., & Dolan, R. J. (1997). Neural mechanisms involved in the processing of global and local aspects of hierarchically organized visual stimuli. *Brain, 120,* 1779–1791.

Frassinetti, F., Angeli, V., Meneghello, F., Avanzi, S., & Làdavas, E. (2002). Long-lasting amelioration of visuospatial neglect by prism adaptation. *Brain, 125,* 608–623.

Gainotti, G. (1968). Les manifestations de négligence et d'inattention pour l'hemispace. *Cortex, 4,* 64–91.

Gainotti, G., Messerli, P., & Tissot, R. (1972). Qualitative analyses of unilateral spatial neglect in relation to laterality of cerebral lesions. *Journal of Neurology, Neurosurgery, and Psychiatry, 35,* 545–550.

Gialanella, B., & Mattioli, F. (1992). Anosognosia and extrapersonal neglect as predictors of functional recovery following right hemisphere stroke. *Neuropsychological Rehabilitation, 2,* 169–178.

Goodrich, S. J., & Ward, R. (1997). Anti-extinction following unilateral parietal damage. *Cognitive Neuropsychology, 14,* 595–612.

Grabowecky, M., Robertson, L. C., & Treisman, A. (1993). Preattentive processes guide visual search: Evidence from patients with unilateral visual neglect. *Journal of Cognitive Neuroscience, 5,* 288–302.

Halligan, P. W., Burn, J. P., Marshall, J. C., & Wade, D. T. (1990). Do visual field deficits exacerbate visuospatial neglect? *Journal of Neurology, Neurosurgery, and Psychiatry, 53,* 487–491.

Halligan, P. W., Manning, L., & Marshall, J. C. (1991). Hemispheric activation vs spatiomotor cueing in visual neglect: A case study. *Neuropsychologia, 29,* 165–176.

Halligan, P. W., & Marshall, J. C. (1989). Laterality of motor response in visuo-spatial neglect: A case study. *Neuropsychologia, 27,* 1301–1307.

Halligan, P. W., & Marshall, J. C. (1991a). Figural modulation of visuo-spatial neglect: A case study. *Neuropsychologia, 29,* 619–628.

Halligan, P. W., & Marshall, J. C. (1991b). Left neglect for near but not far space in man. *Nature, 350,* 498–500.

Halligan, P. W., & Marshall, J. C. (1993). When two is one: A case study of spatial parsing in visual neglect. *Perception, 22,* 309–312.

Halligan, P. W., & Marshall, J. C. (1994a). Focal and global attention modulate the expression of visuo-spatial neglect: A case study. *Neuropsychologia, 32,* 13–21.

Halligan, P. W., & Marshall, J. C. (1994b). Toward a principled explanation of unilateral neglect. *Cognitive Neuropsychology, 11,* 167–206.

Halligan, P. W., Marshall, J. C., & Wade, D. T. (1989). Visuospatial neglect: Underlying factors and test sensitivity. *Lancet, 2,* 908–910.

Harvey, M., Hood, B., North, A., & Robertson, I. H. (2003). The effects of visuomotor feedback training on the recovery of hemispatial neglect symptoms: Assessment of a 2–week and follow-up intervention. *Neuropsychologia, 41,* 886–893.

Heilman, K. M., Bowers, D., Valenstein, E., & Watson, R. T. (1987). Hemispace and hemispatial neglect. In M. Jeannrod (Ed.), *Neurophysiological and neuropsychological aspects of spatial neglect.* Amsterdam: Elsevier Science.

Heilman, K. M., & Valenstein, E. (1972). Frontal lobe neglect in man. *Neurology, 22,* 660–664.

Heilman, K. M., & Valenstein, E. (1979). Mechanisms underlying hemispatial neglect. *Annals of Neurology, 5,* 166–170.

Heir, D. B., Mondlock, J., & Caplan, L. R. (1983). Recovery of behavioral abnormalities after right hemisphere stroke. *Neurology, 33,* 345–350.

Husain, M., & Kennard, C. (1996). Visual neglect associated with frontal lobe infarction. *Journal of Neurology, 243,* 652–657.

Ivry, R. B., & Robertson, L. C. (1998). *The two sides of perception.* Cambridge, MA: MIT Press.

Joanette, Y., Brouchon, M., Gauthier, L., & Samson, M. (1986). Pointing with left vs right hand in left visual field neglect. *Neuropsychologia, 24,* 391–396.

Karnath, H.-O. (1988). Deficits of attention in acute and recovered visual hemi-neglect. *Neuropsychologia, 26,* 27–43.

Karnath, H.-O., Christ, K., & Hartje, W. (1993). Decrease of contralateral neglect by neck muscle vibration and spatial orientation of trunk midline. *Brain, 116,* 383–396.

Karnath, H.-O., Ferber, S., & Himmelbach, M. (2001). Spatial awareness is a function of the temporal not the parietal lobe. *Nature, 411,* 950–953.

Karnath, H.-O., & Hartje, W. (1987). Residual information processing in the neglect half-field. *Journal of Neurology, 234,* 180–184.

Karnath, H.-O., & Himmelbach, M. (2002). Strategies of lesion localization. Reply to Marshall, Fink, Halligan, and Vallar. *Cortex, 38,* 258–260.

Karnath, H.-O., Himmelbach, M., & Rorden, C. (2002). The subcortical anatomy of human spatial neglect: Putamen, caudate nucleus and pulvinar. *Brain, 125,* 350–360.

Karnath, H.-O., Schenkel, P., & Fischer, B. (1991). Trunk orientation as the determining factor of the "contralateral" deficit in the neglect syndrome and as the physical anchor of the internal representation of body orientation in space. *Brain, 114,* 1997–2014.

Kartsounis, L. D., & Warrington, E. K. (1989). Unilateral visual neglect overcome by cues implicit in stimulus arrays. *Journal of Neurology, Neurosurgery, and Psychiatry, 52,* 1253–1259.

Kinsbourne, M. (1987). Mechanisms of unilateral neglect. In M. Jeannerod (Ed.), *Neurophysiological and neuropsychological aspects of spatial neglect.* Amsterdam: Elsevier Science.

Kinsbourne, M. (1993). Orientational bias model of unilateral neglect: Evidence from attentional gradients within hemispace. In I. H. Robertson & J. C. Marshall (Eds.), *Unilateral neglect: Clinical and experimental studies.* East Sussex, UK: Erlbaum.

Kinsbourne, M. (1994). Mechanisms of neglect: Implications for rehabilitation. *Neuropsychological Rehabilitation, 4,* 151–154.

Làdavas, E. (1987). Is the hemispatial deficit produced by right parietal lobe damage associated with retinal or gravitational coordinates? *Brain, 110,* 167–180.

Làdavas, E., Berti, A., Ruozzi, E., & Barboni, F. (1997). Neglect as a deficit determined by an imbalance between multiple spatial representations. *Experimental Brain Research, 116,* 493–500.

Làdavas, E., Carletti, M., & Gori, G. (1994). Automatic and voluntary orienting of attention in patients with visual neglect: Horizontal and vertical dimensions. *Neuropsychologia, 32,* 1195–1208.

Làdavas, E., Del Pesce, M., & Provinciali, L. (1989). Unilateral attention deficits and hemispheric asymmetries in the control of visual attention. *Neuropsychologia, 27,* 353–366.

Làdavas, E., Paladini, R., & Cubelli, R. (1993). Implicit associative priming in a patient with left visual neglect. *Neuropsychologia, 31,* 1307–1320.

Làdavas, E., Petronio, A., & Umilta, C. (1990). The deployment of visual attention in the intact field of hemineglect patients. *Cortex, 26,* 307–317.

Maguire, A. M. (2000). Reducing neglect by introducing ipsilesional global cues. *Brain and Cognition, 43,* 328–332.

Maguire, A. M., & Ogden, J. A. (2002). MRI brain scan analyses and neuropsychological profiles of nine patients with persisting unilateral neglect. *Neuropsychologia, 40,* 879–887.

Manly, T. (2002). Cognitive rehabilitation for unilateral neglect: Review. *Neuropsychological Rehabilitation, 12,* 289–310.

Manly, T., Hawkins, K., Evans, J., Woldt, K., & Robertson, I. H. (2002). Rehabilitation of executive function: Facilitation of effective goal management on complex tasks using auditory alerts. *Neuropsychologia, 40,* 271–281.

Marr, D. (1982). *Vision.* San Francisco: W. H. Freeman.

Marshall, J. C., & Halligan, P. W. (1988). Blindsight and insight in visuo-spatial neglect. *Nature, 336,* 766–767.

Marshall, J. C., & Halligan, P. W. (1994a). Left in the dark: The neglect of theory. *Neuropsychological Rehabilitation, 1,* 161 168.

Marshall, J. C., & Halligan, P. W. (1994b). The yin and the yang of visuo-spatial neglect: A case study. *Neuropsychologia, 32,* 1037–1057.

Mattingley, J. B. (2002). Visuomotor adaptation to optical prisms: A new cure for spatial neglect? *Cortex, 38,* 277–283.

Mattingley, J. B., Robertson, I. H., & Driver, J. (1998). Modulation of covert visual attention by hand movement: Evidence from parietal extinction after right-hemisphere damage. *Neurocase, 4,* 245–253.

McGlinchey-Berroth, R., Milberg, W. P., Verfaellie, M., Grande, L., D'Esposito, M., & Alexander, M. (1996). Semantic processing and orthographic specificity in hemispatial neglect. *Journal of Cognitive Neuroscience, 8,* 291–304.

McIntosh, R. D., Rossetti, Y., & Milner, A. D. (2002). Prism adaptation improves chronic visual and haptic neglect: A single case study. *Cortex, 38,* 309–320.

Meichenbaum, D., & Goodman, J. (1971). Training impulsive children to talk to themselves: A means of developing self-control. *Journal of Abnormal Psychology, 77,* 115–126.

Mesulam, M.-M. (1981). A cortical network for directed attention and unilateral neglect. *Annals of Neurology, 10,* 309–329.

Michel, C., Pisella, L., Halligan, P. W., Luaute, J., Rode, G., Boisson, D., & Rossetti, Y. (2003). Simulating unilateral neglect in normals using prism adaptation: Implications for theory. *Neuropsychologia, 41,* 25–39.

Milner, A. D., & Goodale, M. A. (1995). *The visual brain in action.* Oxford: Oxford University Press.

Motomura, N., Yamadori, A., Mori, E., Ogura, J., Sakai, T., & Sawada, S. (1986). Unilateral spatial neglect due to haemorrhage in the thalamic region. *Acta Neurologica Scandinavica, 74,* 190–194.

Navon, D. (1977). Forest before trees: The precedence of global features in visual perception. *Cognitive Psychology, 9,* 353–383.

Ogden, J. A. (1985a). Anterior-posterior interhemispheric differences in the loci of lesions producing visual hemineglect. *Brain and Cognition, 4,* 59–75.

Ogden, J. A. (1985b). Contralesional neglect of constructed visual images in right and left brain-damaged patients. *Neuropsychologia, 23*, 273–277.

Ogden, J. A. (1987). The 'neglected' left hemisphere and its contribution to visuospatial neglect. In M. Jeannerod (Ed.), *Neurophysiological and neuropsychological aspects of spatial neglect.* Amsterdam: Elsevier Science.

Paolucci, S., Antonucci, G., Guariglia, C., Magnotti, L., Pizzamiglio, L., & Zoccolotti, P. (1996). Facilitatory effect of neglect rehabilitation on the recovery of left hemiplegic stroke patients: A cross-over study. *Journal of Neurology, 243*, 308–314.

Pardo, J. V., Fox, P. T., & Raichle, M. E. (1991). Localisation of a human system for sustained attention by positron emission tomography. *Nature, 349*, 61–64.

Perani, D., Vallar, G., Paulesu, E., Alberoni, M., & Fazio, F. (1993). Left and right hemisphere contribution to recovery from neglect after right hemisphere damage: An [18F]FDG PET study of two cases. *Neuropsychologia, 31*, 115–125.

Petersen, S. E., Corbetta, M., Miezin, F. M., & Shulman, G. L. (1994). PET studies of parietal involvement in spatial attention: Comparison of different task types. *Canadian Journal of Experimental Psychology, 48*, 319–338.

Pizzamiglio, L., Antonucci, G., Judica, A., Montenero, P., Razzano, C., & Zoccolotti, P. (1992). Cognitive rehabilitation of the hemineglect disorder in chronic patients with unilateral right-brain damage. *Journal of Clinical and Experimental Neuropsychology, 14*, 901–923.

Pizzamiglio, L., Frasca, R., Guariglia, C., Incoccia, C., & Antonucci, G. (1990). Effect of optokinetic stimulation in patients with visual neglect. *Cortex, 26*, 535–540.

Posner, M. I. (1995). Attention in cognitive neuroscience: An overview. In M. S. Gazzaniga (Ed.), *The cognitive neurosciences.* Cambridge, MA: MIT Press.

Posner, M. I., Inhoff, A. W., Friedrich, F. J., & Cohen, A. (1987). Isolating attentional systems: A cognitive-anatomical analysis. *Psychobiology, 15*, 107–121.

Posner, M. I., & Petersen, S. E. (1990). The attention system of the human brain. *Annual Review of Neuroscience, 13*, 25–42.

Posner, M. I., Walker, J. A., Friedrich, F. J., & Rafal, R. D. (1984). Effects of parietal injury on covert orienting of attention. *Journal of Neuroscience, 4*, 1863–1874.

Posner, M. I., Walker, J. A., Friedrich, F. J., & Rafal, R. D. (1987). How do the parietal lobes direct covert attention. *Neuropsychologia, 25*, 135–145.

Rafal, R., & Robertson, L. C. (1995). The neurology of visual attention. In M. S. Gazzaniga (Ed.), *The cognitive neurosciences.* Cambridge, MA: MIT Press.

Reuter-Lorenz, P. A., Kinsbourne, M., & Moscovitch, M. (1990). Hemispheric control of spatial attention. *Brain and Cognition, 12*, 240–266.

Riddoch, M. J., & Humphreys, G. W. (1983). The effect of cueing on unilateral neglect. *Neuropsychologia, 21*, 589–599.

Riddoch, M. J., & Humphreys, G. W. (1987). Perceptual and action systems in unilateral visual neglect. In M. Jeannerod (Ed.), *Neurophysiological and neuropsychological aspects of spatial neglect.* Amsterdam: Elsevier Science.

Rizzolatti, G., & Berti, A. (1993). Neural mechanisms of spatial neglect. In I. H. Robertson & J. C. Marshall (Eds.), *Unilateral neglect: Clinical and experimental studies.* Hove, UK: Erlbaum.

Rizzolatti, G., & Camarda, R. (1987). Neural circuits for spatial attention and unilateral neglect. In M. Jeannerod (Ed.), *Neurophysiological and neuropsychological aspects of neglect.* Amsterdam: Elsevier Science.

Rizzolatti, G., & Gallese, V. (1988). Mechanisms and theories of spatial neglect. In F. Boller & J. Grafman (Eds.), *Handbook of neuropsychology* (Vol. 1). Amsterdam: Elsevier Science.

Robertson, I., & Cashman, E. (1991). Auditory feedback for walking difficulties in a case of unilateral neglect: A pilot study. *Neuropsychological Rehabilitation, 1,* 175–183.

Robertson, I. H. (1999). The rehabilitation of attention. In D. T. Stuss, G. Winocur, & I. H. Robertson (Eds.), *Cognitive neurorehabilitation.* Cambridge, UK: Cambridge University Press.

Robertson, I. H., Halligan, P. W., & Marshall, J. C. (1993). Prospects for the rehabilitation of unilateral neglect. In I. H. Robertson & J. C. Marshall (Eds.), *Unilateral neglect: Clinical and experimental studies.* Hove, UK: Erlbaum.

Robertson, I. H., & Hawkins, K. (1999). Limb activation and unilateral neglect. *Neurocase, 5,* 153–160.

Robertson, I. H., Hogg, K., & McMillan, T. M. (1998). Rehabilitation of unilateral neglect: Improving function by contralesional limb activation. *Neuropsychological Rehabilitation, 8,* 19–29.

Robertson, I. H., Mattingley, J. B., Korden, C., & Driver, J. (1998). Phasic alerting of neglect patients overcomes their spatial deficit in visual awareness. *Nature, 395,* 169–172.

Robertson, I. H., McMillan, T. M., MacLeod, E., Edgeworth, J., & Brock, D. (2002). Rehabilitation by limb activation training reduces left-sided motor impairment in unilateral neglect patients: A single-blind randomised control trial. *Neuropsychological Rehabilitation, 12,* 439–454.

Robertson, I. H., & Murre, J. M. J. (1999). Rehabilitation of brain damage: Brain plasticity and principles of guided recovery. *Psychological Bulletin, 125,* 544–575.

Robertson, I. H., & North, N. (1992). Spatio-motor cueing in unilateral left neglect: The role of hemispace, hand and motor activation. *Neuropsychologia, 30,* 553–563.

Robertson, I. H., & North, N. (1993). Active and passive activation of left limbs: Influence on visual and sensory neglect. *Neuropsychologia, 31,* 293–300.

Robertson, I. H., & North, N. T. (1994). One hand is better than two: Motor extinction of left hand advantage in unilateral neglect. *Neuropsychologia, 32,* 1–11.

Robertson, I. H., North, N. T., & Geggie, C. (1992). Spatiomotor cueing in unilateral left neglect: Three case studies of its therapeutic effects. *Journal of Neurology, Neurosurgery, and Psychiatry, 55,* 799–805.

Robertson, I. H., Ridgeway, V., Greenfield, E., & Parr, A. (1997). Motor recovery after stroke depends on intact sustained attention: A 2-year follow-up study. *Neuropsychology, 11,* 290–295.

Robertson, I. H., Tegnér, R., Tham, K., Lo, A., & Nimmo-Smith, I. (1995). Sustained attention training for unilateral neglect: Theoretical and rehabilitation implications. *Journal of Clinical and Experimental Neuropsychology, 17,* 416–430.

Robertson, I. H., Ward, T., Ridgeway, V., & Nimmo-Smith, I. (1994). *The test of everyday attention (TEA).* Bury St. Edmunds, UK: Thames Valley Test Company.

Robertson, L. C. (1996). Attentional persistence for features of hierarchical patterns. *Journal of Experimental Psychology: General, 125,* 227–249.

Robertson, L. C., Egly, R., Lamb, M. R., & Kerth, L. (1993). Spatial attention and cueing to global and local levels of hierarchical structure. *Journal of Experimental Psychology, 19,* 471–487.

Robertson, L. C., & Lamb, M. R. (1991). Neuropsychological contributions to theories of part/whole organisation. *Cognitive Psychology, 23,* 299–330.

Robertson, L. C., Lamb, M. R., & Knight, R. T. (1988). Effects of lesions of temporal-parietal junction on perceptual and attentional processing in humans. *Journal of Neuroscience, 8,* 3757–3769.

Robertson, L. C., Lamb, M. R., & Knight, R. T. (1991). Normal global-local analysis in patients with dorsolateral frontal lobe lesions. *Neuropsychologia, 29,* 959–967.

Robinson, R. G. (1985). Lateralized behavioral and neural chemical consequences of unilateral brain injury in rats. In S. G. Glick (Ed.), *Cerebral lateralization in nonhuman species.* Orlando, FL: Academic Press.

Rorden, C., Mattingley, J. B., Karnath, H.-O., & Driver, J. (1997). Visual extinction and prior entry: Impaired perception of temporal order with intact motion perception after unilateral parietal damage. *Neuropsychologia, 35,* 421–433.

Rossetti, Y., Rode, G., Pisella, L., Farne, A., Li, L., Boisson, D., & Perenin, M. (1998). Prism adaptation to a rightward optical deviation rehabilitates left hemispatial neglect. *Nature, 395,* 166–169.

Rubens, A. B. (1985). Caloric stimulation and unilateral visual neglect. *Neurology, 35,* 1019–1024.

Samuelsson, H., Jensen, C., Ekholm, S., Naver, H., & Blomstrand, C. (1997). Anatomical and neurological correlates of acute and chronic visuospatial neglect following right hemisphere stroke. *Cortex, 33,* 271–285.

Schenkenberg, T., Bradford, D. C., & Ajax, E. T. (1980). Line bisection and unilateral visual neglect in patients with neurologic impairment. *Neurology, 30,* 509–517.

Schindler, I., Kerkhoff, G., Karnath, H.-O., Keller, I., & Goldenberg, G. (2002). Neck muscle vibration induces lasting recovery in spatial neglect. *Journal of Neurology, Neurosurgery, and Psychiatry, 73,* 412–419.

Seron, X., Coyette, F., & Bruyer, R. (1989). Ipsilateral influences on contralateral processing in neglect patients. *Cognitive Neuropsychology, 6,* 475–498.

Söderback, I., Bengtsson, I., Ginsburg, E., & Ekholm, J. (1992). Video feedback in occupational therapy: Its effect in patients with neglect syndrome. *Archives of Physical Medicine and Rehabilitation, 73,* 1140–1146.

Sterzi, R., Bottini, G., Celani, M., Righetti, E., Lamassa, M., Ricci, M., & Vallar, G. (1993). Hemianopia, hemianaesthesia and hemiplegia after right and left hemisphere damage: A hemisphere difference. *Journal of Neurology, Neurosurgery, and Psychiatry, 56,* 308–310.

Stone, S. P., Patel, P., Greenwood, R. J., & Halligan, P. W. (1992). Measuring visual neglect in acute stroke and predicting its recovery: The visual neglect recovery index. *Journal of Neurology, Neurosurgery, and Neuropsychiatry, 55,* 431–436.

Sturm, W., Willmes, K., Orgass, B., & Hartje, W. (1997). Do specific attention deficits need specific training? *Neuropsychological Rehabilitation, 7,* 81–103.

Vallar, G. (1993). The anatomical basis of spatial hemineglect in humans. In I. H. R. J. C. Marshall (Ed.), *Unilateral neglect: Clinical and experimental studies.* East Sussex, UK: Erlbaum.

Vallar, G. (1998). Spatial hemineglect in humans. *Trends in Cognitive Sciences, 2,* 87–97.

Vallar, G., Bottini, G., Rusconi, M. L., & Sterzi, R. (1993). Exploring somatosensory hemineglect by vestibular stimulation. *Brain, 116,* 71–86.

Vallar, G., & Perani, D. (1986). The anatomy of unilateral neglect after right-hemisphere stroke lesions. A clinical/CT-scan correlation study in man. *Neuropsychologia, 24,* 609–622.

Vallar, G., & Perani, D. (1987). The anatomy of spatial neglect in humans. In M. Jeannerod (Ed.), *Neurophysiological and neuropsychological aspects of spatial neglect.* Amsterdam: Elsevier Science.

Vallar, G., Perani, D., Cappa, S. F., Mesa, C., Lenzi, G. L., & Fazio, F. (1988). Recovery from aphasia and neglect after subcortical stroke: Neuropsychological and cerebral perfusion study. *Journal of Neurology, Neurosurgery, and Psychiatry, 51,* 1269–1276.

Vallar, G., Rusconi, M. L., Bignamini, L., Geminiani, G., & Perani, D. (1994). Anatomical correlates of visual and tactile extinction in humans: A clinical CT scan study. *Journal of Neurology, Neurosurgery, and Psychiatry, 57,* 464–470.

Vallar, G., Sterzi, R., Bottini, G., Cappa, S., & Rusconi, M. L. (1990). Temporary remission of left hemianesthesia after vestibular stimulation. *Cortex, 26,* 123–131.

Volpe, B. T., Ledoux, J. E., & Gazzaniga, M. S. (1979). Information processing of visual stimuli in an "extinguished" field. *Nature, 282,* 722–724.

Walker, R., Findlay, J. M., Young, A. W., & Welch, J. (1991). Disentangling neglect and hemianopia. *Neuropsychologia, 29,* 1019–1027.

Weinberg, J., Diller, L., Gordon, W., Gertsman, L., Lieberman, A., Lakin, O., et al. (1977). Visual scanning training effects of reading-related tasks in acquired right brain damage. *Archives of Physical Medicine and Rehabilitation, 58,* 479–486.

Weintraub, S., & Mesulam, M.-M. (1987). Right cerebral dominance in spatial attention: Further evidence based on ipsilateral neglect. *Archives of Neurology, 44,* 621–625.

Wilson, B., Cockburn, J., & Halligan, P. W. (1987). *Behavioural Inattention Test.* Fareham, UK: Thames Valley Test Company.

Zoccolotti, P., Guariglia, C., Pizzamiglio, L., Judica, A., Razzano, C., & Pantano, P. (1992). Good recovery in visual scanning in a patient with persistent anosognosia. *International Journal of Neuroscience, 63,* 93–104.

7

■ ■ ■ ■

Disorders of Executive Functioning and Self-Awareness

Gary R. Turner
Brian Levine

Executive functions and self-awareness are among the highest achievements of brain evolution. These capacities allow us to willfully transcend the immediate moment, to imagine nonexistent states of being, to make and execute plans, and to flexibly adjust these plans when necessary. In short, they are a major part of what distinguishes humans from other species. Because of their dependence on multiple interacting brain structures, they are highly sensitive to brain injury and therefore of interest to all clinicians involved in neurobehavioral assessment and treatment.

Imprecision and inconsistency in the definition and assessment of these strategies create unique clinical challenges. Although recent neuroscience research has advanced understanding of executive and self-aware abilities, these advances have not been consistently implemented in theoretically based, empirically testable rehabilitation programs.

In this chapter, we briefly review models of executive functioning and self-awareness, discuss the acquired neuropathologies most commonly associated with deficits in these areas, and describe the behavioral correlates of these disorders. We then report a systematic review of literature on interventions for these disorders, with suggestions that may help to narrow the gap between knowledge and practice in rehabilitation of executive functioning and self-awareness.

MODELS OF EXECUTIVE FUNCTIONING AND SELF-AWARENESS

Defining Executive Functions and Self-Awareness

Before going further, readers should pause for a moment to reflect on the sequence of activities that brought them to this point in the day. When did you first decide that you would take time from your schedule to pick up this particular text? Can you recall where you were, what was going on around you, what your thoughts were or what considerations may have gone into planning for this activity? What did you have to arrange in your schedule to make this time available? Perhaps you had to purchase the text from the bookstore or search for it on a library shelf. Maybe you had to prepare lunches for the kids, get them off to school, check your e-mail, and then rummage through your own bookshelves before being able to pick up the text and read to this section. Now think ahead to the next item on your agenda. Do you have any appointments for later today or tomorrow? How are you planning to get to there? Is there sufficient fuel in the car? What route are you going to take? Do the kids need to be retrieved from day care before or after your appointment? Will you be preparing a meal? Do you have all the ingredients? What shops will be open after your meeting?

Executive functions can be defined as a collection of abilities that map on to this example, including setting a personal goal (i.e., reading this chapter), weighing alternatives (e.g., Do I go to the gym? Read the chapter? Visit mom?), selecting a particular course of action (i.e., deciding on the chapter), sequencing intervening events (e.g., get kids to school, read e-mail, and find text) and regulating behavior to ensure the attainment of the goal (e.g., ignoring the phone or rejecting a lunch invitation) (Tranel, Anderson, & Benton, 1994). All these abilities share a common element of control and direction of more basic, lower-level abilities (Stuss & Levine, 2002).

Overlapping and supporting these is the uniquely human ability to maintain a consistent sense of self across time, from past to present to future, defined as autonoetic (literally, self-knowing) awareness (Tulving, 1985, 2002; Wheeler, Stuss, & Tulving, 1997). Stuss (1991) noted a relationship between this ability and frontal lobe function. He characterized the patients with frontal leukotomy/lobotomy as "having lost awareness of themselves as a continuing and changing entity with personal responsibility for such change" (p. 66). The notion of personal agency, or awareness of the self as separate from the environment yet free to act on it (Kihlstrom & Tobias, 1991), is commonly invoked in accounts of awareness deficits following brain damage, especially involving the prefrontal cortex (McGlynn & Schacter, 1989; Prigatano, 1999; Stuss, 1991; Stuss & Alexander, 2000a).

In this chapter, we review selected models of executive functioning and self-awareness that have been most influential in neuropsychological research. Our presentation is roughly chronological to illustrate the constructs' evolution over the past two decades. Each of these models is useful, yet none alone fully accounts for this collection of mental capacities. While considerable heterogeneity exists among the models, each deals in some way with the prefrontal cortex (i.e., the region of the frontal lobes anterior to the motor strip), the most recently evolved and least understood area of the brain, occupying about 30% of the human cortical mantle (Semenderferi, Lu, Schenker, & Damasio, 2002). The study of brain–behavior relationships in this domain has had a unique history with respect to other mental abilities described in this text. Whereas attention, language, memory, and visuospatial processes have been studied as psychological constructs in their own right, then mapped to brain function, the study of executive processes has taken a somewhat opposite path. Executive and self-related functions have historically been defined in relation to patients with damage to the frontal lobes, usually with dramatic deficits, with executive and prefrontal functions treated mainly as synonymous.

This state of affairs has proven problematic for both theory and clinical practice. For theory, defining executive functions as "what the frontal lobes do" creates an infinite regression. Given the functional heterogeneity of the frontal lobes, adherence to the frontal = executive doctrine makes one vulnerable to shifting constructs depending on location of damage within the frontal lobes. Moreover, the prefrontal cortex is widely and reciprocally interconnected with the rest of the brain. Posterior, subcortical, and diffuse damage can therefore mimic prefrontal cortical damage through frontal systems disconnection (Kolb & Cioe, Chapter 1, this volume). In a clinical setting, patients with neurobehavioral deficits can have any or all of these in combination with focal prefrontal damage, complicating estimates of lesion–behavior specificity.

While our approach is to treat executive functions and self-awareness as viable constructs in their own right, their historical relationship to the frontal lobes cannot be avoided; practically all the empirical evidence reviewed here is drawn from either studies of patients with frontal damage or functional neuroimaging studies focusing on prefrontal function. The reader is advised to keep in mind that prefrontal damage is likely to cause a deficit in executive functions or self-awareness of one form or another, but also that these deficits are not solely the domain of the prefrontal cortex.

Models of Executive (Prefrontal) Function

Supervisory Attention System (Norman & Shallice, 1986; Shallice, 1982)

Norman and Shallice (1986) proposed that thought and action are controlled by distinct processing mechanisms in routine versus novel situations. In routine situations, where responses are considered to be automatic (i.e., without conscious awareness), action is controlled by individual schemas: automated programs capable of achieving relevant goal-states effectively and efficiently once initiated by environmental triggers (Shallice & Burgess, 1993). Routine action selection is controlled by a contention scheduling mechanism whereby any schema whose activation value exceeds an established threshold is brought online and all other competing schemata are suppressed through lateral inhibition processes.

The supervisory attentional system (SAS) is engaged when deliberate attention is needed for planning or decision making, troubleshooting, novel or technically difficult action, or resisting habitual response tendencies and temptations (Norman & Shallice, 1986). In such situations, routine environmental triggering of thought and action schemata are insufficient to generate an appropriate response (Shallice, 1988). The SAS involves multiple processes that guide behavior through three stages of action control: strategy generation, implementation, and monitoring (Shallice & Burgess, 1996). Disturbances of the SAS can account for the seemingly paradoxical behavior of patients with frontal lobe lesions: behavioral rigidity (i.e., perseveration) and distractibility. Unmodulated contention scheduling (resulting from diminished SAS control), following frontal lobe pathology, would produce perseverative behavior in situations whenever a single action schema is highly activated as a result of salient environmental triggers, represented in the extreme by utilization behavior (Lhermitte, 1983). Distractibility, on the other hand, results when multiple environmental triggers are similarly activated (Shallice, 1988, p. 336).

This model has proven fruitful in the analysis of behavior in patients (Shallice & Burgess, 1991) and test development (Burgess & Shallice, 1996a, 1996b). It has been particularly useful in the analysis of "strategy application disorder," the syndrome in which patients' behavior in naturalistic, unstructured situations is not governed by higher-level control mechanisms (Burgess, 2000; Goldstein, Bernard, Fenwick, Burgess, & McNeil, 1993; Levine et al., 1998; Shallice & Burgess, 1991). One problem with this model, however, has been the underspecification of the SAS, typically represented as a single box in diagrams. Supervisory attention is rather more likely to reflect a collection of control processes that modulate contention scheduling in different ways as proposed by Stuss, Shallice, Alexander, and Picton (1995), who fractionated the SAS into five discrete control processes, including the energization or inhibition of action schemata, adjustment of contention scheduling, monitoring of schema activity, and control of "if–then" logical processes. An important contribution of this model was the ability to associate discrete control mechanisms with frontal and posterior subregions. In Shallice's (2002) formulation, four discrete supervisory processes mediate behavior in nonroutine situations: (1) top-down modulation of schemata in contention scheduling—localized within left dorsolateral prefrontal cortex (PFC); (2) monitoring of behavior—mediated by right dorsolateral PFC; (3) specification of a required memory trace (i.e., retrieval mode)—associated with right ventrolateral PFC; and (4) establishment of future intentions—localized within the frontal pole (Brodmann's area 10).

Goal Selection and Goal Neglect (Duncan, 1986; Duncan, Emslie, Williams, Johnson, & Freer, 1996)

Duncan (1986) has argued that a principal function of the PFC involves the control of action by its desired result, observing that the disorganization of cognition and action is a common outcome following frontal lobe lesions. Drawing from early reports of patients with frontal lobe lesions (Bianchi, 1922; Luria, 1966) and approaches to machine-based problem solving (Newell & Simon, 1963), this model posits a central role for the PFC in the processes of goal formulation, action selection, and goal monitoring. Specifically, action is assumed to be directed by goal lists, series of task requirements that must be completed to achieve a desired goal state. These lists, in turn, guide the formation of action structures, which consist of component actions and mental operations that essentially provide a procedural map to the desired goal state. Finally, a continual "means–ends analysis" is carried out to assess the discrepancy that exists between current and desired goal states. This latter stage, in turn, guides the selection of new goal lists and action structures.

In keeping with this model, Duncan et al. (1996) suggest that a fundamental aspect of frontal lobe dysfunction may be "goal neglect"—the tendency of frontal patients to disregard the requirements of a given task even though they are able to retain these requirements throughout task performance. More recently, Duncan et al. (2000) have argued that goal neglect may be inversely correlated with the ability to pursue multiple goals simultaneously (i.e., dual-task performance) as well as measures of fluid intelligence (i.e., Spearman's g) and that these psychological constructs may share a common neuroanatomical substrate within the dorsolateral prefrontal cortex. Although this latter notion is controversial, Duncan's behavioral analysis of goal management has practical implications for clinical work and rehabilitation (Levine, Robertson, et al., 2000).

Working Memory (Baddeley, 1986; Fuster, 1997; Goldman-Rakic, 1987)

The maintenance and manipulation of information online has been central to models of prefrontal function since Jacobsen's (1936) discovery that monkeys with prefrontal lesions could not perform delayed-response tasks requiring the storage, maintenance, and use of spatial location information after a brief delay. The term "working memory" (Baddeley, 1986) has been applied to subsequent animal research as well as to research in humans involving the use of information held online in the service of more complex goals.

Fuster and Alexander (1970, 1971) identified prefrontal "memory cells" that fire only during the delay portion of a standard delay-task paradigm, providing a physiological basis for online storage of information. Later work identified separate "ramp-up" cells in which firing coincides with the upcoming response rather than the onset of the delay period (Quintana & Fuster, 1999). This line of research led to the conception of prefrontal function as cross-temporal mediation of behavior, with a neuronal architecture dedicated to online maintenance of past events and a second dedicated to anticipatory attentional (or motor) set (Fuster, 2000). By this view, the dorsolateral prefrontal cortex sits atop the perception–action cycle and acts as a bridge for the temporal separation of perception and action particularly in situations marked by novelty, ambiguity, and complexity (Fuster, 1997). This model of executive functioning is teleological in that it represents an ability to use information and knowledge drawn from past experience to influence future actions.

Goldman-Rakic (1987, 1996) has suggested that representational memory (the online maintenance of information no longer in the environment) and its use are properties distributed throughout the PFC in modality-specific working-memory circuits (e.g., dissociable "what" and "where" systems for working memory; Goldman-Rakic, 1996). This domain-specific view of prefrontal representational memory has been supported by intracellular recordings (Funahashi, Bruce, & Goldman-Rakic, 1993) and functional neuroimaging studies in humans (Courtney, Ungerleider, Keil, & Haxby, 1996) but has been contested by evidence in support of process specificity (i.e., online maintenance, manipulation, and inhibition; D'Esposito et al., 1998).

Although originating in animal work, this research has informed conceptualizations of executive disorders in humans by specifying basic building blocks of prefrontal function in ways that could not be accomplished in humans. Much of the work in humans has been done in the context of Baddeley's (1986) executive-slave systems model, in which auditory–linguistic and visuospatial slave systems (i.e., the articulatory loop and the visuospatial sketchpad) maintain representations in posterior cortices, while the central executive, located in the PFC, coordinates working-memory activity. More recently, Baddeley and Hitch (2000) have added a fourth component, the episodic memory buffer: an integrative, temporary store for multimodal, temporally extended "episodic" representations that serve as a conduit between long-term episodic memory and the online operation of working memory. While the authors suggest that this additional component may be considered as a fractionation of the central executive, as with the SAS (to which it has been directly related), the specific mechanisms of the central executive are underspecified.

Executive Knowledge (Structured Event Complexes)

Grafman (1995) has described neural representations of knowledge or symbols as the principal domain of the PFC. According to this model, higher-order cognition is controlled by hierarchically organized knowledge domains in the PFC. The basic knowledge unit in this system represents a set of events, actions, or ideas that are sequentially linked. These are, in turn, linked to each other in more temporally extended structured event complexes (SECs) that contain event themes, boundaries, and consequences. These SECs are analogous to the action schema of the model discussed earlier (Norman & Shallice, 1986). The SEC specified for cognitive planning, social behavior, and the management of knowledge is designated the managerial knowledge unit (MKU). MKUs themselves are hierarchically organized from the abstract (for guiding behavior in novel situations) to those that direct behavior in increasingly specified contexts. Research based on this model has used a script generation task (Sirigu et al., 1996; Sirigu et al., 1995; Zalla, Plassiart, Pillon, Grafman, & Sirigu, 2001) in which participants generate an action sequence describing a novel or familiar event and/or build coherent, logical action sequences from a list of actions. Although this model is differentiated from the others in its detailed description of the content (the "what") of executive operations, it lacks similar detail in its description of processes (the "how").

Somatic Markers (Damasio, 1994; Damasio, Tranel, & Damasio, 1991)

The ventromedial prefrontal cortex is uniquely positioned to integrate information from all sensory modalities (the external world) with information about body states (visceral, autonomic, endocrine, and musculoskeletal; the internal world; Nauta, 1971) that can be used to mark future outcomes as advantageous or disadvantageous. These "somatic markers" bias decision making by narrowing the decision space (Damasio, 1994; Damasio, Tranel, & Damasio, 1990). Individuals deprived of this capacity beacuse of ventromedial prefrontal damage are prone to inappropriate, risky, and socially inappropriate behavior due to a failure of somatic markers heralding negative outcomes to influence behavior. This model and the accompanying notion of "acquired sociopathy" has been invoked to account for the remarkable behavior syndrome of patients with ventromedial prefrontal damage described in the case study literature (e.g., Eslinger & Damasio, 1985; Harlow, 1868).

Support for this model has been garnered from a card-game gambling task that mimics the ambiguity inherent in real-life risky situations (e.g., Bechara, Damasio, Damasio, & Anderson, 1994; Bechara, Damasio, & Damasio, 2000; Bechara, Damasio, Tranel, & Damasio, 1997). Decks in this game are stacked such that certain decks provide low rewards and low penalties and other decks provide high rewards and high penalties. Healthy adults quickly learn that the latter decks are too risky in spite of their high rewards. Patients with ventro-medial prefrontal damage and acquired sociopathy tend to select from the risky decks. Perhaps most important, when selecting from the risky decks, the pa-tients do not show the normal electrodermal responses that are presumed to reflect the autonomic signal that should bias them against the risky response (Bechara et al., 1997), providing a convincing link to the importance of somatic markers in this behavior.

The dissociations between these decision-making deficits and other "executive"-type functions presumed to be mediated by other prefrontal re-gions (Bechara, Damasio, Tranel, & Anderson, 1998) provide strong evidence for intraprefrontal functional specificity of executive processes (as opposed to a unitary model). Although dorsolateral prefrontal cortical cognitive reasoning functions are included in this model, these processes are not addressed in de-tail.

Transcending the Default Mode (Mesulam, 2002)

Mesulam (2002) has proposed a central role for the PFC in overcoming the "default mode," a state in which actions are dictated by drive-related stimulus-response linkages unmodified by either context or experience. In the default mode, actions are driven by the need for immediate gratification, choices are minimized, hard-wired responses are promoted, and the appearance of a stim-ulus cannot be differentiated from its significance. The executive functions of the frontal lobes overcome the default mode to allow more context-driven and less stimulus-bound responses to occur. These executive processes, including working memory, inhibition, significance mapping, and the encoding of context and perspective, all operate by inserting a buffer between stimulus and re-sponse, allowing for the consideration of alternatives and therefore behavioral flexibility. In short, the frontal lobes (as well as other heteromodal association cortices) free the individual from the rigid binding of stimulus and response.

Models of Self-Awareness

The past 10 years have seen a sharp increase in empirical investigations con-cerning self-awareness, including lesion studies (e.g., Stuss & Alexander,

2000a, 2000b), neuroimaging (e.g., Craik et al., 1999; Tulving, Kapur, Marko-witsch, et al., 1994), developmental studies (e.g., Zelazo & Zelazo, 1998), and animal studies (Gallup, 1994). Nonetheless, few models of self-awareness have been described in the literature. An important distinction in this literature is that between modality-specific unawareness or anosognosias (such as that seen in association with hemispatial neglect) and more general unawareness of cognitive and behavioral deficits across multiple modalities. The former has been associated with a monitoring disturbance in cognitive operations downstream from more basic sensory processing, possibly in association with inferior parietal damage, whereas the latter is more likely seen in association with prefrontal damage (Bisiach, Vallar, Perani, Papagno, & Berti, 1986; McGlynn & Schacter, 1989; Nauta, 1971)

Stuss (1991) and Stuss and Alexander (2000a) have described a hierarchical model of self-awareness in which the frontal lobes are the site of the highest level of processing in an integrated system for the interpretation of and response to incoming information. The first stage involves basic arousal. At the second level, a model of the self and its environs emerges from the mapping of emotional processing onto unelaborated perceptual information within the association cortices of the posterior cortex. At the next level, executive functions, mediated by the frontal lobes, moderate between the outputs of posterior processes. The weaving of emotion with these executive control processes is presumed to result in a broader world model—one that can guide behavior in novel situations or generate socially or psychologically adaptive behaviors. At the highest level of integration, highly processed perceptual information, elaborated by associative processes (i.e., experience and expectation), is integrated with emotional input, transforming an objective experience into a subjective one that can be used to guide future behavior. It is this extended temporality, a subjective sense of a personal continuity, the ability to draw emotionally laden events from the past and use them to guide future behavior that is disturbed following damage to the PFC and, perhaps more specifically, the frontal poles (see Stuss & Alexander, 2000a). This capacity, described by Tulving (1985) as autonoetic consciousness, draws on the subjective reexperiencing of, in James's words, the warmth, intimacy, and immediacy of past, personal history.

DISSOCIATING PREFRONTAL ANATOMY AND FUNCTION

The PFC can be subdivided according to gyral anatomy, vascular zones, corticocortical connections, thalamic projections, cytoarchitecture, or neurotransmitter systems. None of these methods used alone is entirely satisfactory. Brain–behavior mapping in prefrontal and other heteromodal cortices is more complex than is the case for more upstream neural operations (Mesulam, 1998). Seemingly distinct behavioral operations are subserved by multiple prefrontal regions, and seemingly discrete prefrontal regions subserve multiple behavioral operations, a state known as degenerate mapping. For clinical purposes, this means that impaired test performance may not be specific to damage in a single region of association cortex, and that deficits observed on more than one task need not necessarily imply multiple lesions (Mesulam, 1998).

While the foregoing suggests that a task-oriented view toward prefrontal functional heterogeneity is perilous, frontal subdivisions can nonetheless be defined based on the following anatomical dimensions: left–right, dorsal–ventral, lateral–medial, and anterior–posterior. Damage to one of these dimensions can be related to syndromes of behavior, impairments on classes of task, and possible rehabilitation outcomes. These dimensions are now briefly reviewed. For more detail, the reader is referred to Mesulam (2002), Stuss and Levine (2002), Passingham (1993), and Petrides and Pandya, (1994, 2002).

The frontal hemispheric distinction mirrors that described for right- and left-lateralized operations in general (for right-handers), with the right prefrontal lobe involved in holistic operations and emotional processes, and the left preferentially involved in sequential (particularly verbal) operations. Material-specific effects can be found for visual (right frontal) and verbal (left frontal) tasks (Glosser & Goodglass, 1990), but in many cases the executive nature of the task overrides material specificity, so that patients with either right or left frontal damage are impaired (e.g., Petrides, 1985). In addition to the obvious functional significance of Broca's area (located in posterior left ventrolateral prefrontal cortex) for speech operations, the left prefrontal cortex mediates semantic processing, particularly in relation to mnemonic encoding (Tulving, Kapur, Craik, Moscovitch, & Houle, 1994). In contrast, the right prefrontal cortex is involved in establishing a mental set for mnemonic retrieval (i.e., retrieval mode; Lepage, Ghaffar, Nyberg, & Tulving, 2000) and output monitoring (Stuss et al., 1994), although additional left prefrontal participation occurs when retrieval tasks involve complex analysis and self-cueing for additional retrieval (Nolde, Johnson, & Raye, 1998).

Evolutionary theory of cortical architectonics, originated by Sanides (1970) and elaborated by Pandya and Yeterian (1996a), describes two cytoarchitectonic trends: dorsal and ventral. The dorsal (archicortical) trend emerges from the entorhinal/hippocampal complex and encompasses the dorsolateral regions of the prefrontal cortex (DLPFC), whereas the ventral (paleocortical) trend emerges from the olfactory cortex and encompasses the orbital and ventral regions of the prefrontal cortex (VPFC). Relative to lateral prefrontal cortex, medial sectors are more closely related to limbic nuclei and thus to internal states (Barbas, 1995).

The DLPFC, particularly the lateral sector, is associated with spatial and conceptual reasoning, certain attentional functions (e.g., switching and response preparation) and monitoring within working memory (Petrides, Alivisatos, Evans, & Meyer, 1993; Stuss, Shallice, Alexander, & Picton, 1995). Because most neuropsychological tests of prefrontal functions emerged from research in patients with DLPFC dysfunction, these are the processes most reliably assessed by tests of executive functioning (e.g., Milner, 1963).

Medial prefrontal cortex arising from the dorsal trend encompasses the cingulate, supplementary motor, and high medial frontal systems involved in activation and initiation (Pandya & Yeterian, 1996b). Damage to these regions disrupts the linkage between intention and behavior (Goldberg, 1985). Acute bilateral damage to these regions can cause akinetic mutism, a syndrome of profound inactivity in which there is no influence of internal drive states on behavior. More subtle manifestations (often seen upon resolution of akinetic mutism) include reduced initiative and drive (i.e., an abulic or "pseudo-depressed" syndrome; Blumer & Benson, 1975). Patients with high medial lesions respond better to external than to internal cues. Accordingly, patients with high medial frontal damage may be more likely to benefit from environmental prosthetics (cues, lists, alarms) than from retraining of internal drive states.

Relative to DLPFC, behaviors associated with VPFC are more impervious to neuropsychological investigation (Stuss & Levine, 2002). As noted previously, this region is intimately connected with the limbic nuclei involved in emotional processing and is involved in establishing and reversing reward associations and inhibition (Rolls, 2002). The association of VPFC with emotion, reward, and inhibition processes also suggests a broader role for this region in higher-order capacities such as decision making (see above) and strategic self-regulation (Levine, 2002; Levine, Dawson, Boutet, Schwartz, & Stuss, 2000). Patients with VPFC damage have impairments in the reversal of prior stimulus–reward associations. Recent functional imaging work has related this function to lateral VPFC (Elliott, Dolan, & Frith, 2000), where damage can cause irritability and impulsivity. Medial VPFC is more directly linked with limbic emotional centers and is involved in the creation and monitoring of stimulus–reward associations in incompletely specified situations (Elliott et al., 2000) and affective biasing of decisions (see earlier section on somatic marker theory, Damasio, 1994).

On the anterior–posterior plane, pyramidal motor output is greatest in the posterior premotor regions and declines with an increasing anterior gradient, where more complex cognitive operations prevail. The frontal poles (i.e., Brodmann area 10), have recently been identified as important to the highest-level introspective processes involved in complex information processing, including self-awareness, humour, and "theory of mind" (Christoff & Gabrieli, 2000; Shammi & Stuss, 1999; Stuss, Gallup, & Alexander, 2001; Stuss & Levine, 2002). Some of these processes are also associated with anterior medial paracingulate regions (Frith & Frith, 1999). In light of these recent findings, a distinction between executive control of cognition and executive control of awareness may begin to be drawn.

DISORDERS OF EXECUTIVE FUNCTION
AND SELF-AWARENESS

As noted previously, executive functions and self-awareness, while historically associated with the PFC, are vulnerable to disruption in any cerebral system, anterior or posterior, cortical or subcortical. They are further sensitive to changes in psychological status (e.g., anxiety) and daily fluctuations (e.g., fatigue). A survey of all disorders potentially affecting executive function and self-awareness would encompass all neurological syndromes affecting the cerebrum, as well as practically all psychiatry. In the following sections we focus on the most prevalent forms of acquired brain injury that have specific effects on prefrontal systems: frontal tumors, strokes, and traumatic brain injury (TBI). Although these are the most common causes of executive dysfunction and self-awareness deficits, this survey should by no means be seen as exhaustive. The clinician should be vigilant for these deficits in all patients.

Certain diagnostic and treatment considerations apply across multiple etiologies. The effects of lesion location often predominate over etiology effects (given similarities in other factors such as time course; Stuss et al., 1995). For example, a patient with a meningioma arising from the cribiform plate may appear more similar to a patient with a ruptured anterior communicating artery aneurysm than to a patient with a meningioma affecting DLPFC in the chronic phase of recovery. Both the former tumor patient and the aneurysm patient are prone to ventral frontal pathology and its associated behavioral disturbance that is less likely to be observed following high dorsolateral damage (see Kolb & Cioe, Chapter 1, this volume, for limitations on this view). In this section, we note factors distinguishing different etiologies rather than commonalities across etiologies, which are dealt with in the previous sections.

In syndromes with a recovering course, factors such as age of onset, time since injury, and individual differences such as intelligence, sex, and handedness may influence recovery (Kolb & Cioe, Chapter 1, this volume). Of these, epoch or time since injury appears to be a critical factor in treatment planning. Interventions may be most effective at a stage at which spontaneous recovery processes can be maximally engaged (Robertson & Murre, 1999). In other words, intervention before basic arousal and attentional mechanisms have recovered, or following the full course of naturalistic recovery, is often less effective than intervention in between these stages.

Stroke

Stroke is one of the leading causes of death from neural injury and represents a major source of chronic functional incapacity (Kandel, Schwartz, & Jessell, 2000; and see Kolb & Cioe, Chapter 1, this volume). A manifestation of cerebrovascular disease, stroke, or cerebrovascular accident (CVA) is the result of two broadly defined pathological processes occurring within the vasculature of the cerebrum: occlusion and hemorrhage. Occlusion is the most common form of disease process and leads to more than 80% of CVAs (Robinson & Starkstein, 1997). A second disease process underlying CVA is hemorrhagic injury including subarachnoid and intracerebral hemorrhage. Hemorrhages may have multiple etiologies, including ruptured aneurysms, arteriovenous malformations, hypertension, or traumatic injury (Kandel et al., 2000). Although hemorrhagic incidents represent a less common cause of CVA, their occurrence is particularly relevant to the study of frontal lobe dysfunction as 85–95% of aneurysms develop at the anterior portion of the cerebral arterial supply (DeLuca & Diamond, 1995). In general, the specific mechanism of injury, while a critical treatment variable, has figured less prominently in the study of chronic-phase neuropsychological syndromes associated with CVA where lesion location has been accorded a more central role.

Disorders of executive functioning and self-awareness after stroke are commonly described within the context of more broadly defined frontal lobe stroke syndromes. Each of these syndromes has been associated with damage to specific frontal brain regions resulting from vascular accidents involving the anterior branches of the middle cerebral artery (MCA), the anterior cerebral artery (ACA), or the anterior communicating artery (ACoA). Strokes involving the distribution of the main trunk or anterior branches of the MCA result in damage to lateral prefrontal brain regions, producing what has been described as a dorsolateral stroke syndrome (Anderson & Damasio, 1995). Damage is commonly unilateral and may involve cortical regions across the entirety of the lateral surface of the PFC, including premotor cortex, frontal operculum, and dorsolateral prefrontal areas. Executive function deficits related to MCA infarcts have been implicated most frequently with pathology of the dorsolateral prefrontal regions in the area of the superior and middle frontal gyri on the lateral surface. Specific deficits include stuck-in-set perseverations, working-memory disorders, and a generalized unawareness of deficient performance in these areas (Anderson & Damasio, 1995).

Mediofrontal syndromes arise as a result of aneurysms of the ACA or ACoA, typically causing bilateral medial frontal damage (Bogousslavsky, 1994). Infarcts arising from ACA aneurysms in the superior medial frontal regions impact the supplementary motor area as well as the anterior cingulate, producing a dorsomedial frontal lobe syndrome (see above, Anderson & Damasio, 1995). Bilateral destruction of the anterior cingulate and the supplementary motor area has been associated with generally slower and incomplete recovery (Anderson & Damasio, 1995).

The ACoA bridges the right and left anterior cerebral arteries (feeding the medial surface of the frontal lobes) as well as sending branches more inferiorly into white matter and basal forebrain regions. It is the source of almost 85% of all ruptured aneurysms within the cerebrum (DeLuca & Diamond, 1995). Specific deficits of executive functioning have been observed in the areas of cognitive inflexibility, poor planning, and concept formation (Bottger, Prosiegel, Steiger, & Yassouridis, 1998); distractibility; poor estimation (DeLuca & Diamond, 1995); perseveration; and reduced verbal fluency (Hillis, Anderson, Sampath, & Rigamonti, 2000; Tidswell, Dias, Sagar, Mayes, & Battersby, 1995). Self-awareness deficits have also been reported following the rupture of ACoA aneurysms, including loss of personal insight (Diamond, DeLuca, & Kelley, 1997), spontaneous (and often wild) confabulations (DeLuca & Diamond, 1995), unawareness of hemineglect (Ellis & Small, 1997), and decision-making deficits (Mavaddat, Kirkpatrick, Rogers, & Sahakian, 2000). While early research suggested that many of these symptoms were attributable to damage to basal forebrain structures, recent findings suggest that damage to this region and the ventromedial frontal region may be necessary to elicit the dense amnesia, confabulation, and personality changes that are the hallmarks of the ACoA syndrome (DeLuca & Diamond, 1995). Concurrent damage to both of these regions has been associated with poor outcomes.

Tumors

Frontal lobe tumors account for one-fifth of all supratentorial tumors (Price, Goetz, & Lovell, 1997). Accordingly, executive function deficits have been consistently reported as behavioral correlates of cerebral tumors (Leimkuhler & Mesulam, 1985; Nakawatase, 1999; Tucha, Smely, Preier, & Lange, 2000). Nonfrontal tumors can also cause deficits through diaschisis (i.e., the impairment of neuronal activity in a functionally related but distant region of the brain; von Monakow, 1914) and disconnection of frontal structures from other cerebral regions (Lezak, 1995; and see Lilja, Salford, Smith, & Hagstadius, 1992).

Neuropsychological assessment of the tumor patients should take into consideration the histological profile and growth rate of the tumor and secondary pathologies. Tumor histology may predict patterns of cognitive dysfunction, as has been observed with gliomas and meningiomas, the most common histological classifications of supratentorial tumors (Nakawatase, 1999). These two tumor classifications may result in different clinical presentation with fast-growing glioblastomas resulting in a poorer cognitive profile than a slower growing meningioma (Price et al., 1997).

In addition to destroying and displacing tissue, intracranial tumors may also produce cognitive dysfunction by inducing seizures, increased intracranial pressure, edema, and paraneoplastic syndrome. As described earlier, the reliance of executive function on extensive neural networks increases the susceptibility of higher cognitive processes to these secondary neuropathological processes (Tucha et al., 2000).

In general, the literature suggests a high frequency of behavioral changes associated with frontal tumors (Price et al., 1997; but see Anderson, Damasio, & Tranel, 1990). A recent study of tumor patients tested prior to the initiation of treatment noted both executive function and attentional deficits. Approximately 78% of patients demonstrated executive dysfunction (especially in the areas of concept formation and verbal fluency; Tucha et al., 2000). Deficits in executive functioning have also been identified in patients following surgery for pituitary tumors (Peace et al., 1997), possibly due to the disruption of ascending attentional systems or to a neurosurgical approach through the frontal lobes.

Traumatic Brain Injury

Owing to its high incidence (80,000–90,000 disabled per year in the United States) and prevalence (5.3 million in the United States disabled by TBI; National Center for Injury Prevention and Control, 1999) and its specific effects on the frontal lobes and their interconnections, TBI is arguably the most important single cause of disorders of executive function and self-awareness. Although interpretation of TBI effects is complicated by the co-occurrence of physical disability, it is the cognitive and behavioral consequences of TBI that are truly enduring, with a greater impact on outcome than physical symptoms (Brooks, Campsie, Symington, Beattie, & McKinlay, 1986; Dikmen, Ross, Machamer, & Temkin, 1995; Jennett, Snoek, Bond, & Brooks, 1981). The chronic disability of TBI is accentuated by its tendency to take place during early adulthood, affecting behavior for decades.

TBI induces a dizzying array of neuropathologies, the interpretation of which is complicated by time course effects and interaction with noninjury factors (e.g., the psychosocial milieu). As TBI pathophysiology is reviewed in detail elsewhere in this volume, this section focuses on aspects of this disorder, specifically pertinent to executive functions and self-awareness. For our purposes, a distinction between diffuse and focal injury provides a useful heuristic (Levine, Katz, Black, & Dade, 2002).

Diffuse axonal injury (DAI) is a crucial neuropathology and cause of coma in TBI (Adams, Graham, Murray, & Scott, 1982; Gennarelli et al., 1982; Povlishock, 1992; Strich, 1956). It is characterized by disconnection and eventual demise of axons, the result of a complex process studied at the molecular level (Maxwell, Povlishock, & Graham, 1997; Povlishock & Christman, 1995; see Kolb & Cioe, Chapter 1, this volume, for a similar description of stroke). When an axon is disconnected, its synaptic field is lost (i.e., it is deafferentated), affecting potentially thousands of neurons for each axon. While clinical radiological assessment focuses on macroscopic DAI lesions in white matter (Gentry, Godersky, Thompson, & Dunn, 1988) microscopic DAI pathology can be found throughout the neuraxis in the absence of macroscopic lesions (Povlishock, 1993). The behavioral consequences of this widespread disconnection syndrome include impaired arousal, inattention, and slowed information processing, particularly on complex tasks (Stuss & Gow, 1992). Owing to the reliance of frontal lobe function on connections to the rest of the brain, DAI also disrupts executive functions. The otherwise intact environment in which DAI occurs (15 per 1,000 axons damaged in a typical motor vehicular accident injury, Povlishock, 1993) is ripe for subsequent neuroplastic changes such as axonal sprouting and synaptogenesis (Christman, Salvant, Walker, & Povlishock, 1997; Povlishock, Erb, & Astruc, 1992; Kolb & Cioe, Chapter 1, this volume). We reported evidence for such changes at the systems level in a recent positron emission tomography (PET) study (Levine, Cabeza, et al., 2002) in which TBI patients demonstrated areas of increased brain activation relative to controls while performing cued recall tasks. These findings, which were present even when task performance was matched to controls, may reflect either cortical disinhibition due to DAI-induced deafferentation or functional compensation for inefficient mnemonic processes. While further work is needed to understand the precise implications of such neuroplastic changes, it is likely that such changes are involved in the recovery process and can be engaged by rehabilitation.

Focal parenchymal injury in TBI is typically due to contusion resulting from inertial forces causing localized damage in ventral and polar frontal and anterior temporal areas where the brain is confined by bony ridges of the inner skull, regardless of the site of impact (Clifton et al., 1980; Courville, 1937; Gentry, Godersky, & Thompson, 1988; Ommaya & Gennarelli, 1974). There is evidence that focal atrophic damage may exist in these regions even when lesions are not visible on conventional MRI (i.e., localized diffuse injury; Berryhill et al., 1995). The location of focal cortical contusions along the ventral trend has specific implications for disorders of executive functioning and self-awareness (Levine, 1999). As described earlier, the ventral trend is concerned with emotional behavior, reward processing, decision making, and self-regulation. In addition, the frontal poles that have been implicated in self-related information processing are vulnerable to contusion in TBI.

Analysis of the neurobehavioral consequences of diffuse and focal pathologies in TBI closely matches the clinical syndromes familiar to workers experienced with this population: information processing and self-regulatory deficits. While the attentional and information processing deficits are usually readily assessed by laboratory tasks, the self-regulatory deficits are more resistant to quantification in the laboratory. As a result, laboratory test results in patients with ventral frontal damage and self-regulatory disorder may not correspond to the degree of real-life disablement due to disinhibited social–emotional functioning and impaired decision making. A major challenge for clinicians is the development of new clinical measures for the identification and subsequent treatment of self-regulatory disorder due to ventral prefrontal damage in TBI (Levine, Dawson, et al., 2000).

REHABILITATION OF EXECUTIVE FUNCTION
AND SELF-AWARENESS DISORDERS

The following literature review includes published, peer-reviewed evidence on structured interventions expressly targeting the remediation of executive or frontal lobe functions and/or disorders of self-awareness following acquired brain injury. Papers were identified through searches of PsycINFO and Medline (using the following terms: "awareness," "executive" or "frontal," "problem solving," "reasoning," "rehabilitation," "remediation") and a review of reference lists from recently published works (e.g., Burgess & Robertson, 2002; Cicerone, 2002; Evans, 2001; Prigatano, 1999; Robertson & Murre, 1999; Sohlberg & Mateer, 2001). We also solicited recently published and submitted works from contributors to this field, which resulted in a list of 40 interventions drawn from 34 papers (Table 7.1). We excluded interventions expressly directed at attention, memory, and behavioral disorders as these are covered elsewhere in this volume. Within the area of awareness, we restricted our focus to those involving higher-order deficits (e.g., insight and judgment) associated with frontal lobe damage. We have not included holistic rehabilitation interventions in this review (see Prigatano, 1999; Ylvisaker & Feeney, 1996; Ylvisaker, Szekeres, & Feeney, 1998, for reviews). Pharmacological interventions have rarely targeted the remediation of executive function and/or self-awareness deficits. We include three such reports in Table 7.1 (McDowell et al., 1998; Powell et al., 1996; Van Reekum et al., 1995) and provide a brief review of this emerging area at the end of the section (for a review of pharmacological interventions and cognitive rehabilitation, see Arnsten & Smith, 1999). We have included single-case studies in our review for completeness, although emphasis is placed on data from group studies. Finally, in keeping with the theme of this volume, we have emphasized those interventions explicitly derived from the theoretical literature wherever possible.

Interventions are organized generally according to the primary categories of rehabilitation targets listed within the papers themselves: cognitive control, planning/problem solving/goal direction, initiation/motivation, self-awareness and self-monitoring (see Table 7.1). Although it would be appealing to adopt a more theory-driven categorization (as described earlier in this chapter), most of the work reviewed here was conducted under constraints of clinical pragmatics rather than theory testing.

Positive results within the training protocol, stability of gains upon cessation of the intervention and generalization of gains to nontrained tasks and daily living activities are tabulated for each intervention (Sohlberg & Mateer, 1989). Fully 100% of our sample reported improvements in target behaviors at the conclusion of treatment, most certainly an artifact of the "file drawer" problem (i.e., treatment failures are not submitted for publication). Nonetheless, nearly a third of the studies reported mixed success (highlighted as +, – in the results section of Table 7.1).

TABLE 7.1. Summary of Executive Function and Self-Awareness Rehabilitation Interventions

Study	Intervention	Participants	Study design	Outcome measure(s)	Results/follow-up	Generalization
Cognitive control processes						
Stablum et al. (2000) - 1	Training on dual-task paradigm	TBI (10)	Controlled group study	Dual-task speed, PASAT	(+) Dual task performance improved; gains stable at 3 months	Improved PASAT performance; anecdotal report of improved real-life tasks
Stablum et al. (2000) - 2	Training on dual-task paradigm	ACoA aneurysm rupture (9)	Controlled group study	Dual-task speed, PASAT and CPT	(+) Dual task performance improved; gains stable at 12 months; improvement on neuropsychological testing at 12 months limited to executive function measures	Improved PASAT/CPT performance
Cicerone (2002)	Cognitive self-monitoring, emotional self-appraisal, and "real-life" scenarios	Mild TBI (4); Control MTBI (4)	Controlled group study (prospective case design)	Pre-post performance on TMT A/B, PASAT, CPT 2 and 7 test, and self-report questionnaire	(+) Greater improvement on neuropsych measures for treatment versus control group (specifically on working memory component of PASAT)	Evidence (self-report) of decreased attentional dysfunction outside of treatment setting
McDowell et al. (1998)	Dopamine administration (bromocriptine)	TBI (24)	Group study (double blind, placebo control)	Dual task, Stroop, delayed response, verbal span, TMT, FAS, control tasks (non-EF)	(+) Bromocriptine = improved performance on all EF measures, no change on control task or working memory maintenance measure	No report
Cicerone & Giacino (1992) - 3	Error monitoring, feedback, correction, and modeling of desired response	TBI (2)	Case study	TOL errors, social behaviors	(+, –) TOL errors and inappropriate behaviors decreased; one required external cueing, one internalized self-monitoring	Clerical task (external cueing still necessary). No spontaneous application of strategy observed
Deacon & Campbell (1991)	Reaction time feedback, limited response windows	ABI closed (12)	Controlled group study	RTs relative to P300 latencies	(+) Reduction of P300 – response time gap	Increased response times maintained after cues removed. Processing speed improved without cost to accuracy

(continued)

241

TABLE 7.1. (*continued*)

Study	Intervention	Participants	Study design	Outcome measure(s)	Results/follow-up	Generalization
Initiation/motivation						
Powell et al. (1996)	Dopaminergic therapy (bromocriptine)	TBI (8); CVA (3)	Case study (reversal design)	Participation, reward responsivity, digit span, recall, verbal fluency, mood rating	(+) Improved performance on all measures; no change observed on mood rating scales; gains maintained 2 weeks after withdrawal in 8 of 11 subjects	No report
van Reekum et al. (1995)	Dopaminergic therapy (amantadine)	TBI (1)	Case study (double blind, placebo control)	Initiation behaviors	(+) Initiation behaviors improved significantly during drug versus placebo administration	No report
Burke et al. (1991) - 2	Self-initiation checklists	TBI (3)	Case study (multiple baseline)	Task completion, verbal initiation cues required	(+) Performance rates approached 100%; initiation cues reduced to near zero; gains stable (without checklists) out to 90 days	No report
Sohlberg et al. (1988)	External cueing	TBI (1)	Case study (multiple baseline)	Verbal initiation, social acknowledgment	(+) Increases in verbal initiation and nonverbal response acknowledgment	Anecdotal report of improved social responding in community setting
Planning/problem solving/goal management						
von Cramon et al. (1991)	Staged problem-solving training (PST)	ABI (20 PST; 17 memory training)	Randomized control design	IQ testing, TOH, planning simulation, behavioral rating	(+) PST group improved on 3/5 IQ subtests, TOH, planning test and behavioral ratings of awareness, goal direction, problem solving, and action style	Improved behavioral ratings of performance in novel situations
von Cramon, Matthes, & von Cramon (1994)	Staged problem-solving training (PST)	TBI (1)	Case study	Vocational performance, problem-solving simulation, awareness ratings (PCRS)	(+, –) Work performance improved; no change in problem-solving simulation or self-awareness ratings (i.e. PCRS discrepancy scores)	No generalization of training to novel situations
Levine, Dawson et al. (2000) - 1	Staged goal-management training (GMT)	TBI (15 GMT; 15 motor-skills training)	Randomized control design	Paper-and-pencil simulations of real-life tasks	(+) GMT group improved performance on all tasks (relative to motor-skills training control group)	Improvement on untrained paper-and-pencil task

242

Study	Intervention	Population	Design	Outcome measure	Results	Generalization
Levine, Robertson et al. (2000) - 2	Staged goal-management training (GMT)	Meningo-encephalitis (1)	Case study	Paper-and-pencil simulations of real-life tasks, meal preparation	(+) Improvement on experimental tasks. Meal preparation errors reduced (formal assessment and self-report). Gains stable at 6 months	Anecdotal report of generalization of training to other activities
Webb & Glueckauf (1994)	Goal-setting training	TBI (8 high, 8 low involvement)	Randomized control design	Goal-setting behavior	(+) Improvement in goal setting observed for both low-/high-involvement groups. Gains stable at 2 months *only for high-involvement group*	No report
Foxx et al. (1989)	Problem-solving training; cueing; feedback and monetary reinforcement	ABI (3)	Controlled group study	Problem-solving questions	(+) Problem-solving responses improved for experimental group after treatment. No change in control groups. Gains stable at 6 months	Problem-solving responses maintained at interviews and in novel, real-life scenarios
Cicerone & Wood (1987)	Self-instructional training	TBI (1)	Case study	Errors and "off-task" behaviors during TOL; WAIS-R subtests; WISC-R mazes; tinker-toy test.	(+, −) TOL errors and off-task behaviors decreased; tinker-toy score improved. No change in WAIS-R or WISC-R maze performance. Gains stable at 4 months	Scores on Self-control Rating Scale improved only after 12 weeks of specific generalization training
Cicerone & Giancino (1992) - 2	Self-instructional training	TBI (5); tumor resection (1)	Case study (multiple baseline)	TOL errors and "off-task" behaviors	(+, −) 5/6 = improvements in TOL, "off-task" behaviors and WISC-R mazes/ WCST perseverations; 1 patient (tumor) = no treatment effects	Spontaneous application in untrained situations observed in 2 patients who received additional generalization training
Burke et al. (1991) - 1	Formulation and usage of task-specific checklists	TBI (1)	Case study (multiple baseline)	Percentage of tasks completed independently	(+) Performance improved to 100% and was maintained upon withdrawal of task checklists. Gains stable at 3 months	Performance on a related but *untrained* task increased to 100%
Delazer et al. (1998)	Task-specific cues to aid in problem solving	TBI (3)	Case study	Correct problem-solving steps; solution accuracy	(+, −) Application of correct problem-solving steps improved; accuracy did not. Gains stable at 10 weeks	Improved problem-solving approach did not generalize to other error-free tests
Giles & Morgan (1990)	Verbal cueing and positive reinforcement	Herpes Encephalitis (1)	Case study	Washing behaviors	(+) Independent washing behaviors increased over course of treatment (with/ without cueing). Gains stable at 3 months	Anecdotal report of increased cooperative behaviors on ward

(continued)

TABLE 7.1. (continued)

Study	Intervention	Participants	Study design	Outcome measure(s)	Results/follow-up	Generalization
Honda (1999)	Self-instruction, problem solving, learning strategies	ACoA aneurysm (3)	Case study	WCST, Tinker-toy, WAIS-R, TMT, significant other interview	(+, −) All subjects improved on TMT & WAIS-R. 2/3 improved on Tinker-toy test. No improvement on WCST	Significant other interviews: positive behavioral change in all subjects following intervention
Hux et al. (1994)	Self-instructional training	Epilepsy (1)	Case study	Arithmetic problems; procedural and computational errors	(+) Accuracy increased without affecting productivity. Procedural errors decreased. Gains stable at 3 weeks	No report
O'Callaghan & Couvadelli (1998)	Self-instructional training	TBI (2); CVA (posterior)	Case study	Problem solving (wheel chair proficiency, table setting)	(+) Performance errors decreased from baseline to zero. Subject # 3 (TBI) performance improvement correlated with stimulant administration (i.e. arousal)	Only for posterior stroke patient
Evans et al. (1998)	Electronic cueing (Neuropage), task-specific checklists	AVM/CVA (1)	Case study	Medication schedule, plant watering, personal hygiene	(+) All target behaviors improved	No report
Manly et al. (2002)	Brief auditory cuing during task performance	TBI (9); CVA (1)	Controlled group study	Six-elements planning task	(+, −) Positive: # of tasks attempted; efficiency of time allocation. Unchanged: prospective memory tasks; time monitoring	No report
Self-awareness and self-monitoring						
Zhou et al. (1996)	TBI knowledge game, positive reinforcement	TBI (2); Anoxia (1)	Case study (multiple baseline)	Knowledge of TBI deficits; self vs. clinician ratings	(+, −) Improved knowledge of TBI deficits. No improvement on insight measure. Similar findings at 4 weeks	Anecdotal reports of improved deficit awareness outside of the treatment setting
Chittum et al. (1996)	Awareness game, positive reinforcement	ABI closed (3)	Case study (multiple baseline)	Responses to awareness questions	(+, −) Participants increased accuracy as compared to pre-game assessments; but accuracy rates ranged from 66 to 100%	Knowledge generalizability highly variable across participants (Range: 33–90%)

Study	Intervention	Population (N)	Design	Outcome measure	Result	Generalization report
Cicerone & Giancino (1992) - 1	Self-prediction paradigm with feedback	TBI (2)	Case study	Performance on TOL; response latencies and error rates	(+, −) Error-free performance. 1 subject spontaneously applied strategy; 1 patient continued to require cueing	1 patient demonstrated generalization to nontreatment environments; 1 required cueing to apply strategy
Youngjohn & Altman (1989)	Self-prediction paradigm with feedback	ABI (6)	Group study	Predicted vs. actual performance ratings	(+) Improved prediction of performance on calculation and verbal recall tasks. Gains maintained (but weakened) one week later	Anecdotal report of moderately improved deficit awareness
Rebmann & Hannon (1995)	Self-prediction paradigm with feedback and monetary reinforcement	TBI (2); AVM (1)	Case study	Predicted vs. actual memory performance	(+) Discrepancy between predicted and actual recall scores decreased (partial effects of lowered predictions and increased performance)	No report
Schlund (1999)	Feedback on performance (recall memory task)	TBI (1)	Case study	Predicted vs. actual memory performance	(+) Improved predicted and actual recall performance. Immediate predictions more reliable than at 24 hours retrospectively/prospectively	No report
Ownsworth, McFarland, & Young (2000)	Group intervention, education, strategy generation, and "real world" exercises	ABI (21)	Group study	Structured interviews and questionnaires (SADI, SRSI, HIBS, SIP)	(+) Improved self-regulation skills (awareness and strategy use); reduction on sickness impact measures (social, emotional, communication). Gains stable at 6 months	Anecdotal report of deficit recognition, anticipation of future consequences and strategy use in daily activities
Sohlberg (2000)	Individual awareness enhancement program (IAEP)	TBI (1)	Case study	Improved awareness and adoption of compensatory strategies	(+) Anecdotal report of improved awareness	No report
Deluca (1992)	Confrontation and feedback	ACoA aneurysm rupture (2)	Case report	Patient observation	(+) Anecdotal report of decreased incidence of confabulation	No report

(continued)

TABLE 7.1. (*continued*)

Study	Intervention	Participants	Study design	Outcome measure(s)	Results/follow-up	Generalization
Cicerone & Tannenbaum (1997)	Structured feedback program, external cueing.	TBI-orbito-medial frontal (1)	Case report	Tests of frontal lobe functioning; social cognition measures; SAI	(+,–) Improvement in emotional regulation (with cueing) and awareness. No improvement in self-monitoring and social cognition	Improvements limited to specific therapeutic context. No evidence of generalization to real-life tasks
Burke et al. (1991) - 3	Structured feedback, self-monitoring techniques	TBI (2)	Case study	Frequency of sexual behaviors	(+) Inappropriate sexual behaviors reduced to near zero for both participants. Gains maintained at 30 days/15 months	No report
Lira et al. (1983)	Self-monitoring program, problem recognition, positive self-verbalization	TBI (1)	Case study	Frequency of impulsive behaviors	(+) Significant decrease in violent outbursts. Gains stable at 5 months	Gains generalized to vocational setting
Alderman et al. (1995) - 2	Self-monitoring training, DRL	Herpes Encephalitis (1)	Case study	Frequency of target behaviors (verbal intrusions outside clinical setting)	(+) Target behaviors reduced with extended intervention (92 sessions). Gains stable at 5 months	Anecdotal report: gains maintained following move to less structured institutional environment
Knight et al. (2002)	Self-monitoring training, DRL	TBI, CVA (3)	Case study	Frequency of target behaviors	(+) DRL resulted in most rapid change; SMT resulted in greatest behavioral change. Gains stable at 3 months	Anecdotal report of spill-over positive effect on other rehabilitation activities

Note. TBI, traumatic brain injury; PASAT, Paced Auditory Serial Addition Task; CPT, Continuous Performance Test; TMT, Trail-Making Test (Parts A & B); FAS, Controlled Oral Word Association Test—Verbal Fluency (letters F, A, S); EF, executive functions; TOL, Tower of London task; ABI, acquired brain injury; RTs, reaction times; CVA, cerebrovascular accident; TOH, Tower of Hanoi task; PCRS, Patient Competency Rating Scale; WAIS-R, Wechsler Adult Intelligence Scale—Revised; WISC-R, Wechsler Intelligence Scale for Children—Revised; WCST, Wisconsin Card Sorting task; AVM, arteriovenous malformation; SADI, Self-Awareness of Deficits Interview; SRSI, Self-Regulation Skills Interview; HIBS, Head-Injury Behavior Scale; SIP, Sickness Impact Profile; DRL, differential reinforcement to low rates of behavior (operant conditioning).

Overall Summary of Research Design Characteristics

Design

The majority of reports are single-case studies. Twenty-six studies (65%) used quantitative single-subject methods while two (5%) reported qualitative data only. Three randomized control trials (RCTs) are reported (7.5%). Seven group studies (17.5%) used matched controls (not randomly allocated). Two group studies (5%) did not have control groups.

Participants

Data are reported for a total of 258 brain-injured patients of varying etiology, with the majority (59%) status post-TBI. For a large percentage of subjects (30%), mechanisms of injury were not specified; these are labeled "acquired brain injury" (ABI). The remainder of the sample consisted primarily of stroke survivors, encephalitis, or frontal tumor resections.

Outcome Measures

Twenty-seven (67%) of the studies used intervention-specific, nonstandardized measures as a component of their outcome efficacy assessment, ranging in complexity from real-world planning simulations to simple records of targeted behavioral change. Thirteen studies (33%) included standard neuropsychological tests or ratings scales as outcome measures.

Results/Follow-Up

All studies reported at least partial success, with mixed results noted in about a third of the studies. Nineteen (47%) interventions included reports of follow-up assessments (ranging from 1 week to 18 months following the cessation of treatment), with 16 of these 19 noting maintenance of positive changes at follow-up. The remainder of the studies reported mixed results at follow-up.

Generalization

Using liberal criteria (i.e., accepting both quantitative and qualitative evidence of skill transference), just under half of our sample (48%) specifically assessed generalizability as defined by performance on tests or in settings that were not specifically trained. Seven studies (18%) provided evidence of skill transference (either cued or spontaneous) to untrained tasks. A further 12 studies (34%) report the application of acquired skills within novel settings such as other rehabilitation programs, institutional settings, or the community. Only six studies (17%) specifically addressed the generalization from rehabilitation gains into real-world activities. Three studies reported failed attempts to generalize treatment gains to other tasks, environments or real-life activities.

Review of Interventions

Cognitive Control

Six interventions addressed deficits in dual-task performance, working memory, decision making, or monitoring. Stablum, Umilta, Mogentale, Carlan, and Guerrini (2000) drew on the model of a fractionated central executive (Shallice & Burgess, 1996) as the basis for their decision to explicitly target one of these—dual-task performance—for remediation following brain damage. The authors conducted a controlled group study to assess the feasibility of improving dual-task performance in patients with TBI through a direct training approach. Although both treatment and control patients improved on the dual-task paradigm, treated patients improved at a greater rate than did controls. Treated patients' larger gains on the Paced Auditory Serial Addition task (PASAT) relative to controls indicated generalization. Dual-task performance remained stable at 3-month follow-up with anecdotal report of improved real-life functioning (e.g., card playing). The authors replicated the intervention with a group of ACoA aneurysm rupture patients with similar success.

Cicerone (2002) suggested that impairments in the anterior attentional component of the central executive, as described by Baddeley (1986), compromised the efficient allocation of attentional resources following brain damage. He speculated that these deficits in "working attention" could be remediated using a staged training program involving increasingly demanding dual-task paradigms. As predicted, the training program improved working memory (as measured by the PASAT) in a group of four subjects with mild traumatic brain injury. In comparison to controls, there was evidence for improved allocation of working-attention resources (i.e., central executive functioning) among the treated patients. Reduced attentional dysfunction in daily activities was also noted.

McDowell, Whyte, and D'Esposito (1998), again drawing on Baddeley's model of the central executive, administered a D_2 dopamine receptor agonist (bromocriptine) to a group of 24 subjects with TBI in an effort to improve working memory and executive control functions in a double-blind, cross-over, placebo-controlled study. The authors report improvement related to drug administration on an experimental measure of dual-task performance and several neuropsychological measures of executive functioning.

No group study explicitly targeted the rehabilitation of error monitoring deficits (although this area is partially subsumed under other categories of intervention described later). Cicerone and Giacino (1992) have described two cases in which a verbal reinstatement strategy was used to improve self-monitoring. In both cases the patients' actions were immediately stopped by the therapist upon recognition of an error, feedback was provided, and the action sequence was repeated with guidance. In the first case, error logs were maintained and used for comparison in subsequent sessions. Improvements in error monitoring were observed on the Tower of London task and in an unrelated clerical task, but performance reverted to baseline on removal of the formal monitoring supports. In the second case, these same authors used immediate external prompting to increase error monitoring and improve feedback utilization. Anecdotal evidence indicated a reduction in socially inappropriate behavior, even when external prompting was ceased.

External cuing was also employed in a group study of decision-making speed (Deacon & Campbell, 1991). Both treated and nontreated patients with TBI improved reaction times when response-time feedback and delimited response windows were added to a choice reaction time task. External cueing preferentially improved reaction times of the patient group without affecting their accuracy rates. Moreover, the discrepancy between stimulus evaluation (as measured by P300 latencies) and reaction time was reduced to within-normal control levels for the patient group. The effect was subsequently demonstrated without external cueing, indicating that the decision-making process had been at least partially automated through the training process.

Initiation/Motivation

Deficits in initiation or motivated behavior are often a hallmark of frontal lobe damage. Clinical syndromes of abulia and, in extreme cases, akinetic mutism have been associated specifically with damage to the superior medial regions of the frontal lobes (Mesulam, 2002). Two interventions in this section used dopaminergic agents to address motivational deficits. In one study, bromocriptine therapy was related to improvements on measures of active rehabilitation participation, reward responsivity, and measures of executive functioning in 11 mixed etiology subjects, with treatment gains stable in 8 of the 11 some 2 weeks after withdrawal of treatment (Powell, al-Adawi, Morgan, & Greenwood, 1996). Additional positive evidence using amantadine (another dopamine agonist) was reported in a double-blind placebo-controlled case study in a patient with a severe abulic and apathetic syndrome (van Reekum et al., 1995). Positive findings appear to be secondary to the reenervation of, or compensation for, damage to dopaminergic projections from subcortical structures to the PFC implicated in behavioral responsivity to motivationally relevant stimuli. Dopaminergic inputs are particularly vulnerable to disruption by frontal lobe contusions and diffuse axonal injury commonly associated with TBI. However, a recent study by Schneider, Drew-Cates, Wong, and Dombovy (1999) questioned the efficacy of amantadine in remediating cognitive deficits following acute TBI. Negative findings were consistent across a broad assessment battery, including a composite measure of executive functioning and cognitive flexibility and contradicted earlier positive reports (Nickels, Schneider, Dombovy, & Wong, 1994).

Other than behavior modification interventions (see Alderman, Chapter 8, this volume), no group studies specifically targeting the remediation of self-initiation deficits were identified in our review. However, positive case study evidence has been reported using checklists (Burke, Zencius, Wesolowski, & Doubleday, 1991—three patients) and external cueing systems (Sohlberg, Sprunk, & Metzelaar, 1988).

Planning, Problem Solving, and Goal Management

The largest category of interventions (15, or 33%) address disturbances in the ability to link action with intention (Duncan, 1986; Luria, 1966). These interventions seek to reestablish internal regulation of behavior through structured, multistage training programs, targeted reinstitution of verbally mediated self-regulation, and external cueing. Problem-solving training (PST; von Cramon, Matthes von Cramon, & Mai, 1991) targeting five therapeutic goals (problem orientation, problem definition and formulation, alternative generation, decision making, and solution verification; D'Zurilla & Goldfried, 1971) was compared to memory training in a randomized control trial of mixed etiology patients. Training was conducted over 6 weeks for an average of 25 sessions, with additional training for patients demonstrating apathetic or abulic symptomotology. The PST group showed gains on various tasks of reasoning, the Tower of Hanoi, and other experimental planning tests. Behavioral ratings by staff members served as the sole indication of training generalization and no follow-up data were reported. A supplemental single-case study (von Cramon & Matthes von Cramon, 1994) also reported success in remediating specific vocational tasks using a variant of PST, but there was no effect on awareness ratings or problem solving in novel situations. Although this is a well-designed study, including a strong theoretical basis and a carefully matched control group, treatment gains were not consistently observed, nor was treatment generalizability reliably demonstrated. It is also problematic certain patients received extra sessions on the basis of their symptomatology.

Webb and Glueckauf (1994) randomly assigned patients with TBI to a high-involvement goal-setting group (including active strategies for prioritization and goal monitoring) or a low-involvement group (including preassigned goal lists but no formal monitoring training). Both groups made equivalent gains on ratings of goal attainment and goal change from pre- to posttesting, but maintenance of gains at 2-month follow-up was restricted to the high-involvement group. Another approach to remediating problem-solving deficits involving the utilization of specific criterion questions as cues to solve real-life problems was supported in a small controlled study of patients with TBI using scenarios and staged interactions (Foxx, Martella, & Marchand-Martella, 1989).

Drawing directly from Duncan's theory of goal neglect, Levine, Robertson, et al. (2000, experiment 1) applied a similar multistage process to that of von Cramon et al. (goal management training, or GMT; Robertson, 1996) in a brief "rehabilitation probe." Thirty subjects with TBI consecutively admitted to a trauma center were randomly assigned to either a GMT or a motor-skills training (MST) group. GMT consisted of five training stages—each relating to a separate goal management process: orienting, goal setting, partitioning goals into subgoals, encoding and retention of goals, and monitoring. Pre- and posttraining performance was assessed by paper-and-pencil tests designed to mimic real-life tasks that pose problems for patients (e.g., proof reading). The results suggested a beneficial effect of GMT training over and above gains demonstrated in the MST group (due to repeated test administration or contact with the trainer). As this was a very brief intervention experiment designed to assess the potential efficacy of GMT, no follow-up data were collected. However, a more extensive application of GMT was successfully applied in a single-case study of a postencephalitic patient, with training adapted to improve meal preparation (Levine, Robertson, et al., 2000, experiment 2). GMT is currently being addressed in larger-scale RCTs.

A second strategy that has been used to bridge the gap between intention and action commonly seen following frontal lobe damage is the targeted reestablishment of verbal self-regulation. Luria and Homskaya (1964) suggested that self-regulation is mediated by covert, "inner speech" which provides a critical bridging mechanism between the general intention to solve a problem and its concrete solution. A case study by Cicerone and Wood (1987) used this approach in an attempt to remediate a planning deficit in a patient with TBI. The authors adapted a self-instructional training program (Meichenbaum & Goodman, 1971) that required the subject to complete the Tower of London (TOL) task, verbalizing each step in the plan of action out loud before and during its completion. Over subsequent trials, this verbalization was gradually reduced to a whisper and finally to covert verbalization—representing a reestablishment of "inner speech." Performance improved on the task and gains were maintained at 4-month follow-up. However, generalization required 12 weeks of further training. A follow-up study replicated these findings in a larger sample of six subjects with mixed etiology, with five out of six showing gains. Two patients who received explicit generalization training spontaneously applied the techniques in novel situations (Cicerone & Giacino, 1992).

Goal-directed behavior may also be facilitated with external cueing, as suggested by case studies involving verbal instruction and task checklists (Burke et al., 1991; Delazer, Bodner, & Benke, 1998; Giles & Morgan, 1990; Hux, Reid, & Lugert, 1994; O'Callaghan & Couvadelli, 1998) and an electronic paging system combined with task-specific checklists (Evans, Emslie, & Wilson, 1998). In this latter study, it was reported that the auditory cueing itself was sufficient to reestablish the connection between intention and action. A similar result is reported in a recent TBI group study in which simulated real-life tasks were administered with and without the provision of random auditory "alerting" cues (Manly, Hawkins, Evans, Woldt, & Robertson, 2002). Their approach was based on the hypothesis that an intention to act establishes a marker to interrupt future activity in order to achieve the desired goal (Shallice & Burgess, 1991). Random auditory cues were used as a prosthetic "marker" to assist patients in completing a complex, lifelike planning task. Patients' performance on the cued version of the task was comparable to that of normal controls, suggesting that the auditory alerts bring higher-order goals into consciousness, facilitating more adaptive goal-directed behavior.[1]

Self-Awareness

Awareness interventions can be divided into two categories: educational (i.e., information provision) and experiential (e.g., comparing prediction with actual task performance; Sohlberg, 2000). Two small group ($n = 3$) studies successfully used awareness board games to educate patients with mixed etiology about expected brain injury sequelae (Chittum, Johnson, Chittum, Guercio, & McMorrow, 1996; Zhou et al., 1996). There was only partial evidence, however, that knowledge of these deficits translated into increased awareness.

Evidence for experiential interventions is also limited to small-group or case studies. These interventions involve highlighting, and thereby reducing, discrepancies between predicted and actual performance as a means of increasing awareness. Performance tasks include the TOL test (Cicerone & Giacino, 1992) and memory tasks (Rebmann & Hannon, 1995; Schlund, 1999). In a study of six patients with unspecified etiology, feedback improved patients' prediction of calculation and verbal recall performance, but these gains weakened on retest a week later, possibly due to the brevity of the training (Youngjohn & Altman, 1989). A combination of education and experiential awareness enhancement techniques have been employed by Ownsworth, McFarland, and Young (2000) to improve awareness in a group of 21 subjects with ABI. The authors report improved awareness of deficits and anticipatory awareness of future consequences that was evident at 6 months posttreatment. Sohlberg (2000) has formalized this two-pronged approach (i.e., individual awareness enhancement program—IAEP), emphasizing the need to tailor interventions based on the degree of patients' unawareness and cognitive deficits. Patients with poor deficit awareness and severely compromised cognitive capacity would likely derive few benefits from more cognitively demanding educational interventions (e.g., allowing patients to review their medical records;

providing media clippings relating to brain injury) whereas experiential treatment (e.g., comparing predicted vs. actual performance on various tasks) could be used as an effective intervention strategy for patients with more severe deficits or who are earlier in their course of treatment. Deluca (1992) has described a similarly "tailored" approach to the remediation of a severe confabulatory disorder following ACoA aneurysm rupture in which treatment team and family members were provided with explicit direction as to when and how to confront patients with respect to their confabulatory behavior. Improved awareness and reduced confabulation following treatment was reported in two patients.

Deficient self-monitoring of inappropriate or maladaptive behavior is a common sequelae of brain injury. These behavioral disorders (e.g., impulsivity, aggression, and sexual disinhibition) are usually long-lasting and may represent one of the primary impediments to successful reintegration into the community (Alderman, Fry, & Youngson, 1995). As this subject is covered comprehensively by Alderman (Chapter 8, this volume) we restrict our review to those interventions where self-monitoring (as a subcategory of self-awareness) was the primary rehabilitation target.

Targeted remediation programs involving structured feedback, cueing, and formal efforts to recognize inappropriate behaviors are often part of the interventions to enhance self-monitoring. In one study (Burke et al., 1991), sexual disinhibition was successfully treated by recording incidents of inappropriate sexual displays, providing structured feedback, and modeling appropriate behaviors in two patients with TBI. Positive effects were maintained at long-term follow-up. The second study used similar methods to treat inappropriate social behavior in a patient with traumatic orbitomedial frontal damage and profoundly disturbed emotional regulation, behavioral rigidity, and obsessive behaviors (Cicerone & Tanenbaum, 1997). The patient learned to self-monitor and correct errors in the specific training situations but behavior in real-life situations was unaffected. Lira, Carne, and Masri (1983) reported successful reduction of impulsive behavior in a subject through introduction of a self-monitoring strategy emphasizing problem identification and positive verbal regulation. Impulse control was maintained at 5 months and generalized to a vocational setting. Alderman et al. (1995) described the case of a herpes encephalitis patient whose disruptive verbal intrusions were successfully reduced through a formal self-monitoring training (SMT) program. SMT aims to both improve subjects' ability to attend to their own behavior and then, through operant conditioning, reduce problem behaviors (Alderman & Burgess, 2002). SMT was also successfully employed in a study by Knight, Rutterford, Alderman, and Swan (2002) to reduce problem behaviors in three brain-injured patients. While operant conditioning methods produced more rapid results (Alderman, Chapter 8, this volume), those obtained through SMT were more lasting.

Pharmacological Interventions

Having categorized our interventions by function rather than technique, we did not include a section on pharmacological approaches in Table 7.1. Yet these investigations are increasingly evident in the literature and deserve brief mention here. The three studies included in Table 7.1 specifically address the remediation of executive function deficits through dopaminergic treatments (McDowell et al., 1998; Powell et al., 1996; van Reekum et al., 1995). More recently, psychostimulant administration (through the modulation of dopaminergic pathways) has been associated with improved decision-making speed (Whyte, Vaccaro, Grieb-Neff, & Hart, 2002). Other neurotransmitter systems have also been targeted. Sertraline, a serotonin reuptake inhibitor, was unsuccessfully employed to enhance arousal following TBI (Meythaler, Depalma, Devivo, Guin-Renfroe, & Novack, 2001). Adrenergic agonists (e.g., clonidine) have been shown to improve executive functions in patients with schizophrenia and Korsakoff syndrome (Arnsten & Smith, 1999). Although comparatively few studies of pharmacological interventions have expressly targeted executive dysfunction or deficits of self-awareness, this literature continues to evolve from early case studies to more recent investigations that employ rigorous experimental techniques (e.g., randomized assignment and placebo controls). The importance of this evolution is aptly illustrated by contradictory reports concerning the efficacy of amantadine (see earlier section "Initiation/Motivation") and we return to this general theme of experimental control in the next section.

Summary and Evaluation

This review, specifically targeting executive function and self-awareness, reflects the issues raised in more broadly focused, recent reviews of the intervention literature for patients with ABI (Chesnut et al., 1999; Cicerone et al., 2000). Few studies contain the design ingredients necessary to draw firm conclusions about treatment effectiveness: control groups, randomization, evidence of real-life generalization, and long-term follow-up (Levine & Downey-Lamb, 2002). Interpretation is further complicated by incomplete description of participants, including etiology, epoch, and lesion location (Kolb, Chapter 2, this volume; Levine & Downey-Lamb, 2002). A majority of the published work in this area involves case studies. Although such studies help to guide future inquiry, they do not provide sufficient empirical basis for clinical decision making or policy.

We have emphasized the theoretical basis of rehabilitation rather than issues of study design per se. Although many of the studies referred to models of executive function or self-awareness, far fewer explicitly framed their interventions, predictions, or results within these theoretical models. Encouraging exceptions (Cicerone, 2002; Cicerone & Giacino, 1992; Deacon & Campbell,

1991; Evans et al., 1998; Levine, Robertson, et al., 2000; Manly et al., 2002; McDowell et al., 1998; Powell et al., 1996; Stablum et al., 2000; von Cramon et al., 1991), although not without methodological constraints and mixed results, are regarded as crucial early studies bridging the gap between theory and practice in this area of rehabilitation.

In spite of the shortcomings in this body of research, some consistent themes can be identified that might be useful in the design of future intervention programs. Although little information is provided on lesion localization, it was evident that patients with activation/initiation problems due to medial frontal systems dysfunction present special challenges. Clearly, patients must show some level of engagement to benefit from rehabilitation. On the positive side, this engagement may be subject to pharmacological (dopaminergic) intervention (McDowell et al., 1998; Powell et al., 1996). Similarly, self-monitoring and awareness deficits often pose particular rehabilitation challenges as reduced awareness has been associated with decreased motivation to engage in treatment. Self-monitoring deficits are often associated with intractable, mal adaptive behaviors resulting from ventromedial frontal dysfunction (Cicerone, 1987; Eslinger & Damasio, 1985). Although environmental modification and operant conditioning have been traditionally used to treat these patients, the work of Alderman et al. (1995) and Knight et al. (2002) suggests that a self-monitoring training intervention may provide more sustainable results. These examples drew on patient characteristics (such as neurobehavioral syndromes) to assist in clinical decision making. Future research should seek to identify other patient characteristics that can be used to influence treatment choices.

Another theme concerns the generalization of treatment effects beyond trained tasks. While this is critical for any intervention, it is of particular relevance to executive impairments, which are by definition maximized in novel situations. Our review has uncovered only anecdotal evidence of training generalized beyond the treatment setting, raising the following question: Can a truly dysexecutive patient be trained to spontaneously apply principles from rehabilitation to novel situations? Or, would it be more efficient to focus such interventions on patients with mild to moderate frontal damage? Treatment of more severely impaired patients should emphasize external aids for compensation (Robertson & Murre, 1999) or constraining intervention targets to those tasks essential to daily living (Sloan & Ponsford, 1995). With less than half the studies in our review reporting generalization effects, it is clear that a more structured approach to the assessment of treatment generalization must be pursued before such determinations can be made reliably.

Another related question pertains to the usefulness of neuropsychological test data relative to real-life functioning (Chesnut et al., 1999). Test data are useful to characterize patients for the purposes of comparison with other studies and as intermediate indicators of treatment effects. However, any study purporting to have an effect on patients' real-life functioning must demonstrate such effects with ecologically valid and reliable assessments of improved per-formance—a standard met by few of the studies in this review (see Foxx et al., 1989; Levine, Robertson et al., 2000; von Cramon et al., 1991).

CONCLUSIONS AND FUTURE DIRECTIONS

It is suggested that future research draw more directly from the literature on frontal lobe and executive function to formulate hypotheses and interventions that balance the demands of clinical efficacy and empirical validity. Although it is often difficult to think theory from the front lines, or to conduct RCTs in re-habilitation settings, more evidence from interventions satisfying these two cri-teria are necessary to firmly establish the efficacy of our interventions. This does not diminish the contribution of more clinically oriented group studies, which can make significant contributions when conducted with careful control subject data. Case studies have always been essential in neuropsychology for theory testing but can never be regarded as sufficient to promote a given inter-vention in the absence of group data.

Our literature review illustrates a disconnection between theory and prac-tice, a disconnection mirrored in this chapter itself, in which the reviewed the-oretical models of executive functions and self-awareness made only rare ap-pearances in the subsequent review of rehabilitation interventions. Given the high correlation between executive functioning and psychosocial and voca-tional outcome following brain damage, it is incumbent upon us to seek the source of this disconnection.

The inherent ambiguity in defining and assessing these disorders may be a central factor. The rehabilitation of neurobehavioral deficits in areas such as language and memory is facilitated by the existence of well-established models and operational definitions. Disorders of these functions are easily observed and measured in the laboratory. Patterns of deficit in higher-order executive control processes, on the other hand, have not been consistently described in the literature, commonly co-occur with preserved intellectual functioning, and may only be observable in novel and nonstructured environments—the anti-thesis of the laboratory or clinical setting. Persons with executive function deficits may only return to the clinic after several months or years of a down-ward spiral in their social or vocational lives. These patients are often unable to meet the demands of an increasingly unstructured environment as they trans-fer from the rehabilitation setting to the home and subsequently into vocational or less structured social settings. Second, the often devastating and disruptive behaviors (ranging from extreme aggression to extreme apathy), particularly in the acute rehabilitation period, may preclude the introduction of more theo-retically based rehabilitation interventions in favor of more immediate behav-ioral management/modification techniques.

Finally, any assessment of rehabilitation in the realm of executive dysfunction must consider the distinction between functional recovery on specific tasks versus generalization of treatment gains to untrained tasks. Table 7.1 documents considerable success in increasing patients' independence in specific functional areas (personal hygiene, household maintenance, etc.). However, higher cognitive deficits which impede the more complex demands of daily living such as social interaction, contingency planning, option weighing, insight, and/or introspection appear to be more refractory to treatment. It is this latter category of functional deficit that is frequently reported by caregivers of brain-injured survivors as posing the most difficult challenges following brain injury (Burgess & Robertson, 2002).

We view Table 7.1 as representative of a field in transition from infancy to adolescence. Although other reviewers have documented the need for more empirically validated rehabilitation approaches, our review aimed to highlight the equally important need for theoretically driven interventions. As noted by Kolb (Chapter 2, this volume) understanding of mechanisms (i.e., exactly what has changed as a result of brain injury) must precede the design of rehabilitation treatments. In a future edition of this volume we hope to able to report on the results of such interventions, some of which are currently under way in our laboratories.

NOTE

1   A recent report by Rath, Dvorah, Langenbahn, Sherr, and Diller (2003) presented results of a problem-solving training intervention using an RCT design in a cohort of 60 TBI subjects. Treatment group subjects were trained in problem-solving skills (von Cramon et al., 1991) and emotional self-regulation while controls received a program of conventional cognitive rehabilitation. Improvements specific to treatment included reduced perseverative responding on the WCST and improved problem solving on self-report and role play measures. Treatment gains were stable at 6 months with anecdotal report of generalization to real-life behaviors.

REFERENCES

Adams, J. H., Graham, D. I., Murray, L. S., & Scott, G. (1982). Diffuse axonal injury due to nonmissile head injury in humans: An analysis of 45 cases. *Annals of Neurology, 12,* 557–563.

Alderman, N., & Burgess, P. W. (2002). Assessment and rehabilitation of the dysexecutive syndrome. In R. Greenwood, T. M. McMillan, M. P. Barnes, & C. D. Ward (Eds.), *Handbook of neurological rehabilitation* (2nd ed.). Hove, East Sussex, UK: Psychology Press.

Alderman, N., Fry, R. K., & Youngson, H. A. (1995). Improvement of self-monitoring skills, reduction of behavior disturbance and the dysexecutive syndrome: Comparison of response cost and a new programme of self-monitoring training. *Neuropsy-chological Rehabilitation, 5*(3), 193–221.

Anderson, S. W., & Damasio, A. R. (1995). Frontal-lobe syndromes. In J. Bogousslavsky & L. Caplan (Eds.), *Stroke syndromes* (pp. 140–144). New York: Cambridge University Press.

Anderson, S. W., Damasio, H., & Tranel, D. (1990). Neuropsychological impairments associated with lesions caused by tumour or stroke. *Archives of Neurology, 47,* 397–405.

Arnsten, A., & Smith, D. H. (1999). Pharmacological strategies for neuroprotection and rehabilitation. In D. T. Stuss, G. Winocur, & I. H. Robertson (Eds.), *Cognitive neurorehabilitation: A comprehensive approach* (pp. 113–135). Cambridge, UK: Cambridge University Press.

Baddeley, A. (1986). *Working memory.* Oxford, UK: Clarendon Press.

Baddeley, A. D., & Hitch, G. J. (2000). Development of working memory: Should the Pascual-Leone and the Baddeley and Hitch models be merged? *Journal of Experimental Child Psychology, 77*(2), 128–137.

Barbas, H. (1995). Anatomic basis of cognitive-emotional interactions in the primate prefrontal cortex. *Neuroscience and Biobehavioral Reviews, 19,* 499–510.

Bechara, A., Damasio, A. R., Damasio, H., & Anderson, S. W. (1994). Insensitivity to future consequences following damage to human prefrontal cortex. *Cognition, 50*(1–3), 7–15.

Bechara, A., Damasio, H., & Damasio, A. R. (2000). Emotion, decision making and the orbitofrontal cortex. *Cerebral Cortex, 10*(3), 295–307.

Bechara A., Damasio, H., Tranel, D., & Anderson, S.W. (1998). Dissociation of working memory from decision making within the human prefrontal cortex. *Journal of Neuroscience, 18*(1), 428–37.

Bechara, A., Damasio, H., Tranel, D., & Damasio, A. R. (1997). Deciding advantageously before knowing the advantageous strategy. *Science, 275*(5304), 1293–1295.

Berryhill, P., Lilly, M. A., Levin, H. S., Hillman, G. R., Mendelsohn, D., Brunder, D. G., et al. (1995). Frontal lobe changes after severe diffuse closed head injury in children: A volumetric study of magnetic resonance imaging. *Neurosurgery, 37*(3), 392–399.

Bianchi, L. (1922). *The mechanism of the brain and the function of the frontal lobes.* Edinburgh, Scotland: Livingstone.

Bisiach, E., Vallar, G., Perani, D., Papagno, C., & Berti, A. (1986). Unawareness of disease following lesions of the right hemisphere: Anosognosia for hemiplegia and anosognosia for hemianopia. *Neuropsychologia, 24,* 471–482.

Blumer, D., & Benson, D. F. (1975). Personality changes with frontal and temporal lobe lesions. In D. F. Benson & D. Blumer (Eds.), *Psychiatric aspects of neurologic disease* (Vol. 1, pp. 151–170). New York: Grune & Stratton.

Bogousslavsky, J. (1994). Frontal stroke syndromes. *European Neurology, 34*(6), 306–315.

Bottger, S., Prosiegel, M., Steiger, H.-J., & Yassouridis, A. (1998). Neurobehavioral disturbances, rehabilitation outcome, and lesion site in patients after rupture and repair of anterior communicating artery aneurysm. *Journal of Neurology, Neurosurgery and Psychiatry, 65*(1), 93–102.

Brooks, N., Campsie, L., Symington, C., Beattie, A., & McKinlay, W. (1986). The five year outcome of severe blunt head injury: a relative's view. *Journal of Neurology, Neurosurgery and Psychiatry, 49*(7), 764–770.

Burgess, P. W. (2000). Strategy application disorder: The role of the frontal lobes in human multi-tasking. *Psychological Research, 63*(3–4), 279–288.

Burgess, P. W., & Robertson, I. H. (2002). Principles of the rehabilitation of frontal lobe function. In D. T. Stuss & R. Knight (Eds.), *Principles of frontal lobe function* (pp. 557–572). New York: Oxford University Press.

Burgess, P. W., & Shallice, T. (1996a). Bizarre responses, rule detection, and frontal lobe lesions. *Cortex, 32*, 241–259.

Burgess, P. W., & Shallice, T. (1996b). Response suppression, initiation, and strategy use following frontal lobe lesions. *Neuropsychologia, 34*, 263–273.

Burke, W. H., Zencius, A. H., Wesolowski, M. D., & Doubleday, F. (1991). Improving executive function disorders in brain-injured clients. *Brain Injury, 5*(3), 241–252.

Chesnut, R. M., Carney, N., Maynard, H., Mann, N. C., Patterson, P., & Helfand, M. (1999). Summary report: Evidence for the effectiveness of rehabilitation for persons with traumatic brain injury. *Journal of Head Trauma Rehabilitation, 14*(2), 176–188.

Chittum, W. R., Johnson, K., Chittum, J. M., Guercio, J. M., & McMorrow, M. J. (1996). Road to awareness: An individualized training package for increasing knowledge and comprehension of personal deficits in persons with acquired brain injury. *Brain Injury, 10*(10), 763–776.

Christman, C. W., Salvant, J. B., Jr., Walker, S. A., & Povlishock, J. T. (1997). Characterization of a prolonged regenerative attempt by diffusely injured axons following traumatic brain injury in adult cat: A light and electron microscopic immunocytochemical study. *Acta Neuropathologica (Berlin), 94*(4), 329–337.

Christoff, K., & Gabrieli, J. D. E. (2000). The frontopolar cortex and human cognition: Evidence for a rostrocaudal hierarchical organization within the human prefrontal cortex. *Psychobiology, 20*(2), 168–186.

Cicerone, K. D. (1987). Planning disorder after closed head injury. A case study. *Archives of Physical Medicine and Rehabilitation, 68*(2), 111–115.

Cicerone, K. D. (2002). The enigma of executive functioning: Theoretical contributions to therapeutic interventions. In P. J. Eslinger (Ed.), *Neuropsychological interventions: Emerging treatment and management models for neuropsychological impairments* (pp. 246–293). New York: Guilford Press.

Cicerone, K. D., Dahlberg, C., Kalmar, K., Langenbahn, D. M., Malec, J. F., Bergquist, T. F., et al. (2000). Evidence-based cognitive rehabilitation: Recommendations for clinical practice. *Archives of Physical Medicine and Rehabilitation, 81*(12), 1596–1615.

Cicerone, K. D., & Giacino, J. T. (1992). Remediation of executive function deficits after traumatic brain injury. *Neurorehabilitation, 2*(3), 12–22.

Cicerone, K. D., & Tanenbaum, L. N. (1997). Disturbance of social cognition after traumatic orbitofrontal brain injury. *Archives of Clinical Neuropsychology, 12*(2), 173–188.

Cicerone, K., & Wood, J. (1987). Planning disorder after closed head injury: A case study. *Archives of Physical Medicine and Rehabilitation, 68*, 111–115.

Clifton, G., Grossman, R., Makela, M., Miner, M. E., Handel, S., & Sadhu, V. (1980). Neurological course and correlated computerized tomography findings after severe closed head injury. *Journal of Neurosurgery, 52*, 611–624.

Courtney, S. M., Ungerleider, L. G., Keil, K., & Haxby, J. V. (1996). Object and spatial visual working memory activate separate neural systems in human cortex. *Cerebral Cortex, 6*(1), 39–49.

Courville, C. B. (1937). *Pathology of the central nervous system, part 4.* Mountain View, CA: Pacific Press.

Craik, F., I.M., Moroz, T. M., Moscovitch, M., Stuss, D. T., Winocur, G., Tulving, E., et al. (1999). In search of the self, a positron emission tomography study. *Psychological Science, 10*(1), 26–34.

Damasio, A. R. (1994). *Descartes' error.* New York: Putnam.

Damasio, A. R., Tranel, D., & Damasio, H. (1990). Individuals with sociopathic behavior caused by frontal damage fail to respond autonomically to social stimuli. *Behavioral Brain Research, 41*(2), 81–94.

Damasio, A. R., Tranel, D., & Damasio, H. C. (1991). Somatic markers and the guidance of behavior: Theory and preliminary testing. In H. Levin, H. Eisenberg, & A. Benton (Eds.), *Frontal lobe function and dysfunction* (pp. 217–229). New York: Oxford University Press.

Deacon, D., & Campbell, K. B. (1991). Decision-making following closed-head injury: Can response speed be retrained? *Journal of Clinical and Experimental Neuropsychology, 13*(5), 639–651.

Delazer, M., Bodner, T., & Benke, T. (1998). Rehabilitation of arithmetical text problem solving. *Neuropsychological Rehabilitation, 8*(4), 401–412.

DeLuca, J. (1992). Cognitive dysfunction after aneurysm of the anterior communicating artery. *Journal of Clinical and Experimental Neuropsychology, 14*(6), 924–934.

DeLuca, J., & Diamond, B. J. (1995). Aneurysm of the anterior communicating artery: A review of the neuroanatomical and neuropsychological sequelae. *Journal of Clinical and Experimental Neuropsychology, 17*, 100–121.

D'Esposito, M., Aguirre, G. K., Zarahn, E., Ballard, D., Shin, R. K., & Lease, J. (1998). Functional MRI studies of spatial and nonspatial working memory. *Cognitive Brain Research, 7*(1), 1–13.

Diamond, B. J., DeLuca, J., & Kelley, S. M. (1997). Memory and executive functions in amnesic and non-amnesic patients with aneurysms of the anterior communicating artery. *Brain, 120*(Pt. 6), 1015–1025.

Dikmen, S. S., Ross, B. L., Machamer, J. E., & Temkin, N. R. (1995). One year psychosocial outcome in head injury. *Journal of the International Neuropsychological Society, 1*, 67–77.

Duncan, J. (1986). Disorganization of behavior after frontal lobe damage. *Cognitive Neuropsychology, 3*, 271–290.

Duncan, J., Emslie, H., Williams, P., Johnson, R., & Freer, C. (1996). Intelligence and the frontal lobe: The organization of goal-directed behavior. *Cognitive Psychology, 30*(3), 257–303.

Duncan, J., Seitz, R. J., Kolodny, J., Bor, D., Herzog, H., Ahmed, A., et al. (2000). A neural basis for general intelligence. *Science, 289*(5478), 457–460.

D'Zurilla, T. J., & Goldfried, M. R. (1971). Problem solving and behavior modification. *Journal of Abnormal Psychology, 78*, 107–126.

Elliott, R., Dolan, R. J., & Frith, C. D. (2000). Dissociable functions in the medial and lateral orbitofrontal cortex: Evidence from human neuroimaging studies. *Cerebral Cortex, 10*(3), 308–317.

Ellis, S., & Small, M. (1997). Localization of lesion in denial of hemiplegia after acute stroke. *Stroke, 28*(1), 67–71.

Eslinger, P. J., & Damasio, A. R. (1985). Severe disturbance of higher cognition after bilateral frontal lobe ablation: Patient EVR. *Neurology, 35*, 1731–1741.

Evans, J. J. (2001). Rehabilitation of the dysexecutive syndrome. In R. L. Wood & T. M. McMillan (Eds.), *Neurobehavioral disability and social handicap following traumatic brain injury* (pp. 3–27). Philadelphia: Psychology Press.

Evans, J. J., Emslie, H., & Wilson, B. A. (1998). External cueing systems in the rehabilitation of executive impairments of action. *Journal of the International Neuropsychological Society, 4*(4), 399–408.

Foxx, R. M., Martella, R. C., & Marchand-Martella, N. E. (1989). The acquisition, maintenance, and generalization of problem-solving skills by closed head-injured adults. *Behavior Therapy, 20*(1), 61–76.

Frith, C. D., & Frith, U. (1999). Interpreting minds— A biological basis. *Science, 286*(5445), 1692–1695.

Funahashi, S., Bruce, C., & Goldman-Rakic, P. (1993). Dorsolateral prefrontal lesions and oculomotor delayed-response performance: Evidence for mnemonic "scotomas." *Journal of Neuroscience, 13*(4), 1479–1497.

Fuster, J. M. (1997). *The prefrontal cortex: Anatomy, physiology, and neuropsychology of the frontal lobe* (3rd ed.). New York: Raven Press.

Fuster, J. M. (2000). Executive frontal functions. *Experimental Brain Research, 133*, 66–70.

Fuster, J. M., & Alexander, G. E. (1970). Delayed response deficit by cryogenic depression of frontal cortex. *Brain Research, 20*(1), 85–90.

Fuster, J. M., & Alexander, G. E. (1971). Neuron activity related to short-term memory. *Science, 173*(997), 652–654.

Gallup, G. G. (1994). Monkeys, mirrors and minds. *Behavioral and Brain Sciences, 17*(3), 572–573.

Gennarelli, T. A., Thibault, L. E., Adams, J. H., Graham, D. I., Thompson, C. J., & Marcincin, R. P. (1982). Diffuse axonal injury and traumatic coma in the primate. *Annals of Neurology, 12*(6), 564–572.

Gentry, L. R., Godersky, J. C., & Thompson, B. (1988). MR imaging of head trauma: Review of the distribution and radiopathologic features of traumatic lesions. *American Journal of Neuroradiology, 9*, 101–110.

Gentry, L. R., Godersky, J. C., Thompson, B., & Dunn, V. D. (1988). Prospective comparative study of intermediate-field MR and CT in the evaluation of closed head trauma. *American Journal of Neuroradiology, 9*, 101–110.

Giles, G. M., & Morgan, J. H. (1990). Self-instruction in the training of functional skills: A single case study. *British Journal of Occupational Therapy, 53*(8), 314–316.

Glosser, G., & Goodglass, H. (1990). Disorders in executive control functions among aphasic and other brain-damaged patients. *Journal of Clinical and Experimental Neuropsychology, 12*(4), 485–501.

Goldberg, G. (1985). Supplementary motor area structure and function: Review and hypothesis. *Behavioral and Brain Sciences, 8*, 567–616.

Goldman-Rakic, P. S. (1987). Circuitry of primate prefrontal cortex and regulation of behavior by representational memory. In F. Plum & V. Mountcastle (Eds.), *Handbook of physiology: The nervous system* (Vol. 5, pp. 373–417). Bethesda, MD: American Physiological Society.

Goldman-Rakic, P. (1996). Prefrontal cortex revisited: A multiple-memory domain model of human cognition. In R. Caminiti, K.-P. Hoffmann, F. Lacquaniti, & J. Altman (Eds.), *Vision and movement: Mechanisms in the cerebral cortex. Workshop II* (Vol. 2, pp. 162–172). Strasbourg: Human Frontier Science Program.

Goldstein, L. H., Bernard, S., Fenwick, P. B., Burgess, P. W., & McNeil, J. (1993). Unilateral frontal lobectomy can produce strategy application disorder. *Journal of Neurology, Neurosurgery and Psychiatry, 56*(3), 274–276.

Grafman, J. (1995). Similarities and distinctions among current models of prefrontal cortical functions. *Annals of the New York Academy of Sciences, 769*, 337–368.

Harlow, J. M. (1868). Recovery after severe injury to the head. *Publication of the Massachusetts Medical Society, 2*, 327–346.

Hillis, A. E., Anderson, N., Sampath, P., & Rigamonti, D. (2000). Cognitive impairments after surgical repair of ruptured and unruptured aneurysms. *Journal of Neurology, Neurosurgery and Psychiatry, 69*(5), 608–615.

Honda, T. (1999). Rehabilitation of executive function impairments after stroke. *Topics in Stroke Rehabilitation, 6*(1), 15–22.

Hux, K., Reid, R., & Lugert, M. (1994). Self-instruction training following neurological injury. *Applied Cognitive Psychology, 8*(3), 259–271.

Jacobsen, C. F. (1936). Studies of cerebral function in primates. *Comparative Psychology Monographs, 13*, 1–68.

Jennett, B., Snoek, J., Bond, M. R., & Brooks, N. (1981). Disability after severe head injury: Observations on the use of the Glasgow Outcome Scale. *Journal of Neurology, Neurosurgery and Psychiatry, 44*(4), 285–293.

Kandel, E. R., Schwartz, J. H., & Jessell, T. M. (2000). *Principles of neural science* (4th ed.). New York: McGraw-Hill.

Kihlstrom, J. F., & Tobias, B. A. (1991). Anosognosia, consciousness, and the self. In G. Prigatano & D. Schacter (Eds.), *Awareness of deficit after brain injury* (pp. 198–222). New York: Oxford University Press.

Knight, C., Rutterford, N. A., Alderman, N., & Swan, L. J. (2002). Is accurate self-monitoring necessary for people with acquired neurological problems to benefit from the use of differential reinforcement methods? *Brain Injury, 16*(1), 75–87.

Leimkuhler, M. E., & Mesulam, M. M. (1985). Reversible go–no go deficits in a case of frontal lobe tumor. *Annals of Neurology, 18*(5), 617–619.

Lepage, M., Ghaffar, O., Nyberg, L., & Tulving, E. (2000). Prefrontal cortex and episodic memory retrieval mode. *Proceedings of the National Academy of Science USA, 97*(1), 506–511.

Levine, B. (1999). Self-regulation and autonoetic consciousness. In E. Tulving (Ed.), *Memory, consciousness, and the brain: The Tallinn conference* (pp. 200–214). Philadelphia: Psychology Press.

Levine, B. (2002). Novel approaches to the assessment of prefrontal brain damage effects: The R-SAT studies (symposium participant). *Journal of the International Neuropsychological Society, 8*, 320.

Levine, B., Cabeza, R., McIntosh, A.R., Black, S.E., Grady, C.L., & Stuss, D.T. (2002).

Functional reorganisation of memory after traumatic brain injury: a study with H(2)(15)0 positron emission tomography. *Journal of Neurology, Neurosurgery and Psychiatry, 73*(2), 173–81.

Levine, B., Dawson, D., Boutet, I., Schwartz, M. L., & Stuss, D. T. (2000). Assessment of strategic self-regulation in traumatic brain injury: Its relationship to injury severity and psychosocial outcome. *Neuropsychology, 14*(4), 491–500.

Levine, B., & Downey-Lamb, M. (2002). Design and evaluation of intervention experiments. In P. J. Eslinger (Ed.), *Neuropsychological interventions: Clinical research and practice* (pp. 80–104). New York: Guilford Press.

Levine, B., Katz, D., Black, S. E., & Dade, L. (2002). New approaches to brain-behavior assessment in traumatic brain injury. In D. T. Stuss & R. Knight (Eds.), *Principles of frontal lobe function* (pp. 448–465). New York: Oxford University Press.

Levine, B., Robertson, I. H., Clare, L., Carter, G., Hong, J., Wilson, B. A., et al. (2000). Rehabilitation of executive functioning: An experimental–clinical validation of goal management training. *Journal of International Neuropsychological Society, 6*(3), 299–312.

Levine, B., Stuss, D. T., Milberg, W. P., Alexander, M. P., Schwartz, M., & Macdonald, R. (1998). The effects of focal and diffuse brain damage on strategy application: Evidence from focal lesions, traumatic brain injury, and normal aging. *Journal of the International Neuropsychological Society, 4*, 247–264.

Lezak, M. D. (1995). *Neuropsychological assessment* (3rd ed.). New York: Oxford University Press.

Lhermitte, F. (1983). "Utilization behavior" and its relation to lesions of the frontal lobes. *Brain, 106*, 237–255.

Lilja, A., Salford, L. G., Smith, G. J., & Hagstadius, S. (1992). Neuropsychological indexes of a partial frontal syndrome in patients with nonfrontal gliomas. *Neuropsychology, 6*(4), 315–326.

Lira, F. T., Carné, W., & Masri, A, M. (1983). Treatment of anger and impulsivity in a brain damaged patient: A case study applying stress innoculation. *Clinical Neuropsychology, 5*(4), 159–160.

Luria, A. R. (1966). *Higher cortical functions in man*. New York: Basic Books.

Luria, A. R., & Homskaya, D. (1964). Disturbance in the regulative role of speech with frontal lobe lesions. In J. M. Warren & K. Akert (Eds.), *The frontal granular cortex and behavior* (pp. 353–371). New York: McGraw-Hill.

Manly, T., Hawkins, K., Evans, J., Woldt, K., & Robertson, I. H. (2002). Rehabilitation of executive function: Facilitation of effective goal management on complex tasks using periodic auditory alerts. *Neuropsychologia, 40*(3), 271–281.

Mavaddat, N., Kirkpatrick, P. J., Rogers, R. D., & Sahakian, B. J. (2000). Deficits in decision-making in patients with aneurysms of the anterior communicating artery. *Brain, 123*(Pt. 10), 2109–2117.

Maxwell, W. L., Povlishock, J. T., & Graham, D. L. (1997). A mechanistic analysis of nondisruptive axonal injury: A review [published erratum appears in J Neurotrauma 1997 Oct;14(10):755]. *Journal of Neurotrauma, 14*(7), 419–440.

McDowell, S., Whyte, J., & D'Esposito, M. (1998). Differential effect of a dopaminergic agonist on prefrontal function in traumatic brain injury patients. *Brain, 121*(Pt. 6), 1155–1164.

McGlynn, S. M., & Schacter, D.M. (1989). Unawareness of deficits in neuropsychological syndromes. *Journal of Clinical and Experimental Neuropsychology, 11*(2), 143–205.

Meichenbaum, D., & Goodman, D. (1971). Training impulsive children to talk to themselves: A means of developing self-control. *Journal of Abnormal Psychology, 77,* 115–126.

Mesulam, M. M. (1998). From sensation to cognition. *Brain, 121*(Pt. 6), 1013–1052.

Mesulam, M. M. (2002). The human frontal lobes: Transcending the default mode through contingent encoding. In D. T. Stuss & R. Knight (Eds.), *Principles of frontal lobe function* (pp. 8–30). New York: Oxford University Press.

Meythaler, J. M., Depalma, L., Devivo, M. J., Guin-Renfroe, S., & Novack, T. A. (2001). Sertraline to improve arousal and alertness in severe traumatic brain injury secondary to motor vehicle crashes. *Brain Injury, 15*(4), 321–331.

Milner, B. (1963). Effects of different brain lesions on card sorting: The role of the frontal lobes. *Archives of Neurology, 9,* 100–110.

Nakawatase, T. Y. (1999). Frontal lobe tumors. In B. L. Miller & J. L. Cummings (Eds.), *Human frontal lobes* (pp. 436–445). New York: Guilford Press.

National Center for Injury Prevention and Control. (1999). *Traumatic brain injury in the United States: A report to congress.* Atlanta, GA: Centers for Disease Control and Prevention.

Nauta, W. J. H. (1971). The problem of the frontal lobe: A reinterpretation. *Journal of Psychiatric Research, 8,* 167–187.

Newell, A., & Simon, H. A. (1963). GPS, a program that simulates human thought. In E. A. Feigenbaum & J. Feldman (Eds.), *Computers and thought* (pp. 279–293). New York: McGraw-Hill.

Nickels, J. L., Schneider, W. N., Dombovy, M. L., & Wong, T. M. (1994). Clinical use of amantadine in brain injury rehabilitation. *Brain Injury, 8*(8), 709–718.

Nolde, S. F., Johnson, M. K., & Raye, C. L. (1998). The role of prefrontal cortex during tests of episodic memory. *Trends in Cognitive Science, 2*(10), 399–406.

Norman, D. A., & Shallice, T. (1986). Willed and automatic control of behavior. In R. J. Davidson, G. E. Schwartz, & D. Shapiro (Eds.), *Consciousness and self regulation* (pp. 1–17). New York: Plenum Press.

O'Callaghan, M. E., & Couvadelli, B. (1998). Use of self-instructional strategies with three neurologically impaired adults. *Cognitive Therapy and Research, 22*(2), 91–107.

Ommaya, A. K., & Gennarelli, T. A. (1974). Cerebral concussion and traumatic unconsciousness. Correlation of experimental and clinical observations of blunt head injuries. *Brain, 97*(4), 633–654.

Ownsworth, T. L., McFarland, K., & Young, R. (2000). Self-awareness and psychosocial functioning following acquired brain injury: An evaluation of a group support program. *Neuropsychological Rehabilitation, 10*(5), 465–484.

Pandya, D. N., & Yeterian, E. H. (1996a). Comparison of prefrontal architecture and connections. *Philosophical Transactions of the Royal Society of London, Part B, 351,* 1423–1432.

Pandya, D. N., & Yeterian, E. H. (1996b). Morphological correlations of human and monkey frontal lobes. In A. R. Damasio, H. Damasio, & Y. Christen (Eds.), *Neurobiology of decision making* (pp. 13–46). New York: Springer.

Passingham, R. (1993). *The frontal lobes and voluntary action.* Oxford, UK: Oxford University Press.

Peace, K. A., Orme, S. M., Thompson, A. R., Padayatty, S., Ellis, A. W., & Belchetz, P. E. (1997). Cognitive dysfunction in patients treated for pituitary tumors. *Journal of Clinical and Experimental Neuropsychology, 19*(1), 1–6.

Petrides, M. (1985). Deficits on conditional associative-learning tasks after frontal- and temporal-lobe lesions in man. *Neuropsychologia, 23*(5), 601–614.

Petrides, M., Alivisatos, B., Evans, A. C., & Meyer, E. (1993). Dissociation of human mid-dorsolateral from posterior dorsolateral frontal cortex in memory processing. *Proceedings of the National Academy of Sciences of the United States of America, 90*(3), 873–877.

Petrides, M., & Pandya, D. N. (1994). Comparative architectonic analysis of the human and the macaque frontal cortex. In F. Boller & J. Grafman (Eds.), *Handbook of neuropsychology* (Vol. 9, pp. 17–58). Amsterdam: Elsevier.

Petrides, M., & Pandya, D. N. (2002). Association pathways of the prefrontal cortex and functional observations. In D. T. Stuss & R. Knight (Eds.), *Principles of frontal lobe function* (pp. 31–50). New York: Oxford University Press.

Povlishock, J. T. (1992). Traumatically induced axonal injury: Pathogenesis and pathobiological implications. *Brain Pathology, 2*(1), 1–12.

Povlishock, J. T. (1993). Pathobiology of traumatically induced axonal injury in animals and man. *Annals of Emergency Medicine, 22*(6), 980–986.

Povlishock, J. T., & Christman, C. W. (1995). The pathobiology of traumatically induced axonal injury in animals and humans: A review of current thoughts. *Journal of Neurotrauma, 12*(4), 555–564.

Povlishock, J. T., Erb, D. E., & Astruc, J. (1992). Axonal response to traumatic brain injury: Reactive axonal change, deafferentation, and neuroplasticity. *Journal of Neurotrauma, 9*(Suppl. 1), S189–200.

Powell, J. H., al-Adawi, S., Morgan, J., & Greenwood, R. J. (1996). Motivational deficits after brain injury: Effects of bromocriptine in 11 patients. *Journal of Neurology, Neurosurgery and Psychiatry, 60*(4), 416–421.

Price, R. P., Goetz, K. L., & Lovell, M. R. (1997). Neuropsychiatric aspects of brain tumors. In S. C. Yodofsky & R. E. Hales (Eds.), *American Psychiatric Press textbook of neuropsychiatry* (3rd ed., pp. 635–643). Washington, DC: American Psychiatric Press.

Prigatano, G. P. (1999). *Principles of neuropsychological rehabilitation.* New York: Oxford University Press.

Quintana, J., & Fuster, J. M. (1999). From perception to action: Temporal integrative functions of prefrontal and parietal neurons. *Cerebral Cortex, 9*(3), 213–221.

Rath, J. F., Dvorah, S., Langenbaum, D. M., Sherr, R. L., & Diller, L. (2003). Group treatment of problem-solving deficits in outpatients with traumatic brain injury: A randomized control study. *Neuropsychological Rehabilitation, 13*(4), 461–488.

Rebmann, M. J., & Hannon, R. (1995). Treatment of unawareness of memory deficits in adults with brain injury: Three case studies. *Rehabilitation Psychology, 40*(4), 279–287.

Robertson, I. H. (1996). *Goal management training: A clinical manual.* Cambridge, UK: PsyConsult.

Robertson, I. H., & Murre, J. M. (1999). Rehabilitation of brain damage: Brain plasticity and principles of guided recovery. *Psychological Bulletin, 125*(5), 544–575.

Robinson, R. G., & Starkstein, S. E. (1997). Neuropsychiatric aspects of cerebrovascular disorders. In S. C. Yodofsky & R. E. Hales (Eds.), *American Psychiatric Press textbook of neuropsychiatry* (3rd ed., pp. 607–614). Washington, DC: American Psychiatric Press.

Rolls, E. T. (2002). The functions of the orbitofrontal cortex. In D. T. Stuss & R. Knight (Eds.), *Principles of frontal lobe function* (pp. 354–375). New York: Oxford University Press.

Sanides, F. (1970). Functional architecture of motor and sensory cortices in primates in the light of a new concept of neocortex development. In C. R. Noback & W. Montana (Eds.), *Advances in primatology* (Vol. 1, pp. 137–208). New York: Appleton-Century-Crofts.

Schlund, M. W. (1999). Self awareness: Effects of feedback and review on verbal self reports and remembering following brain injury. *Brain Injury, 13*(5), 375–380.

Schneider, W. N., Drew-Cates, J., Wong, T. M., & Dombovy, M. L. (1999). Cognitive and behavioral efficacy of amantadine in acute traumatic brain injury: An initial double-blind placebo-controlled study. *Brain Injury, 13*(11), 863–872.

Semendeferi K., Lu A., Schenker N., & Damasio, H. (2002). Humans and great apes share a large frontal cortex. *Nature Neuroscience. 5*(3), 272–276.

Shallice, T. (1982). Specific impairments in planning. *Philosophical Transactions of the Royal Society of London, Series B, 298,* 199–209.

Shallice, T. (1988). *From neuropsychology to mental structure.* Cambridge, UK: Cambridge University Press.

Shallice, T. (2002). Fractionation of the supervisory system. In D. T. Stuss & R. Knight (Eds.), *Principles of frontal lobe function* (pp. 261–277). New York: Oxford University Press.

Shallice, T., & Burgess, P. W. (1991). Deficits in strategy application following frontal lobe damage in man. *Brain, 114,* 727–741.

Shallice, T., & Burgess, P. W. (1993). Supervisory control of action and thought selection. In A. Baddeley & L. Weiskrantz (Eds.), *Attention: selection, awareness, and control: A tribute to Donald Broadbent* (pp. 171–187). Oxford, UK: Clarendon Press.

Shallice, T., & Burgess, P. (1996). The domain of supervisory processes and temporal organization of behavior. *Philosophical Transactions of the Royal Society of London. Series B, Biological Sciences, 351*(1346), 1405–1411.

Shammi, P., & Stuss, D. T. (1999). Humour appreciation: A role of the right frontal lobe. *Brain, 122*(Pt. 4), 657–666.

Sirigu, A., Zalla, T., Pillon, B., Grafman, J., Agid, Y., & Dubois, B. (1996). Encoding of sequence and boundaries of scripts following prefrontal lesions. *Cortex, 32,* 297–310.

Sirigu, A., Zalla, T., Pillon, B., Grafman, J., Dubois, B., & Agid, Y. (1995). Planning and script analysis following prefrontal lobe lesions. *Annals of the New York Academy of Sciences, 769,* 277–288.

Sloan, S., & Ponsford, J. (1995). Assessment of cognitive difficulties following TBI. In J. Ponsford, S. Sloan, & P. Snow (Eds.), *Traumatic brain injury: Rehabilitation for everyday adaptive living* (pp. 65–101). Hillsdale, NJ: Erlbaum.

Sohlberg, M. M. (2000). Assessing and managing unawareness of self. *Seminars in Speech and Language, 21*(2), 135–150.

Sohlberg, M. M., & Mateer, C. A. (1989). *Introduction to cognitive rehabilitation: Theory and practice.* New York: Guilford Press.

Sohlberg, M. M., & Mateer, C. A. (2001). *Cognitive rehabilitation: An integrative neuropsychological approach*. London: Guilford Press.

Sohlberg, M. M., Sprunk, H., & Metzelaar, K. (1988). Efficacy of an external cuing system in an individual with severe frontal lobe damage. *Cognitive Rehabilitation, 6*, 36–41.

Stablum, F., Umilta, C., Mogentale, C., Carlan, M., & Guerrini, C. (2000). Rehabilitation of executive deficits in closed head injury and anterior communicating artery aneurysm patients. *Psychological Research, 63*(3–4), 265–278.

Strich, S. (1956). Diffuse degeneration of the cerebral white matter in severe dementia following head injury. *Journal of Neurology, Neurosurgery and Psychiatry, 19*, 163–185.

Stuss, D. T. (1991). Disturbance of self-awareness after frontal system damage. In G. Prigatano & D. Schacter (Eds.), *Awareness of deficit after brain injury* (pp. 63–83). New York: Oxford University Press.

Stuss, D. T., & Alexander, M. P. (2000a). Affectively burnt in: A proposed role of the right frontal lobe. In E. Tulving (Ed.), *Memory, consciousness and the brain:The Tallin Conference* (pp. 215–227). Philadelphia: Psychology Press.

Stuss, D. T., & Alexander, M. P. (2000b). Executive functions and the frontal lobes: A conceptual view. *Psychological Research, 63*(3–4), 289–298.

Stuss, D. T., Alexander, M. P., Palumbo, C. L., Buckle, L., Sayer, L., & Pogue, J. (1994). Organizational strategies of patients with unilateral or bilateral frontal lobe injury in word list learning tasks. *Neuropsychology, 8*, 355–373.

Stuss, D. T., Gallup, G. G., & Alexander, M. P. (2001). The frontal lobes are necessary for "theory of mind." *Brain, 124*(Pt. 2), 279–286.

Stuss, D. T., & Gow, C. A. (1992). "Frontal dysfunction" after traumatic brain injury. *Neuropsychiatry, Neuropsychology, and Behavioral Neurology, 5*(4), 272–282.

Stuss, D. T., & Levine, B. (2002). Adult clinical neuropsychology: Lessons from studies of the frontal lobes. *Annual Review of Psychology, 53*, 401–433.

Stuss, D. T., Shallice, T., Alexander, M. P., & Picton, T. (1995). A multidisciplinary approach to anterior attentional functions. *Annals of the New York Academy of Sciences, 769*, 191–212.

Tidswell, P., Dias, P. S., Sagar, H. J., Mayes, A. R., & Battersby, R. D. (1995). Cognitive outcome after aneurysm rupture: Relationship to aneurysm site and perioperative complications. *Neurology, 45*(5), 875–882.

Tranel, D., Anderson, S. W., & Benton, A. (1994). Development of the concept of "executive function" and its relationship to the frontal lobes. In F. Boller & J. Grafman (Eds.), *Handbook of neuropsychology* (Vol. 9, pp. 125–148). Amsterdam: Elsevier.

Tucha, O., Smely, C., Preier, M., & Lange, K. W. (2000). Cognitive deficits before treatment among patients with brain tumors. *Neurosurgery, 47*(2), 324–334.

Tulving, E. (1985). Memory and consciousness. *Canadian Psychology, 26*, 1–12.

Tulving, E. (2002). Episodic memory: From mind to brain. *Annual Review of Psychology, 53*, 1–25.

Tulving, E., Kapur, S., Craik, F. I. M., Moscovitch, M., & Houle, S. (1994). Hemispheric encoding/retrieval asymmetry in episodic memory: Positron emission tomography findings. *Proceedings of the National Academy of Sciences of the United States of America, 91*, 2016–2020.

Tulving, E., Kapur, S., Markowitsch, H. J., Craik, F. I. M., Habib, R., & Houle, S. (1994).

Neuroanatomical correlates of retrieval in episodic memory: Auditory sentence recognition. *Procedings of the National Academy of Sciences of the United States of America, 91,* 2012–2015.

van Reekum, R., Bayley, M., Garner, S., Burke, I. M., Fawcett, S., Hart, A., et al. (1995). N of 1 study: Amantadine for the amotivational syndrome in a patient with traumatic brain injury. *Brain Injury, 9*(1), 49–53.

von Cramon, D. Y., & Matthes von Cramon, G. (1994). Back to work with a chronic dysexecutive syndrome? (A case report). *Neuropsychological Rehabilitation, 4*(4), 399–417.

von Cramon, D. Y., Matthes von Cramon, G., & Mai, N. (1991). Problem-solving deficits in brain-injured patients: A therapeutic approach. *Neuropsychological Rehabilitation, 1*(1), 45–64.

von Monakow, C. (1914). *Localization in the cerebrum and the degeneration of functions through cortical sources.* Wiesbaden, Germany: J.F. Bergman.

Webb, P. M., & Glueckauf, R. L. (1994). The effects of direct involvement in goal setting on rehabilitation outcome for persons with traumatic brain injuries. *Rehabilitation Psychology, 39*(3), 179–188.

Wheeler, M. A., Stuss, D. T., & Tulving, E. (1997). Toward a theory of episodic memory: The frontal lobes and autonoetic consciousness. *Psychological Bulletin, 121,* 331–354.

Whyte, J., Vaccaro, M., Grieb-Neff, P., & Hart, T. (2002). Psychostimulant use in the rehabilitation of individuals with traumatic brain injury. *Journal of Head Trauma Rehabilitation, 17*(4), 284–299.

Ylvisaker, M., & Feeney, T. J. (1996). Executive functions after traumatic brain injury. *Seminars in Speech & Language, 17*(3), 217–232.

Ylvisaker, M., Szekeres, S. F., & Feeney, T. J. (1998). Cognitive rehabilitation: Executive functions. In M. Ylvisaker (Ed.)., *Traumatic brain injury rehabilitation: Children and adolescents* (2nd ed., pp. 221–269). Woburn, MA: Butterworth-Heinemann.

Youngjohn, J. F., & Altman, I. M. (1989). A performance-based group approach to the treatment of anosagnosia and denial. *Rehabilitation Psychology, 34,* 217–222.

Zalla, T., Plassiart, C., Pillon, B., Grafman, J., & Sirigu, A. (2001). Action planning in a virtual context after prefrontal cortex damage. *Neuropsychologia, 39*(8), 759–770.

Zelazo, P. R., & Zelazo, P. D. (1998). The emergence of consciousness. *Advances in Neurology, 77,* 149–163.

Zhou, J., Chittum, R., Johnson, K., Poppen, R., Guercio, J., & McMorrow, M. (1996). The utilization of a game format to increase knowledge of residuals among people with acquired brain injury. *Journal of Head Trauma Rehabilitation, 11*(1), 51–61.

8

Disorders of Behavior

Nick Alderman

Disorders of behavior are well known among people with acquired brain injury (ABI), and are especially characteristic of survivors of traumatic brain injury (TBI). Behavior disorders that typify the acute stage (confusion, agitation) will change in nature with the resolution of consciousness. Postacute behavior disturbance may take varied forms, including passivity and aggression, whereas others mimic a range of symptoms consistent with psychiatric disorders. A worrying trend is that not only are postacute behavior disorders a likely sequelae of TBI, particularly when these are classified as severe, but they may become chronic, increasing in both frequency and severity with the passage of time (Brooks, McKinlay, Symington, Beattie, & Campsie, 1987; Johnson & Balleny, 1996). Understandably, they constitute an enormous source of stress within families (McKinlay, Brooks, Bond, Martinage, & Marshall, 1981); in addition, these disorders persist far longer that the severity of injury (as measured by duration posttraumatic amnesia) suggest (Weddell, Oddy, & Jenkins, 1980).

While there is considerable diversity in the form behavior disorders take, some are more characteristic. For example, Wood (2001) refers to problems of labile mood, impulse control, and personality change typifying the clinical picture associated with TBI among a wider constellation of cognitive and behavioral symptoms that constitute what he labels "neurobehavioral disability." The development of aggressive behavior disorders has been especially highlighted, not only because it is a major contributing factor regarding stress in families but because its presence can lead to individuals failing to achieve their maximum potential in rehabilitation (Burke, Wesolowski, & Lane, 1988) or even exclusion from this process altogether (Prigatano, 1987). As well as the more obvious example of aggression, Alderman (2001) has argued that a whole range of postacute behavior disorders fall under the umbrella of "challenging behavior," that is, behaviors that jeopardize the safety of the person exhibiting them, or limit access to ordinary community facilities (Emerson et al., 1987). While this concept is well known among other clinical populations, Alderman expressed the view that when applied to people with ABI it should be extended to include any behaviors that constrain the ability to participate in postacute rehabilitation programs. In this way, disorders of initiation and passivity, which characterize some forms of brain injury, for example, are also classified as "challenging" as their outcome is equal to that attained by some of the more obvious behavior disorders, such as aggression.

ETIOLOGY OF BEHAVIOR DISORDERS

ABI encompasses a wide variety of neurological conditions. Among the most prevalent are TBI, stroke, degenerative diseases, cerebral tumor, infection, and anoxia. Others are less frequent, for example, Korsakoff's syndrome. Because of the range of differing conditions, neurological patients do not constitute a homogeneous group (Wilson, 1991).

Consequently, behavioral manifestations lack uniformity and vary between conditions because of differences in underlying neuropathology. However, lack of homogeneity is further compounded by other factors. For example, the prevalence of some conditions varies between age cohorts; thus, stroke is more common among older people, whereas TBI is observed more frequently among children and young adults. Premorbid factors mean that no two brains are identical; similarly, no two brains are damaged in exactly the same way (Mateer & Ruff, 1990). The sequelae of brain injury may be extensive and include cognitive, emotional, physical, and functional impairments, as well as behavioral problems. However, Wilson (1991) makes the point that people are almost certain to present with a combination of these difficulties, and that these are rarely identical. Thus, although the location and extent of the neuropathology may initially dictate the form a behavior disorder takes, it will be subjected to many secondary influences which modify how it is subsequently manifested. Attempting to isolate a single cause for a defined behavior is therefore not only simplistic but fraught with methodological difficulties, as this will seldom be univariate but instead the result of complex interactions between many factors.

While this is a daunting task, it is nevertheless one that needs to be attempted. Eames (1990, 2001) makes the point that organic brain disorders primarily underlie some behavior problems, and that these may superficially resemble primary or reactive psychiatric disorders. He argues that it is necessary to attempt to isolate and distinguish these if subsequent treatment is to be successful. Similarly, although there are now a wide range of treatment options available for the management of postacute behavioral problems, attempts should be made to isolate (as far as possible) those factors that drive them in order that appropriate interventions be put in place as opposed to subjecting patients to the lottery of educated guesswork. In this respect, a number of practitioners have advocated that the area of behavioral assessment is of special relevance given the difficulties imposed by neurological damage on other forms of appraisal (see, for example, Wood, 1987; Davis, Turner, Rolinder, & Cartwright, 1994; Treadwell & Page, 1996; von Cramon & Matthes-von Cramon, 1994). Within this domain, single-case experimental design has much to offer (Alderman, 2002).

It is therefore necessary for the clinician to be aware of the range of factors that may interact to drive and maintain behavior disorders. A number of these have been discussed in the literature, and in the following sections I attempt to briefly consider some of the principal ones.

Organic Factors

Correlating specific lesion sites to particular behavioral symptoms exhibited by patients has been the subject of medical and scientific scrutiny for some time. One of the earliest, and best known, examples of this was the account given by Broca in 1861 regarding a patient who could not speak intelligibly (Barlow & Hersen, 1984). At autopsy, Broca identified the brain area responsible and established a tradition that continues today of mapping brain–behavior relationships.

It is within this tradition that study of the cerebral basis of behavior disorders has become equally well established. It is beyond the scope of this chapter to provide more than passing acknowledgment to some of this work. However, reference will be made to those brain areas implicated in some of the more frequently documented postacute behavioral problems.

Severe brainstem injuries have been associated with drive disorders in which the sufferer experiences low arousal, excessive sleepiness, and fatigability: This will typically occur alongside spasticity and rigidity of the limbs, dysarthria, and problems with swallowing. The condition may improve with increased stimulation but return when it is withdrawn (Eames, 2001). Damage to the dopaminergic mesocingulate system has been noted to result in the condition of abulia (Fisher, 1983). The clinical picture is characterized by normal alertness and sleep pattern, but the individual shows lack of initiative and is slow to respond to commands. Destruction of cells in the cingulate gyrus itself can manifest itself behaviorally as retarded depression; however, when asked, patients typically deny any depression of mood. A further feature may be that while patients are able to verbalize interests and goals, they do not pursue them (Eames, 2001).

Midbrain lesions may result in periods of either easily provoked tearfulness or excessive and inappropriate laughter. These symptoms may be respectively mistaken for depression and euphoria; however, there is usually a dissociation between this behavior and the person's subjective emotional state (Eames, 1990).

Lesions of the corpus callosum may result in behaviors characterized by "opposite effort" in which the patient is unable to perform an action to specific command, although it is preserved when it forms part of a wider behavioral sequence (Eames, 1990). In addition to ideomotor dyspraxia, symptoms consistent with psychoses and severe behavior disturbance may also be present (David, Wacharasindhu, & Lishman, 1993).

Damage to the hypothalamus is associated with persistent food-seeking behavior in the absence of normal hunger (Childs, 1987). Hypersexuality may follow either medial basal-frontal or diencephalic injury, while sexual preference may change when limbic system structures are damaged (Miller, Cummings, McIntyre, Ebers, & Grode, 1986).

Intermittent explosive anger and aggression has been associated with electrophysiological disturbances in function in medial temporal lobe structures, or in diencephalic limbic structures with which they are connected. Aggressive behavior typically occurs in response to trivial provocation, there may be a patchy amnesia for events during outbursts, and remorse may follow. Such behavior is of short duration and seen as "out of character." This variant of the so-called temperolimbic disorders (Monroe, 1970, 1986) has become known as episodic dyscontrol syndrome (EDS). Its development parallels that of post-traumatic epilepsy in that its onset is marked by a delay (sometimes years) after insult and it shows little tendency to improve over time (see Miller, 1994; Eames, 1990, 2001).

There is some evidence to suggest that some forms of mood disorder may have a similar mechanism because they, like EDS, are characterized by paroxysmal changes. While they mimic symptoms of anxiety and depression, they are distinguishable from classic affective disorder by their temporal pattern and short duration (Monroe, 1986; Hellekson, Buckland, & Price, 1979).

"Frontal Lobe Syndrome"

There is no doubt that that area of the brain that has received the most attention regarding cerebral correlates of behavior disorders comprises that of the frontal lobes. The range of anecdotal social changes that are associated with damage to anterior brain structures is conspicuous and has been comprehensively documented in the literature. The case of Phineas Gage (see Kimble, 1963) represents perhaps one of the earliest and certainly one of the most striking documented descriptions of the behavior and personality changes that illustrate such social change. This followed a penetrating injury of the brain that resulted in a large bilateral lesion of the ventromedial prefrontal cortex.

However, damage to anterior structures does not result in a consistent range of handicaps (including disorders of behavior). Instead, different clusters of behavioral problems and personality abnormalities characterize outcome: This is undoubtedly because the frontal lobes are tasked with a wide variety of complex integrative functions, and because of the myriad, rich number of connections between them and posterior brain structures. Consequently, these clusters of diverse behavioral symptoms will be driven by different underlying mechanisms (Eslinger & Damasio, 1985).

Despite the variety, complexity, and richness of frontal lobe functioning, brain–behavior mapping suggests that specific disorders of behavior are characteristic of damage to particular areas. Much of this evidence comes from study of survivors of road traffic accidents in which rapid acceleration/deceleration forces cause both diffuse axonal shearing and focal lesions to frontal and temporal lobe structures (see Bigler, 1990). In addition to anecdotal correlation of the onset of behavior disorders and frontal lobe injury, advances in scanning technology have helped confirm this relationship. For example, Langfitt et al. (1986) demonstrated that extensive hypometabolism of the frontal region was related to those deficits of cognition and behavior typically associated with frontal lobe damage using positron emission tomography (PET). Using single photon emission computerized tomography (SPECT), Oder, Goldenberg, Spatt, Binder, and Deecke (1992) found a high correlation between frontal flow indices and the presence of disinhibition; severity of disinhibition increased with lower frontal flow rates. Because circumscribed lesions are less likely as a result of TBI, survivors tend to present with a range of behavior disorders characterized by emotional lability, impulsive behavior, social disinhibition, and altered personality, in addition to cognitive impairment (Bigler, 1984, 1990). The aggregate of coarse behavioral symptoms that often result from nonspecific damage to anterior brain structures has perhaps contributed to the oversimplification of what has become known as the frontal lobe syndrome.

However, study of individuals with localized cortical and subcortical lesions confirms what was mentioned earlier, that rather than being a single "syndrome," different types and combinations of behavior disorders arise from damage to localized parts of the frontal lobes. Typically, the frontal lobes are themselves divided into three main subareas, the dorsal lateral, medial, and orbital cortices (Uytdenhoef et al., 1983). Damage to orbital prefrontal cortex is associated with poor impulse control and aggression (Grafman et al., 1996). Grafman, Vance, and Weingaiter (1986) demonstrated a laterality effect in that left orbital damage may result in agitated anxiety and depression, while that inflicted to the right is especially related to increased anger and hostility. Eames (1990) highlights the role of orbital prefrontal cortex in increased social disinhibition, as well as egocentricity, immaturity, and poor insight. Furthermore, increased irritability is attributed (in part) to specific orbitofrontal lesion, or through disruption of the connections between frontal and limbic systems. Starkstein and Robinson (1991) also highlighted this latter point. They attributed mania to damage to the orbito–temporal–limbic feedback loop, in which the inhibitory function of the cortex over the amygdala is disrupted, thereby depriving the cognitive functions of any ability to suppress instinctive emotional reactions. Interference in the processing of facial expressions because of damage to the connections between the amygdala and the temporal lobes contributes to problems of excessive friendliness and lack of ability to recognize that behavior is unwanted (Adolphus, 1999; Davidson & Irwin, 1999). Lesions to medial prefrontal cortex are associated with apathy especially when connections to the limbic system are involved (Cummings, 1993; Eames, 1990). Finally, dorsal lateral lesions are associated with poor executive functioning, impairment of which skills we will see later may drive a range of behavior disorders (Dolan et al., 1993). The specificity of these three main areas of the frontal lobes regarding behavior and emotional disturbance has again been recently confirmed (Paradiso, Chemerinski, Yazici, Tartaro, & Robinson, 1999).

Exacerbation of Premorbid Features

There is much evidence to suggest that preexisting characteristics may increase the likelihood of TBI, not least of which are premorbid personality traits and a tendency to engage in increased risk-taking behavior (see, e.g., Naugle, 1990; Jacobs, 1990). London (1967) argued that behavioral changes represented an exaggeration of premorbid personality traits, while McAllister (1992) suggested that one effect of TBI was to exacerbate premorbid problems with impulse control. Thus, people who had a tendency to be aggressive prior to injury may have this trait inflated as a consequence. These hypotheses have some face validity given that the population is characterized by the presence of behavioral problems prior to injury. Conversely, Thomsen (1990) warns that the presence of behavior disorders should not be taken as prima facie evidence of brain injury if it can be shown that these were present beforehand.

Reactive Disorders

Behavior disorders may be a function of coping with the level of handicap acquired through brain injury. Bond (1984) argued that premorbid traits help shape postinjury emotional reactions. Eames (2001) stressed that reactive emotional disorders may develop in response to perceived loss of abilities, skills, and status. In some cases, that may lead to denial and the development of dissociative hysterical disorders. Major depressive disorder is a common outcome of TBI, occurring in approximately 25% of survivors (Fedoroff et al., 1992;

Jorge et al., 1993). The presence of major mood disorder may underlie some behavior problems (e.g., aggression and noncooperation) when attempts are made to engage the depressed patient in rehabilitation.

Denial and Poor Awareness

Denial of problems and difficulties following brain injury, or poor awareness of these, is a well-documented phenomenon: This denial includes unawareness of behavior disorders (Prigatano, 1991; Wood, 1988; Sazbon & Groswasser, 1991). Wilson, Alderman, Burgess, Emslie, and Evans (1996) and Alderman, Dawson, Rutterford, and Reynolds (2001) found significant discrepancies between ratings of a range of problems characteristic of brain injury made by patients regarding themselves and relatives and/or carers regarding the patients: Typically, patients rated themselves as being less impaired than those who knew them well. Denial and poor awareness may persist in the long term (Groswasser, Mendelson, Stern, Schecter, & Najenson, 1977; Prigatano, Altman, & O'Brien, 1990). Etiology may be organic (see, e.g., Hier, Mondlock, & Caplan, 1983) or as a result of cognitive impairment (e.g., in monitoring; McGlynn & Schacter, 1989). In addition, denial may persist as a means of protecting the individual from what for them are the devastating consequences of their brain injury (Manchester and Wood, 2001). Lack of awareness may explain the presence of uncooperative and aggressive behaviors observed in rehabilitation as individuals may not perceive the need to engage in therapy. For example, data from a study by Alderman, Knight, and Henman (2002) found a negative and significant correlation between staff ratings of patients' insight and the frequency of physical aggression against people.

Postinjury Learning

Some behavior disorders may be acquired through operant learning. When exposed to activities for which there is little enthusiasm (e.g., rehabilitation sessions), people may spontaneously engage in a range of behaviors that staff find unpleasant or threatening (Miller & Cruzat, 1981). Rehabilitation staff may learn to reduce demands on such patients in order to avoid such behavior; consequently, these behaviors become negatively reinforced as patients learn they result in escape or avoidance of similar situations in the future (for examples of this, see Alderman, 1991; Alderman, Shepherd, & Youngson, 1992).

Environmental Factors

The environment, or more accurately, the social systems that operate within it, may work to inadvertently reinforce behavior disorders. For example, within the context of a busy, underresourced rehabilitation unit, there may be insufficient time to give people regular quality social contact. However, when an individual begins to engage in inappropriate behavior (e.g., to shout, scream, masturbate, or be aggressive), staff may rapidly engage in attempts that result in cessation of such conduct. People may be told, "Don't do that." Unfortunately, within an environment devoid of positive and empathic social contact, such attention, even when it is delivered in the form of criticism, may be welcome. Staff may thereby unwittingly reinforce behavior disorders (Alderman, 2001).

Cognitive Deficits

Problems with language, memory, attention, executive, and intellectual functions are characteristic of TBI. It can easily be appreciated how behavior disorders may arise when one or more of these cognitive modalities is grossly impaired (for an example regarding amnesia, see Alderman & Burgess, 1994).

Impairments in attention and working memory have been especially highlighted in relation to the evolution and maintenance of behavioral problems, and some sophisticated cognitive models have been developed regarding such impairments. Those proposed by Shallice (1982) and Baddeley (1986) are particularly relevant. Both models attempt to account for these problems in terms of a breakdown in the allocation of attentional controls that exercise important executive functions. Shallice (1982) argued the pattern of functional deficits was attributable to impairment in attentional control mechanisms. Baddeley (1986) identified the supervisory system proposed by Shallice with the central executive component of his own model of working memory. Both models attempt to account for these problems in terms of a breakdown in the allocation of attentional controls which exercise important executive functions, loss or impairment of which may result in behavior that becomes labeled "problematic."

In Shallice's model, overlearned units of behavior, or schemata, are activated by social and other stimuli. It is envisaged that the process of activation is mainly automatic and outside the realm of consciousness, controlled by a system called contention scheduling. Because this process is relatively automatic, it is envisaged that it frees up resources for other cognitive activity. For example, as I type this manuscript, I am not having to think too much about the process of typing: These skills (knowing the position of the various keys, pressing them in the correct sequence so that meaningful sentences appear on the computer monitor, etc.) represent the various schemata that, because they are well practiced, have become overlearned. These schemata are activated as thoughts I wish to add to the manuscript are formed in my mind. This process of creativity would be grossly impaired if the mechanics of typing had to be consciously controlled. Under Shallice's model, contention scheduling largely takes care of the technical aspects of operating the computer leaving me free sufficient cognitive resources to (ideally!) engage in a little original thinking. Monitoring the whole process is another structure Shallice labeled the "supervisory attentional system" (SAS). This interrupts contention scheduling when an inappropriate schema is triggered, or in novel situations for which no schema exists. It enables existing but inappropriate schemata to be overridden or selects new combinations of schemata appropriate to the change in circumstances. When this happens, control of behavior returns to conscious command, and by necessity information processing and response selection becomes slow and deliberate. This model has been used by Burgess and Wood (1990) and Burgess and Alderman (1990) to explain some behavior disorders including inappropriate speech content, shouting, aggression, and disinhibited sexual behavior.

The second model which highlights the role of a breakdown in attentional controls in the etiology and maintenance of behavior disorders comes from the concept of working memory proposed by Baddeley and Hitch (1974). Working memory is conceptualized as consisting of several temporary storage systems whose activities are coordinated by a central executive (CE), aided by a number of subsystems which include the articulatory loop (which deals with verbal information) and the visuospatial sketchpad (which processes nonverbal material). The CE allocates attentional resources to these subsystems: Baddeley (1986) identified the SAS proposed by Shallice (1982) with the CE component of working memory. Impairment of the CE will consequently result in inefficiencies in the allocation of attentional resources which are evidenced in a range of behavioral and other symptoms seen in patients, which together constitute a "dysexecutive syndrome" (DES; Baddeley, 1986; Baddeley & Wilson, 1988). Impairment of CE functioning may result in difficulties in scheduling two or more concurrent tasks, distractibility, poor monitoring of performance, problems utilizing feedback, and attention and memory problems.

Alderman and colleagues (Alderman, 1996; Alderman, Fry, & Youngson, 1995) proposed that some behavior disorders shown by people with acquired neurological damage are directly attributable to deficits in CE function, whereby difficulties with attending to multiple events is evident functionally through problems in monitoring one's self, one's own performance, and changes in the external environment. The consequence of this is that opportunities to receive and process feedback are reduced, which results in failure to modify behavior as a response to changing circumstances: Individuals with the dysexecutive syndrome therefore present as impulsive, distractible, and unresponsive to cues from others and behave inappropriately in social situations. Alderman (1996) argued that when CE deficit is very severe only one stimulus set at a time may be routinely attended to. This may explain why a characteristic feature of the dysexecutive syndrome is a reduced ability to change behavior in an adaptive, flexible way, in response to changes in the environment. For example, if a person's attention is solely directed to what he or she is saying, that person will not be able to routinely and simultaneously monitor the response of the individual to whom it is directed. The nonverbal and other cues the latter generate will not be available in the form of feedback that is normally used to assess the appropriateness of speech content. Typically, people are able to simultaneously attend to both their own behavior and the response of the environment to it: Under normal circumstances, perception of positive feedback will contribute to continuation of that behavior, whereas negative feedback will result in modification of action. This may be one reason why some people who have sustained brain injury tend to "talk over" others and dominate conversation. Hartmann, Pickering, and Wilson (1992) and Alderman (1996) have demonstrated experimental evidence for a CE deficit in people with ABI (predominately TBI). As with Shallice's (1982) SAS model, it has been used to account for a range of behavior problems characteristic of this populations (see, e.g., Alderman et al., 1995).

Multivariate Etiology of Behavior Disorders

While all the foregoing factors have a role to play (to a greater or lesser extent) in driving the types of behavior disorder observed in people with ABI, the reader will be asked to consider again that the origin of such problems is necessarily more complicated. Any of the foregoing are unlikely to occur in isolation because of the wide range of additional problems that also arise from neurological damage (cognitive, functional, and physical). These, and lack of homogeneity within this clinical population, mean the relevance of each possible cause will vary, sometimes greatly, between people. Finally, the environment may also seriously influence the extent of any behavior disorder. Ultimately, behavior disorders will be the consequence of complex and bewildering interactions between a considerable number of contributing variables.

As an example, consider aggression. Miller (1994) summarized three frequently cited causes of aggressive behavior among people with TBI. First, it may be attributable to an EDS, in which disturbance of mood and behavior is a consequence of electrophysiological brain disturbance. Second, damage to frontal brain structures decreases ability to inhibit or regulate emotional responses, leading to a lower threshold for aggressive behavior. Third, brain injury exacerbates negative premorbid personality traits: People who were aggressive are likely to be more so as a consequence of neurological damage. Each of these three factors has been considered here. However, as we have seen, other reasons may also contribute to aggression—for example, inadvertent reinforcement of challenging behavior in environments where positive contingencies for desirable conduct arc not routinely available (see, e.g., the description of patient NR in Alderman, 2003). Recently, Alderman et al. (2002) have also highlighted the role of language dysfunction in the case of physically aggressive behavior that lacks identifiable antecedents.

To illustrate the multivariate origins of aggressive behavior disorders, consider the following examples. A patient who sustained a very severe closed head injury is admitted to a rehabilitation center for assessment and treatment.

He attends physiotherapy for treatment of upper-limb contractures. As a result of his injury he has little awareness of the serious nature of the handicaps acquired and consequently does not appreciate the need for rehabilitation. Treatment of his contractures is painful. Lack of insight and the discomfort experienced do not render him a willing participant. The organic consequences of his injury have disrupted connections between frontal and limbic brain structures: He is therefore irritable and his ability to tolerate frustration is low. He also has a history of violent behavior prior to injury and this aspect of his personality is exacerbated as a consequence. He thus cannot tolerate the pain he experiences in physiotherapy and because of the preceding factors, he engages in a spontaneous bout of aggressive behavior directed at the therapist, who he perceives as the source of his discomfort. The therapist backs away and discontinues treatment. The patient thus learns that in order to avoid or escape an activity perceived as irrelevant and painful, he displays aggression toward the therapist, who subsequently withdraws and reinforces this behavioral response. Consider a second example. A patient with monitoring difficulties is unaware that his social behavior is considered by others to be rude and domineering: His cognitive handicap means he cannot readily receive the normal range of social cues from others that would otherwise lead him to modify his behavior. He is thus unpopular and avoided by rehabilitation staff and his peers. However, because he is irritable as a result of the organic component of his brain injury, he is prone to explosive outbursts which occur when others walk away from him (he considers them to be rude!). Unfortunately, his aggressive behavior encourages other people to avoid him all the more. However, the patient subsequently learns that the social attention he craves is given him in abundance when he begins to bang his head on the wall (a behavior which itself was primarily a consequence of his irritability and social isolation). The frequency of this behavior subsequently increases.

TREATMENT APPROACHES

The Need for Individual Assessment

In the case of persistent and severe behavior disorders, treatment within a specialized neurorehabilitation center is desirable (McMillan & Oddy, 2001), because it will be organized in such a way to sustain the admission of patients whose behavior is challenging. Furthermore, the complex interaction of variables that drive such disorders requires detailed assessment, which is unlikely to be available within other services. Given the complex range of individual contributing factors, and the nature of their interactions under different circumstances, such assessment is essential to deliver effective treatment interventions that have been designed to meet the unique needs of each person.

The range and effectiveness of those treatments available for behavior disorders for people with ABI is considerable and includes both pharmacological and rehabilitative interventions (Rao & Lyketsos, 2000). The importance of rehabilitation being designed to facilitate plastic changes at the cellular level discussed by Kolb (Chapter 2, this volume) and Kolb and Cioe (Chapter 1, this volume) has particular relevance for psychological and other therapies that have the potential to shape the experience of the person with ABI. This experience can alter brain organization and function, and promote recovery, which suggests that people with ABI be given appropriate therapy from as early a stage in their recovery as possible. It is clearly beyond the scope of a single chapter to attempt a comprehensive review of all of these (see Wood & McMillan, 2001, for a recent and comprehensive appraisal). However, some of the principal means of treatment will be considered here in light of the contributing factors and theories of behavior disorder outlined earlier.

Pharmacological Approaches

In a recent review of the literature, Rao and Lyketsos (2000) highlighted the difficulties in evaluating the impact of pharmacological therapy in the treatment of neuropsychiatric sequelae of TBI, which includes behavior disorders, because of lack of methodologies that enable objective scientific study of effectiveness to be made. Alderman, Knight, and Morgan (1997) previously made the same point regarding treatment of aggression. Lack of proper methodologies to evaluate outcome, and poor homogeneity within the brain-injury population, renders only tentative conclusions to be reached regarding efficacy of drug treatments. Determining outcome is further complicated because neurological patients are reported to be very sensitive to medications, and undesirable side effects can in themselves prove debilitating. A major problem highlighted by Eames (1990, 2001) is that symptoms of organic brain injury can be mistaken for functional mental illness (e.g., paroxysmal mood disorder can mimic a primary depressive illness; for further discussion regarding this area, see Halligan & Marshall, 1996). The consequence of this is that inappropriate conclusions will be drawn regarding efficacy of the pharmacological therapy prescribed, or that little is achieved beyond the sedation of behavior. It is therefore essential that an assessment is made by an experienced neuropsychiatrist (Alderman, 2001). Furthermore, the success of other nonpharmacological therapies may be in part dependent on first successfully identifying and treating organic brain disorders which themselves underlie behavior disorders (Eames, 1990).

The literature contains successful accounts (within the constraints of variable methods of scientific scrutiny being employed) of a range of medications used with behaviorally disturbed brain-injured patients, including psychostimulants, dopaminergic agents, antidepressants, and anticonvulsants (Rao & Lyketsos, 2000). No more than a passing reference will be made to some of these here.

TBI is especially associated with long-term disturbance of dopamine transmission. In particular, the frontal lobes are rich in dopamine and as a consequence of TBI, dopamine activity characteristically decreases with obvious implications for behavior disorders. Dopamine agents may therefore have special relevance. For example, amantadine has been shown to be beneficial in the reduction of agitation, emotional lability, and aggression (Gualtieri, 1991) while bromocriptine has helped patients with abulia (Eames, 1989). Other drive disorders typical of brainstem injuries have responded to use of psychostimulants such as methylphenidate (Glenn, 1998).

Anticonvulsants may be especially relevant in the treatment of EDS and other paroxysmal mood disorders. There are reports in the literature regarding management of EDS which testify to the successful reduction of aggressive behavior using anticonvulsants, within the constraints of the methodological issues highlighted earlier (Hirsch, 1993; Mooney & Hass, 1993; Giakas, Seibyl, & Mazure, 1990); carbamazepine appears to have special relevance (Foster, Hillbrand, & Chi, 1989; Mattes, 1990). Eames (1988) and Wood (1987) recommend a combination of carbamazepine and behavior modification methods as providing the optimal route for the treatment of aggression secondary to EDS. They argue that whereas medication exerts control over underlying seizure activity, behavior modification methods are used to teach adaptive forms of behavior and new skills (for an example of this, see patient MD described by Alderman, Davies, Jones, & McDonnell, 1999). Anticonvulsants have also been successfully employed in the treatment of other paroxysmal mood disorders whose presence may contribute to more challenging behavior disorders (see Eames, 1990, 2001).

Psychotherapy

Psychotherapy has been used with some success in the remediation of behavioral disorders following brain damage. Psychotherapy is in itself a broad and multiply defined concept (Jackson & Gouvier, 1992) which encompasses various therapies that have arisen from different models of psychopathology (Patterson, 1986). One of the earliest attempts at using psychotherapy with brain-injured people was reported by Ben-Yishay and his colleagues during the early 1970s (see, e.g., Ben-Yishay et al., 1985). Faced with the task of attempting to rehabilitate soldiers injured in the Arab–Israeli wars, they developed an intensive social milieu approach employing psychotherapeutic techniques, within which combinations of cognitive and emotional problems are addressed. The results of this program suggested that the potential level of social recovery for patients with brain injury was greater than had previously been anticipated.

George Prigatano (1986) has described successful outcomes with this population using psychotherapy within a general rehabilitation program to facilitate awareness and acceptance. Successful employment of various psychotherapeutic techniques, including individual and family counseling within a social milieu treatment program, have been reported as leading to improvement of insight and psychosocial problems (Prigatano et al., 1984; Prigatano, 1986).

Successful outcomes have also been reported regarding the use of insight psychotherapy (Stern & Stern, 1985; Geva & Stern, 1985; Tadir & Stern, 1985), group psychotherapy conducted on both an inpatient and outpatient basis (Carberry & Burd, 1983; Corrigan, Arnett, Houck, & Jackson, 1985; Leer, 1986; Leer & Sonday, 1986; Jackson & Gouvier, 1992), and family therapy (Power & Dell Orto, 1980) in the treatment of psychosocial problems following brain injury.

Unfortunately, psychotherapeutic methods are not suitable for all people with ABI. Jackson and Gouvier (1992) pointed out that successful participation in group psychotherapy is usually dependent on the brain-injured person having already made a "moderately good cognitive and behavioral recovery" (p. 322). People who have sustained severe brain injury are often not amenable to psychotherapy for a number of reasons. For example, Wood (1988) agrees that while methods such as counseling and group therapy can improve the behavior and social adaptability of individuals with minor brain injury, they are generally not helpful in cases in which damage is more severe. One reason for this is that as a consequence of brain injury, some individuals lack awareness, have poor insight, are inaccurate in their self-report, and have motivational problems. These issues will interfere with participation in psychotherapy (Burgess & Wood, 1990) and are extremely difficult to overcome (Sazbon & Groswasser, 1991). A second reason is that challenging behavior exhibited by the brain-injured person may be so severe it excludes that person from treatment (Wood, 1987). Wood and Worthington (2001a) argue that those methods advocated by Ben Yishay and Prigatano are only employed with more articulate patients with less debilitating handicaps. By definition, those with severe behavior disorders, especially those who lack insight, are almost certain to be excluded from therapeutic milieu programs in which psychotherapeutic techniques are used. Consequently, such programs fail to adequately address the complex interaction of cognitive and behavior disorders apparent in severe brain injuries.

Cognitive Therapy

A specific form of psychotherapy is cognitive therapy, an approach fundamentally concerned with information processing—how people perceive and interpret their experience and how this in turn alters and shapes their behavior. Events are processed through preexisting cognitive schemata (beliefs, knowledge, and prepositions) which effectively bias interpretation of experience. Emotional disorders can arise through cognitive distortion whereby the interpretation of experience is colored to reflect the nature of these schemata. For example, in depression events are processed through schemata, that reflect hopelessness, helplessness, and failure (Beck, 1976) while in anxiety they are concerned with threat (Clark, 1989). Furthermore, bias in interpretation of experience maintains these maladaptive schemata which are evident from the automatic thoughts triggered by events. The cognitive therapies embrace this "information processing" approach to the interpretation of experience by attempting to help patients understand the link between beliefs, thinking, and behavior; identify their own thinking distortions; and generate more rational interpretations of events. Patients are helped to become their own "therapist" and encouraged to test the validity of their automatic thoughts through participation in behavioral experiments. Cognitive distortions are transformed or replaced altogether by altering the underlying belief systems that generate them through this process of hypothesis testing. Furthermore, therapy is very much a collaborative venture between the cognitive therapist and the patient. In this way dysfunctional emotion and behavior which are shaped by the perception of experience are successfully modified to the benefit of the individual.

The cognitive therapies continue to be successfully employed with many client groups, covering a broad range of disorders (Scott, 1997), and represent the preferred and most efficacious intervention available in some cases (see, e.g., Clark et al., 1994).

Given the success of these methods, and the prevalence and severity of behavioral disorders among people with ABI, application of the cognitive therapies to this group has inherent appeal. However, those factors that impede participation in psychotherapy may also constitute a special challenge to overcome when using cognitive therapy (Burgess & Wood, 1990; Sazbon & Groswasser, 1991; Alderman, 2003). The first is the problem of lack of awareness; the second is impairment of those cognitive skills necessary to engage in the hypothesis-testing process that is central to cognitive therapy.

We have seen already that problems of reduced awareness are well documented following brain trauma. Reduced awareness of behavioral disorders may be a persistent problem which is the result of either psychological defense mechanisms (Lewis, 1991) or directly attributable to neurological damage itself (e.g., McGlynn & Schacter, 1989). Problems with monitoring discussed earlier can also contribute to impairment of awareness as patients may not consistently detect social cues that would otherwise inform them that their behavior is causing concern. Central tenets within cognitive therapy are that patients are aware of the need to change their behavior, are motivated to do so, and become fully engaged in the therapeutic process (Manchester & Wood, 2001). Thus in the case of patients who lack awareness of their behavior disorders, efforts must be made to increase their insight and then harness sufficient motivation to undertake therapy. Manchester and Wood (2001) have written an extensive account of how this may be achieved using Prochaska and DiClemente's (1982) six-stage model of change. Crucial to overcoming the barrier of poor awareness are the first two stages of this model, precontemplation and contemplation. Here, the task of the therapist is to increase awareness by encouraging patients to recognize the discrepancy between their own goals and the increased perception of risks of not achieving these goals associated with their behavior. Through a process of elaborate collaborative working, patients are guided to the point where this discrepancy is understood and the need to change, in order to achieve their goals, arrived at. This process requires a highly skilled therapist. Increasing awareness which has a neurological basis must have a poorer prognosis than that which is the product of impaired monitoring, while there are obvious dangers in removing psychological barriers that have evolved in order to protect people from unpleasant, anxiety-evoking truths. For example, Fordyce, Roueche, and Prigatano (1983) highlighted the increase in incidence of depression that occurs following development of greater self-awareness among people with ABI.

The second challenge to overcome concerns impairment of those cognitive functions necessary to engage in this process. Attention, monitoring skills, memory, the ability to think abstractly, and the ability to generate alternatives are all crucial. Yet deficits in memory and executive functioning are almost routine following brain injury. Manchester and Wood (2001) acknowledge these difficulties and highlight the need for repeated practice and internalization of new cognitive schemata (via a "verbal script" taught in sessions) at very frequent intervals to encourage skill acquisition through procedural learning. They advocate employing brief, highly structured, repetitive sessions within which role play is used to encourage assimilation of new, adaptive automatic thoughts. Again, the approach is highly skilled and almost certainly requires inpatient treatment within a specialized environment that can sustain such sessions at the frequency necessary for learning to take place. Another cognitive impairment that may impede cognitive therapy is that of concrete, inflexible thinking. Within cognitive therapy, the process of subjecting maladaptive automatic thoughts that drive behavior is undertaken by the patient and facilitated by the therapist. Once these thoughts have been identified, it is the patient who appraises them and seeks to generate more rational alternatives. When the ability to think in abstract terms and generate alternatives is grossly impaired, this process, which is central to cognitive therapy, may be untenable. However, in the case of the behaviorally disturbed patient who is both aware of and motivated to change, so-called concrete cognitive restructuring strategies (CCRS) may be used in which alternatives to dysfunctional automatic beliefs are identified by the therapist and taught through mass practice. The patient is encouraged to state alternatives taught in this way at very frequent intervals, both in and out the presence of those triggers associated with the target behavior. When used in conjunction with behavior modification techniques, CCRS can enable substitution of dysfunctional for functional cognitive schemata, despite concrete and inflexible thinking. For an example of this, see the account of patient SJ given by Burgess and Alderman (1990) in which CCRS was used along with the behavior modification techniques of exposure and mastery, to reduce duration of shouting that prevented acquisition of independent hygiene skills.

Despite its appeal, there may be considerable challenges to surmount in using cognitive therapy with people who have severe brain injury and behavior disorders. Patients whose poor awareness is a direct function of neurological damage may simply not be amenable to the sort of techniques described by Manchester and Wood (2001), while those with very severe memory impairment and other cognitive deficits may be similarly excluded. The presence of language and communication problems is also a challenge to overcome. Furthermore, the nature of underlying neurological damage may interfere with the presumed relationship between adaptive thinking and behavior. For example, while it may be perfectly possible to replace negative automatic thoughts with more functionally desirable ones, damage to the orbito–temporal–limbic feedback loop, in which the inhibitory function of the cortex over the amygdala is disrupted, will render the expression of spontaneous instinctive emotion (such as aggression) beyond the previously suppressing control of intellectual function (Starkstein & Robinson, 1991). When this is the case, the influence of thinking on behavior is obviously more tenuous.

Because of the sequelae of ABI it may be that the proportion of people who may engage in and benefit from cognitive therapy is somewhat less than other clinical populations. Although advice for how it can be modified so it can be used in ABI is available (see, e.g., Kinney, 2001), its application remains underresearched to date so conclusions cannot be reliably drawn about efficacy just yet (Manchester & Wood, 2001). However, cognitive therapy has been successfully applied to people with learning difficulties, a clinical population that has much in common with ABI (although it must also be acknowledged there are important differences; Alderman, 2001). Methods are selected that best circumvent whatever language and cognitive handicaps a patient has in order to meet his or her needs. Similar rules for selecting what methods may work best according to the challenges set by these handicaps may also be possible for people with ABI (see Williams & Jones, 1997; Jones, Williams, & Lowe, 1993).

Behavior Modification

Use of behavior modification techniques in the remediation of behavior disorders following brain injury has received much attention in the rehabilitation literature during the last two decades. There are many advantages to using this approach (see Powell, 1981; Wilson, 1989), including the availability of techniques to both increase and decrease behaviors of interest, the ability to objectively evaluate treatment outcome, and the fact that interventions are purposely tailored to meet the needs of the individual.

However, there are particular reasons that advocate the use of behavior modification with this clinical population. One of the most obvious reasons to employ it is because people have been excluded from psychotherapy and cognitive therapy through lack of awareness, poor motivation, cognitive impairment, or the severity of behavior disorder. However, the presence of these problems does not necessarily prevent effective use of behavior therapy.

A problem which should be now clear to readers of this chapter is the complexity of the reasons driving behavior disorders: They may be attributable to a wide range of causal factors including organic, neuropsychological, and environmental factors. Assessment of what drives behavior disorders can therefore be highly problematic. Wood and Eames (Wood, 1987, 1990; Wood & Eames, 1981) have previously argued that for the process of assessment, the brain should be considered a dependent variable, subjected to environmental manipulation, and the effects studied. In this way, using an inductive approach that stresses objectivity, the nature of causative factors which underlie behavior disorders are more likely to be determined and understood. In an extension of this model, principles borrowed from operant conditioning, cognitive psychology, and behavioral neurology are combined to form what Wood has labeled the neurobehavioral paradigm (Wood, 1987, 1990; Wood & Worthington, 2001a, 2001b). Neurobehavioral rehabilitation encompasses systems that address cognitive and physical sequelae of brain injury, in addition to targeting behavior disorders. Furthermore, it may be practiced with patients in any stage of their recovery, and on an outpatient or inpatient basis.

It is clearly beyond the scope of this chapter to provide a full account of the neurobehavioral model or specific details of how different therapy disciplines operate within it. Instead, the reader is referred to Wood (1987, 1990) and Wood and Worthington (2001a, 2001b) regarding the assumptions underlying the model and details of how it is achieved within rehabilitation, and to Fussey and Giles (1988) with respect to discipline-specific approaches to wider therapy conducted within a neurobehavioral framework. Alderman (2001) has recently described how the principles of the neurobehavioral paradigm can be specifically operationalized for the purpose of managing challenging behavior.

Concepts central to neurobehavioral practice differentiate it significantly from both the medical model and traditional clinical rehabilitation (Wood & Worthington, 2001a). These concepts include that it happens postacutely (i.e., when medical management is no longer the priority), is transdisciplinary, and demands a structured environment. Within this environment, behavior modification techniques are used, including stimulus-control methods, chaining and shaping, and response–consequence learning technologies (Wood, 1990).

The principles of behavior modification are fundamental. They are used to create conditions that encourage motivation and success, by reinforcing appropriate behavior and skills. Whenever possible, the desirable consequence of appropriate behavior is to withdraw attention using "time out on the spot" from positive reinforcement, (Wood, 1987; Burgess & Wood, 1990). Thus, the treatment philosophy actively encourages management of behavior disorders using the least intrusive approach possible. Behavior modification techniques are not only used to promote prosocial behavior but also incorporated into discipline-specific skill-building approaches concerned with promoting physical and functional independence (see Fussey & Giles, 1988).

It will be recalled from earlier that some categories of behavior disorder have been thought to arise through breakdown in the allocation of attentional controls. Baddeley's central executive model has not only been influential in accounting for behavior disorders but has also generated the development of a number of treatment interventions. It will be recalled that one consequence of damage to the CE component of working memory is that the ability to monitor two or more events concurrently becomes impaired. Behavior disorders arise when problems with monitoring mean that social cues that signal that it is appropriate to change behavior are missed. On the basis of this model, Alderman and colleagues (Alderman, 1996; Alderman, Fry, & Youngson, 1995) suggest that when this is the case, alternative systems must be employed whose purpose is to alert people of cues they otherwise miss. Behavior modification programs delivered within a highly structured environment fulfill this role as they facilitate delivery of feedback in this way and could be the reason that some interventions are particularly effective (see, e.g., Wood, 1987; Alderman & Ward, 1991; Alderman & Burgess, 1994; Alderman & Knight, 1997). Alderman et al. (1995) used the CE model to successfully develop what is arguably a cognitive rehabilitation technique used for the treatment of behavior disorders that are secondary to severe impairment of monitoring function.

There is little doubt that behavior modification programs delivered within a highly structured environment have produced good outcomes. There are many individual case studies that have employed good experimental methodology in the literature to support this. However, the approach is not without its critics. First, to obtain the necessary consistency of approach, behavior modification interventions may not be easily accommodated outside specialized neurobehavioral rehabilitation units because of the amount of resources and specialized knowledge required (Alderman, 2001). Watson, Rutterford, Shortland, Williamson, and Alderman (2001) described a case study in which significant reduction in aggressive behavior was achieved using behavior modification techniques in a patient 10 years after injury within a "traditional" neurorehabilitation center. However, these authors point out that the speed at which gains were made was slower than would have been the case in a specialized center, and that the service had to undergo a degree of reorganization in order to accommodate the intervention (thus achieving a degree of "specialization"). Second, although there are a large number of published case studies that testify to the efficacy of the approach, they tend to be concerned with very specific aspects of behavior: The contribution of any successful intervention to rehabilitation as a whole is sometimes unclear. This is more obvious when the behavior disorder has great impact on the environment, such as aggression, when it can be shown that its presence leads to partial or full exclusion from the rehabilitation process. In these cases, behavior modification delivered within a wider neurobehavioral program has much to offer (see Alderman et al., 1999). Third, leading from the second possible criticism, there have been few studies with larger patient cohorts examining outcome from services which are organized on neurobehavioral principles for behaviorally disordered patients; however, those that have generally confirm the efficacy of this approach (Eames & Wood, 1985a, 1985b; Eames, Cotterill, Kneale, Storrar, & Yeomans, 1996). Fourth, behavior modification interventions have been criticized in that they fail to generalize to other environments beyond those in which treatment was delivered (McGlynn, 1990). However, it may be the case that when cognitive impairment is the major contributing factor to the maintenance of behavior disorders, the highly structured environment acts as a prosthetic in that it facilitates the effective delivery of feedback through operation of behavior modification interventions. When people are discharged and this prosthetic is no longer available, problems with monitoring return and behavior deteriorates. It may be that once discharged from the specialized environment of a neurobehavioral unit, contingencies change in such a way that behavior disorders are reinforced again (Alderman, 2001). When cognitive systems are severely damaged, people may be dependent for life on systems that are placed around them which circumvent the difficulties arising from their breakdown. If so, generalization is unrealistic; instead, finding the least intrusive level of support that enables the best quality of life becomes the goal rather than preoccupation with the idealistic aim of completely removing all structure, including behavioral programs.

SUGGESTIONS FOR FUTURE RESEARCH

There is no doubt that behavior disorders that arise as a result of ABI constitute a major handicap to the person concerned, their family, and the wider community. In this chapter, some of the reasons to account for the pervasiveness of these disorders have been considered and some of the treatment options available described and reviewed. Some treatment methods are clearly driven by theory, but for many the link is less well defined. Of course, the information contained in this chapter is by no means a definitive review of the area. However, it is hoped that sufficient detail will have been imparted to persuade the reader that the issues pertaining to causative factors are by no means simple. Lack of homogeneity within this clinical population, the presence of multiple handicaps resulting from brain lesion, and the multitude of single factors that may contribute all serve to cloud the clinical picture as behavior disorders arise from complex interactions involving these and other variables. Attempting to formulate a single causal model for behavior disorder, or even subtypes (such as aggression), would clearly be foolhardy. Because of the richness and variety of contributory factors and their interactions, behavior disorders will seldom be the expression of a single underlying cause; a thorough assessment should be undertaken in order to understand what factors underlie behavior problems and how they work to maintain them. All this points to the study of the individual as probably providing the most valid source of information to contribute to theory, and definitely that which will give the clinician the knowledge necessary to enable optimal rehabilitation (see Alderman, 2002).

Given the complexity of the issues, the potential for future research and the directions such research may take are considerable. Some of these issues include the following.

First, it is clear that more methodical studies concerning the relative efficacy of pharmacological interventions are required. For example, in a review of the literature, Alderman et al. (1997) found that most accounts they sampled concerning pharmacological treatment of aggression were descriptive. The contribution such studies make in attempting to evaluate the usefulness of these drugs with broadly similar patients presenting with generally similar behavior disorders is obviously poor. Instead, use of appropriate single-case experimental methodologies should enable much more robust and helpful conclusions to be drawn regarding efficacy. Within this context, a comprehensive and scientifically robust study of the use of carbamazepine and valproic acid in the treatment of EDS and other paroxysmal mood disorders remains long overdue (Rao & Lyketsos, 2000).

The second proposed area for research concerns assessment of behavior disorders, particularly when treatment occurs within the context of the neurobehavioral paradigm. The importance of a good functional analysis of behavior has been highlighted by a number of authors and strategies suggested in an effort to best appreciate the myriad complex interactions that contribute to behavior disorders; without a thorough functional analysis, ineffective treatment interventions may be implemented (see Treadwell & Page, 1996). However, successful developments in the use of computers in functional assessment within the area of developmental disabilities (Oliver, Hall, & Nixon, 1999) almost certainly have much to contribute to the appraisal of behavior disorders with complex etiology among people with ABI. This is a line of inquiry that is currently being investigated by Oliver, Alderman, and their colleagues; early results look extremely encouraging.

A third area for research concerns application of the cognitive therapies to people with ABI. It may be recalled that there is acknowledgement from practitioners who use these methods that evidence-based outcomes are lacking (Manchester & Wood, 2001). In this respect, the area parallels the need highlighted regarding efficacy of pharmacological approaches. Development of outcome protocols, again using appropriate single-case study experimental designs, would be welcomed. Furthermore, the relative utility of these therapies in comparison to other methods of treatment (a well-researched line of inquiry regarding other clinical populations and problems) needs to be determined. Knowledge of which factors exclude people from participating in cognitive therapies is also important. It may be a relatively easy matter to identify some of the more obvious ones, such as type and severity of cognitive impairment. However, a more ambitious study could be considered to examine whether the underlying neuropathology contraindicates use of this therapy. For example, with the development of appropriate methodologies, functional neuroimaging could be used to demonstrate the integrity of the orbito–temporal–limbic feedback loop. Compromise of this system could have implications for the efficacy of cognitive therapy if it can be demonstrated that patients may be unable to purposefully and successfully suppress spontaneous instinctive emotion: If this is the case, substitution of dysfunctional automatic thoughts with rational alternatives may have little impact on behavior. Investigating treatment outcome from cognitive therapy and relating this to results from functional neuroimaging could prove highly educative.

Finally, more knowledge regarding efficacy of neurobehavioral services is required. This type of rehabilitation is often costly, time-consuming, and intensive (McMillan & Oddy, 2001), yet comparatively little is known about the effectiveness of specialized neurobehavioral units. While individual outcome regarding specific problems continues to be well researched and represented in the rehabilitation literature, more needs to be known about the nature of the long-term benefits (social, clinical, and economic) resulting from participation in such programs. Furthermore, although there is some evidence that those structures necessitated by the neurobehavioral paradigm can be replicated with some success within less specialized services (see, e.g., Davis et al., 1994; Goll & Hawley, 1988; Watson et al., 2001; Alderman, 2003), there is little documented to demonstrate that it is possible to employ its principles within community settings. Although some advocates of the approach argue that social rehabilitation is community based (i.e., it does not take place in the hospital), it still takes place within the confines of a specialized center (Wood & Worthington, 2001a). Specialized knowledge and resources will also be required (Alderman, 2001). Though not impossible in some cases, it is unlikely that this type of rehabilitation can be conducted within a home environment. For example, when cognitive impairment is the major contributing factor to the maintenance of behavior disorder, the highly structured environment of a specialized center acts as a prosthetic that facilitates effective delivery of feedback through operation of behavior modification interventions. When people are discharged and this prosthetic is no longer available, problems with monitoring return and behavior deteriorates. It may be that when people are no longer within a specialized environment contingencies change in such a way that behavior disorders are reinforced again (Alderman, 2001). It may also be that when cognitive systems are severely damaged, people will be dependent for life on systems that are placed around them which circumvent the difficulties arising from their breakdown. If so, generalization and the ability to replicate such systems in the home are unrealistic expectations; the goal will be to determine the minimum level of support that maximizes the best quality of life. When this proves to be the case, those environmental modifications necessary to achieve this aim must be implemented and maintained in order to support appropriate behavior.

The range of options available in order to successfully manage behavior disorders is increasing. In the future it may be that progress in areas such as intracerebral and fetal brain cell implantation will have radical consequences for outcome after neurological insult (see, e.g., Elsayed, Hogan, Shaw, & Castro, 1996; Barami, Hao, Lotoczky, Diaz, & Lyman, 2001), including behavior problems. In the meantime, the existing range of treatment methods available continues to provide clinicians with methods to ensure optimum quality of life for people with ABI.

REFERENCES

Adolphus, R. (1999). Social cognition and the human brain. *Trends in Cognitive Science, 3,* 469–479.

Alderman, N. (1991). The treatment of avoidance behaviour following severe brain injury by satiation through negative practice. *Brain Injury, 5,* 77–86.

Alderman, N. (1996). Central executive deficit and response to operant conditioning methods. *Neuropsychological Rehabilitation, 6,* 161–186.

Alderman, N. (2001). Management of challenging behaviour. In R. L. Wood & T. McMillan (Eds.), *Neurobehavioural disability and social handicap following traumatic brain injury.* Hove, East Sussex, UK: Psychology Press.

Alderman, N. (2002). Individual case studies. In S. Priebe & M. Slade (Eds.), *Evidence in mental health care.* Hove, East Sussex, UK: Brunner-Routledge.

Alderman, N. (2003). Contemporary approaches to the management of irritability and aggression following traumatic brain injury. *Neuropsychological Rehabilitation, 13,* 211–240.

Alderman, N., & Burgess, P. (1994). A comparison of treatment methods for behaviour disorders following herpes simplex encephalitis. *Neuropsychological Rehabilitation, 4,* 31–48.

Alderman, N., Davies, J. A., Jones, C., & McDonnell, P. (1999). Reduction of severe aggressive behaviour in acquired brain injury: Case studies illustrating clinical use of the OAS–MNR in the management of challenging behaviours. *Brain Injury, 13,* 669–704.

Alderman, N., Dawson, K., Rutterford, N. A., & Reynolds, P. J. (2001). A comparison of the validity of self-report measures among people with acquired brain injury: A preliminary study of the efficacy of the Euroqol-5D. *Neuropsychological Rehabilitation, 11,* 529–537.

Alderman, N., Fry, R. K., & Youngson, H. A. (1995). Improvement of self–monitoring skills, reduction of behaviour disturbance and the dysexecutive syndrome: Comparison of response cost and a new program of self–monitoring training. *Neuropsychological Rehabilitation, 5,* 193–221.

Alderman, N., & Knight, C. (1997). The effectiveness of DRL in the management and treatment of severe behaviour disorders following brain injury. *Brain Injury, 1*, 79–101.

Alderman, N., Knight, C., & Henman, C. (2002). Aggressive behaviours observed within a neurobehavioural rehabilitation service: Utility of the OAS–MNR in clinical audit and applied research. *Brain Injury, 16*, 469–489.

Alderman, N., Knight, C., & Morgan, C. (1997). Use of a modified version of the Overt Aggression Scale in the measurement and assessment of aggressive behaviours following brain injury. *Brain Injury, 11*, 503–523.

Alderman, N., Shepherd, J., & Youngson, H. A. (1992). Increasing standing tolerance and posture quality following severe brain injury using a behaviour modification approach. *Physiotherapy, 78*, 335–343.

Alderman, N., & Ward, A. (1991). Behavioural treatment of the dysexecutive syndrome: Reduction of repetitive speech using response cost and cognitive overlearning. *Neuropsychological Rehabilitation, 1*, 65–80.

Baddeley, A. D. (1986). *Working memory*. Oxford: Clarendon Press.

Baddeley, A. D., & Hitch, G. J. (1974). Working memory. In G. Bower (Ed.), *Recent advances in learning and motivation* (Vol. VIII). New York: Academic Press.

Baddeley, A. D., & Wilson, B. (1988). Frontal amnesia and the dysexecutive syndrome. *Brain and Cognition, 7*, 212–230.

Barami, K., Hao, H. N., Lotoczky, G. A., Diaz, F. G., & Lyman, W. D. (2001). Transplantation of human fetal brain cells into ischemic lesions of adult gerbil hippocampus. *Journal of Neurosurgery, 95*, 308–15.

Barlow, M., & Hersen, P. H. (1984). *Single case experimental designs: Strategies for studying behaviour change* (2nd ed.). New York: Pergamon Press.

Beck, A. T. (1976). *Cognitive therapy and the emotional disorders*. Madison, CT: International Universities Press.

Ben-Yishay, Y., Rattock, J., Lakin, P., Piasetsky, E. B., Ross, B., Silver, S., et al. (1985). Neuropsychologic rehabilitation: Quest for a holistic approach. *Seminars in Neurology, 5*, 252–258.

Bigler, E. D. (1984). *Diagnostic clinical neuropsychology*. Austin: University of Texas Press.

Bigler, E. D. (1990). Neuropathology of traumatic brain injury. In E. D. Bigler (Ed.), *Traumatic brain injury: Mechanisms of damage, assessment, intervention, and outcome*. Austin, Texas: Pro-Ed.

Bond, M. R. (1984). The psychiatry of closed head injury. In D. N. Brooks (Ed.), *Closed head injury: Psychological, social and family consequences*. Oxford, UK: Oxford University Press.

Brooks, D. N., McKinlay, W., Symington, C., Beattie, A., & Campsie, L. (1987). The effects of severe head injury upon patient and relative within seven years of injury. *Journal of Head Trauma Rehabilitation, 2*, 1–13.

Burgess, P. W., & Alderman, N. (1990). Rehabilitation of dyscontrol syndromes following frontal lobe damage: A cognitive neuropsychological approach. In R. L. Wood & I. Fussey (Eds.), *Cognitive rehabilitation in perspective*. Basingstoke, UK: Taylor & Francis.

Burgess, P. W., & Wood, R. L. (1990). Neuropsychology of behaviour disorders following brain injury. In R. L. Wood (Ed.), *Neurobehavioural sequelae of traumatic brain injury*. London: Taylor & Francis.

Burke, H. H., Wesolowski, M. D., & Lane, I. (1988). A positive approach to the treatment of aggressive brain injured clients. *International Journal of Rehabilitation
Research, 11,* 235–241.

Carberry, H., & Burd, B. (1983). Social aspects of cognitive retraining in an outpatient
group setting for head trauma patients. *Cognitive Rehabilitation, 1,* 5–7.

Childs, A. (1987). Naltrexone in organic bulimia: A preliminary report. *Brain Injury, 1,*
49–55.

Clark, D. M. (1989). Anxiety states: Panic and generalized anxiety. In K. Hawton, P. M.
Salkovskis, J. Kirk, & D. M. Clark (Eds.), *Cognitive behaviour therapy for psychiatric problems: A practical guide.* Oxford, UK: Oxford University Press.

Clark, D. M., Salkovskis, P. M., Hackmann, A., Middleton, H., Anastasiades, P., &
Gelder, M. (1994). A comparison of cognitive therapy, applied relaxation and
imipramine in the treatment of panic disorder. *British Journal of Psychiatry, 164,*
759–769.

Corrigan, J. D., Arnett, J. A., Houck, L. J., & Jackson, R. D. (1985). Reality orientation
for brain injured patients. Group treatment and monitoring of recovery. *Archives
of Physical Medicine and Rehabilitation, 66,* 626–630.

Cummings, J. L. (1993). Frontal–subcortical circuits and human behavior. Archives of
Neurology, 50, 873–880.

David, A. S., Wacharasindhu, A., & Lishman, W. A. (1993). Severe psychiatric disturbance and abnormalities of the corpus callosum: Review and case studies. *Journal
of Neurology, Neurosurgery, and Psychiatry, 56,* 85–93.

Davidson, R. J., & Irwin, W. (1999). The functional neuroanatomy of emotion and affective style. *Trends in Cognitive Science, 3,* 11–21.

Davis, J. R., Turner, W., Rolinder, A., & Cartwright, T. (1994). Natural and structured
baselines in the treatment of aggression following brain injury. *Brain Injury, 8,*
589–597.

Dolan, R. J., Bench, C. J., Liddle, P. F., Friston, K. J., Frith, C. D., Grasby, P. M., et al.
(1993). Dorsolateral prefrontal cortex dysfunction in the major psychoses: Sympto-
m or disease specificity? *Journal of Neurology, Neurosurgery, and Psychiatry, 56,*
1290–1294.

Eames, P. (1988). Behavior disorders after severe brain injury: Their nature, causes and
strategies for management. *Journal of Head Trauma Rehabilitation, 3,* 1–6.

Eames, P. (1989). The use of sinemet and bromocriptine. *Brain Injury, 3,* 319–322.

Eames, P. G. (1990). Organic bases of behaviour disorders after traumatic brain injury.
In R. L. Wood (Ed.), *Neurobehavioural sequelae of traumatic brain injury.* London:
Taylor & Francis.

Eames, P. G. (2001). Distinguishing the neuropsychiatric, psychiatric, and psychological
consequences of acquired brain injury. In R. L. Wood & T. McMillan (Eds.),
Neurobehavioural disability and social handicap following traumatic brain injury.
Hove, East Sussex, UK: Psychology Press.

Eames, P., Cotterill, G., Kneale, T. A., Storrar, A. L., & Yeomans, P. (1996). Outcome of
intensive rehabilitation after severe brain injury: A long-term follow-up study.
Brain Injury, 10, 631–650.

Eames, P., & Wood, R. L. (1985a). Rehabilitation after severe brain injury: A follow-up
study of a behaviour modification approach. *Journal of Neurology, Neurosurgery,
and Psychiatry, 48,* 613–619.

Eames, P., & Wood, R. L. (1985b). Rehabilitation after severe brain injury: A special-unit approach to behaviour disorders. *International Rehabilitation Medicine, 7*, 130–133.

Elsayed, M. H., Hogan, T. P., Shaw, P. L., & Castro, A. J. (1996). Use of fetal cortical grafts in hypoxic–ischemic brain injury in neonatal rats. *Experimental Neurology, 137*, 127–41.

Emerson, E., Barrett, S., Bell, C., Cummings, R., McCool, C., Toogood, A., et al. (1987). *Developing services for people with severe learning difficulties and challenging behaviours.* Canterbury, Kent, UK: University of Kent at Canterbury, Institute of Social and Applied Psychology.

Eslinger, P. J., & Damasio, A. R. (1985). Severe disturbances in higher cognition following bilateral frontal lobe ablation: Patient EVR. *Neurology, 35*, 1731–1741.

Fedoroff, J. P., Starkstein, S. E., Forrester, A. W., Geisler, F. H., Jorge, R. E., Arndt, S. V., et al. (1992). Depression in patients with acute traumatic brain injury. *American Journal of Psychiatry, 7*, 918–923.

Fisher, C. M. (1983). Abulia minor vs. agitated behaviour. *Clinical Neurosurgery, 31*, 9–31.

Fordyce, D., Roueche, J., & Prigatano, G. (1983). Enhanced emotional reactions in chronic head trauma patients. *Journal of Neurology, Neurosurgery, and Psychiatry, 46*, 620–624.

Foster, H. G., Hillbrand, M., & Chi, C. C. (1989). Efficacy of carbamazepine in assaultive patients with frontal lobe dysfunction. *Progress in Neuro-Psychopharmacology and Biological Psychiatry, 13*, 865–874.

Fussey, I., & Giles, G. M. (Eds.). (1988). *Rehabilitation of the severely brain injured adult: A practical approach.* London: Croom Helm.

Geva, N., & Stern, J. M. (1985). The mourning process with brain injured patients. *Scandinavian Journal of Rehabilitation Medicine, Supplement No. 12*, 50–52.

Giakas, W. J., Seibyl, J. P., & Mazure, C. M. (1990). Valporate in the treatment of temper outburst. *Journal of Clinical Psychiatry, 51*, 525.

Glenn, M. B (1998). Methylphenidate for cognitive and behavioral dysfunction after traumatic brain injury. *Journal of Head Trauma Rehabilitation, 13*, 87–90.

Goll, S., & Hawley, K. (1988). Social rehabilitation: The role of the transitional living center. In R. L. Wood & P. G. Eames (Eds.), *Models of brain injury rehabilitation.* London: Chapman & Hall.

Grafman, J., Schwab, K., Warden, D., Pridgen, A., Brown, H. R., & Salazar, A. M. (1996). Frontal lobe injuries, violence, and aggression: A report of the Vietnam head injury study. *Neurology, 46*, 1231–1238.

Grafman, J., Vance, S. C., & Weingarter, H. (1986). The effects of lateralised frontal lesions on mood regulation. *Brain, 109*, 1127–1148.

Groswasser, Z., Mendelson, L., Stern., Schecter, I., & Najenson, T. (1977). Re-evaluation of prognostic factors in rehabilitation after severe head injury: Assessment 30 months after trauma. *Scandinavian Journal of Rehabilitation Medicine, 9*, 147–149.

Gualtieri, C. T. (1991). *Neuropsychiatry and behavioral pharmacology.* New York: Springer-Verlag.

Halligan, P. W., & Marshall, J. C. (Eds.). (1996). *Method in madness: Case studies in cognitive neuropsychiatry.* Hove, East Sussex, UK: Psychology Press.

Hartmann, A., Pickering, R. M., & Wilson, B. A. (1992). Is there a central executive deficit after severe head injury? *Clinical Rehabilitation, 6*, 133–140.

Hellekson, C. Buckland, R., & Price, T. (1979). Organic personality disturbance: A case of apparent atypical cyclic affective disorder. *American Journal of Psychiatry, 136,* 833–835.

Hier, D. B., Mondlock, J., & Caplan, L. R. (1983), Behavioural abnormalities after right hemisphere stroke. *Neurology, 33,* 337–344.

Hirsch, J. (1993, March/April). Promising drugs for neurobehavioural treatment. *Headlines,* pp. 10–11.

Jackson, W. T., & Gouvier, W. D. (1992). Group psychotherapy with brain-damaged adults and their families. In C. J. Lang & L. K. Ross (Eds.), *Handbook of head trauma, acute care to recovery.* New York: Plenum Press.

Jacobs, H. E. (1990). Identifying posttraumatic behavior problems: Data from psychosocial follow-up studies. In R. L. Wood (Ed.), *Neurobehavioural sequelae of traumatic brain injury.* London: Taylor & Francis.

Johnson, R., & Balleny, H. (1996). Behaviour problems after brain injury: Incidence and need for treatment. *Clinical Rehabilitation, 10,* 173–181.

Jones, R. S. P., Williams, H., & Lowe, F. (1993). Verbal self-regulation. In I. Fleming & B. Stenfert-Krocso (Eds.), *People with severe learning disability and challenging behaviour: New developments in services and therapy.* Manchester: Manchester University Press.

Jorge, R. E., Robinson, R. G., Arndt, S. V., Forrester, A. W., Geisler, F., & Starkstein, S. E. (1993). Comparison between acute- and delayed-onset depression following traumatic brain injury. *Journal of Neuropsychiatry, 5,* 43–49.

Kimble, D. P. (1963). *Physiological psychology.* Reading, MA: Addison-Wesley.

Kinney, A. (2001). Cognitive therapy and brain injury: Theoretical and conceptual issues. *Journal of Contemporary Psychotherapy, 31,* 89–102.

Langfitt, T. W, Obrist, W. D., Alavi, A., Grossman, R. I., Zimmerman, R., Jaggi, J., et al. (1986). Computerized tomography, magnetic resonance imaging, and positron emission tomography in the study of brain trauma. *Journal of Neurosurgery, 64,* 760–767.

Leer, W. B. (1986). Brain injured activity group for cognitive retraining in a rehabilitation setting. Abstract, Proceedings of the 5th annual meeting of the National Academy of Neuropsychology. *Archives of Clinical Neuropsychology, 1,* 55.

Leer, W. B., & Sonday, W. E. (1986). Brain injured client coping skills group in a rehabilitation setting. Abstract, Proceedings of the 6th annual meeting of the National Academy of Neuropsychology. *Archives of Clinical Neuropsychology, 1,* 277.

Lewis, L. (1991). Role of psychological factors in disordered awareness. In G. Prigatano & D. Schacter (Eds.), *Awareness of deficit after brain injury: Clinical and theoretical issues.* New York: Oxford University Press.

London, P. S. (1967). Some observations on the course of events after severe injury of the head. *Annals of the Royal College of Surgeons of England, 41,* 460–479.

Manchester, D., & Wood, R. L. (2001). Applying cognitive therapy in neuropsychological rehabilitation. In R. L. Wood & T. M. McMillan (Eds.), *Neurobehavioural disability and social handicap following traumatic brain injury.* Hove, East Sussex, UK: Psychology Press.

Mateer, C. A., & Ruff, R. M. (1990). Effectiveness of behavioral management procedures in the rehabilitation of head-injured patients. In R. L. Wood (Ed.), *Neurobehavioural sequelae of traumatic brain injury.* New York: Taylor & Francis.

Mattes, J. A. (1990). Comparative effectiveness of carbamazepine and propranolol for rage outburst. *Journal of Neuropsychiatry and Clinical Neuroscience, 2,* 159–164.

McAllister, T. W. (1992). Neuropsychiatric sequelae of head injuries. *Psychiatric Clinics of North America, 15,* 395–413.

McGlynn, S. M. (1990). Behavioural approaches to neuropsychological rehabilitation. *Psychological Bulletin, 108,* 420–441.

McGlynn, S. M., & Schacter, D. L. (1989). Unawareness of deficits in neuropsychological syndromes. *Journal of Clinical and Experimental Neuropsychology, 11,* 143–205.

McKinlay, W. W., Brooks, D. N., Bond, M. R., Martinage, D. P., & Marshall, M. M. (1981). The short term outcome of severe blunt head injury as reported by the relatives of the injured person. *Journal of Neurology, Neurosurgery and Psychiatry, 44,* 527–533.

McMillan, T. M., & Oddy, M. (2001). Service provision for social disability and handicap after acquired brain injury. In R. L. Wood & T. M. McMillan (Eds.), *Neurobehavioural disability and social handicap following traumatic brain injury.* Hove, East Sussex, UK: Psychology Press.

Miller, E., & Cruzat, A. (1981). A note on the effects of irrelevant information on task performance after mild and severe head injury. *British Journal of Social and Clinical Psychology, 20,* 69–70.

Miller, L. (1994). Traumatic brain injury and aggression. *Journal of Offender Rehabilitation, 2,* 91–103.

Miller, B. L., Cummings, J. L., McIntyre, H., Ebers, G., & Grode, M. (1986). Hypersexuality or altered sexual preference following brain injury. *Journal of Neurology, Neurosurgery and Psychiatry, 49,* 867–873.

Monroe, R. R. (1970). *Episodic behavioral disorders.* Cambridge, MA: Harvard University Press.

Monroe, R. R. (1986). Episodic behavioral disorders and limbic ictus. In B. K. Doane & K. E. Livingston (Eds.), *The limbic system: Functional organization and clinical disorders.* New York: Raven Press.

Mooney, G. F., & Hass, L. J. (1993). Effect of methylphenidate on brain injury-related anger. *Archives of Physical Medicine and Rehabilitation, 74,* 153–160.

Naugle, R. I. (1990). Epidemiology of traumatic brain injury in adults. In E. D. Bigler (Ed.), *Traumatic brain injury: mechanisms of damage, assessment, intervention, and outcome.* Austin, TX: Pro-Ed.

Oder, W., Goldenberg, G., Spatt, I., Binder, H., & Deecke, L. (1992). Behavioural and psychosocial sequelae of severe closed head injury and regional cerebral blood flow: A SPECT study. *Journal of Neurology, Neurosurgery, and Psychiatry, 55,* 475–480.

Oliver, C., Hall, S., & Nixon, J. (1999). A molecular to molar analysis of communicative and problem behaviors. *Research in Developmental Disabilities, 20,* 197–213.

Paradiso, S., Chemerinski, E., Yazici, K. M., Tartaro, A., & Robinson, R. G. (1999). Frontal lobe syndrome reassessed: Comparison of patients with lateral or medial frontal brain damage. *Journal of Neurology, Neurosurgery, and Psychiatry, 67,* 664–667.

Patterson, C. H. (1986). *Theories of counselling and psychotherapy* (4th ed.). New York: Harper & Row.

Powell, G. E. (1981). *Brain function therapy*. Aldershot, UK: Gower Press.

Power, P. W., & Dell Orto, A. E. (1980). Approaches to family intervention. In P. W. Power & A. E. Dell Orto (Eds.), *Role of the family in the rehabilitation of the physically disabled*. Baltimore: University Park Press.

Prigatano, G. P. (1986). Psychotherapy after brain injury. In G. P. Prigatano, D. J. Fordyce, H. K. Zeiner, J. R. Roeche, M. Pepping, & B. C. Wood (Eds.), *Neuropsychological rehabilitation after brain injury*. Baltimore: Johns Hopkins University Press.

Prigatano, G. P. (1987). Psychiatric aspects of head injury: Problem areas and suggested guidelines for research. *BNI Quarterly, 3*, 2–9.

Prigatano, G. P. (1991). Disturbances of self awareness of deficit after traumatic brain injury. In G. P. Prigatano & D. L. Schacter (Eds.), *Awareness of deficit after brain injury: Clinical and theoretical issues*. New York: Oxford University Press.

Prigatano, G. P., Altman, I. M., & O'Brien, K. P. (1990). Behavioural limitations that brain injured patients tend to underestimate. *Clinical Neuropsychologist, 4*, 163–176.

Prigatano, G. P., Fordyce, D. J., Zeiner, H. K., Roueche, J. R., Pepping, M., & Wood, B. C. (1984). Neuropsychological rehabilitation after closed head injury in young adults. *Journal of Neurology, Neurosurgery and Psychiatry, 47*, 505–513.

Prochaska, J. O., & DiClemente, C. C. (1982). Transtheoretical therapy: Towards a more integrative model of change. *Psychotherapy: Theory, research and practice, 19*, 276–288.

Rao, V. R., & Lyketsos, M. D. (2000). Neuropsychiatric sequelae of traumatic brain injury. *Psychosomatics, 41*, 95–103.

Sazbon, L., & Groswasser, Z. (1991). Time-related sequelae of TBI in patients with prolonged post-comatose unawareness (PC-U) state. *Brain Injury, 5*, 3–8.

Scott, J. (1997). Advances in cognitive therapy. *Current Opinion in Psychiatry, 10*, 256–260.

Shallice, T. (1982). Specific impairments of planning. *Philosophical transactions of the Royal Society of London, B, 298*, 199–209.

Starkstein, S. E., & Robinson, R. G. (1991). The role of the human lobes in affective disorder following stroke. In H. S. Levin, H. M. Eisenberg, & A. L. Benton (Eds.), *Frontal lobe function and dysfunction*. Oxford, UK: Oxford University Press.

Stern, B., & Stern, J. M. (1985). On the use of dreams as a means of diagnosis of brain-injured patients. *Scandinavian Journal of Rehabilitation Medicine, Supplement No. 12*, 44–46.

Tadir, M., & Stern, J. M. (1985). The mourning process with brain injured patients. *Scandinavian Journal of Rehabilitation Medicine, Supplement No. 12*, 50–52.

Thomsen, I. V. (1990). Recognising the development of behaviour disorders. In R. L. Wood (Ed.), *Neurobehavioural sequelae of traumatic brain injury*. London: Taylor & Francis.

Treadwell, K., & Page, T. J. (1996). Functional analysis: identifying the environmental determinants of severe behavior disorders. *Journal of Head Trauma Rehabilitation, 11*, 62–74.

Uytdenhoef, P., Portelange, P., Jacquy, J, Charles, G., Linkowski, P., & Mendlewicz, J. (1983). Regional cerebral blood flow and lateralized hemispheric dysfunction in depression. *British Journal of Psychiatry, 143*, 128–132.

von Cramon, D. Y., & Matthes-von Cramon, G. (1994). Back to work with a chronic dysexecutive syndrome? *Neuropsychological Rehabilitation, 4,* 399–417.

Watson, C., Rutterford, N., Shortland, D., Williamson, N., & Alderman, N. (2001). Reduction of chronic aggressive behaviour ten years after brain injury. *Brain Injury, 15,* 1003–1015.

Weddel, R., Oddy, M., & Jenkins, D. (1980). Social adjustment after rehabilitation: A two year follow-up of patients with severe head injury. *Psychological Medicine, 10,* 257–263.

Williams, W. H., & Jones, R. S. P. (1997). Teaching cognitive self-regulation of independence and emotion control skills. In B. Stenfert-Kroese, D. Dagnan, & K. Loumidis (Eds.), *Cognitive behaviour therapy for people with learning disabilities.* London: Routledge.

Wilson, B. (1989). Injury to the central nervous system. In S. Pearce & J. Wardle (Eds.), *The practice of behavioural medicine.* Oxford, UK: University Press.

Wilson, B. A. (1991). Behavior therapy in the treatment of neurologically impaired adults. In P. R. Martin (Ed.), *Handbook of behavior therapy and psychological science: An integrative approach.* New York: Pergamon Press.

Wilson, B. A., Alderman, N., Burgess, P. W., Emslie, H., & Evans, J. J. (1996). *Behavioural assessment of the dysexecutive syndrome.* Bury St Edmunds, UK: Thames Valley Test Company.

Wood, R. L. (1987). *Brain injury rehabilitation: A neurobehavioural approach.* London: Croom Helm.

Wood, R. L. (1988). Management of behaviour disorders in a day treatment setting. *Journal of Head Trauma Rehabilitation, 3,* 53–62.

Wood, R. L. (1990). Conditioning procedures in brain injury rehabilitation. In R. L. Wood (Ed.), *Neurobehavioural sequelae of traumatic brain injury.* London: Taylor & Francis.

Wood, R. L. (2001). Understanding neurobehavioural disability. In R. L. Wood & T. McMillan (Eds.), *Neurobehavioural disability and social handicap following traumatic brain injury.* Hove, East Sussex, UK: Psychology Press.

Wood, R. L., & Eames, P. (1981). Application of behaviour modification in the rehabilitation of traumatically brain injured patients. In G. Davey (Ed.), *Applications of conditioning theory.* London: Methuen.

Wood, R. L., & McMillan, T. M. (Eds.). (2001). *Neurobehavioural disability and social handicap following traumatic brain injury.* Hove, East Sussex, UK: Psychology Press.

Wood, R. L., & Worthington, A. D. (2001a). Neurobehavioural rehabilitation: A conceptual paradigm. In R. L. Wood & T. McMillan (Eds.), *Neurobehavioural disability and social handicap following traumatic brain injury.* Hove, East Sussex, UK: Psychology Press.

Wood, R. L., & Worthington, A. D. (2001b). Neurobehavioural rehabilitation in practice. In R. L. Wood & T. McMillan (Eds.), *Neurobehavioural disability and social handicap following traumatic brain injury.* Hove, East Sussex, UK: Psychology Press.

9

Rehabilitation Following Traumatic Brain Injury and Cerebrovascular Accident

Jennie Ponsford

A great deal of information has been presented regarding biological bases of neurobehavioral injury and recovery. This chapter attempts to further bridge the gap between researcher and clinician by discussing the application of these therapeutic approaches to the two most common causes of disability following neuronal injury: traumatic brain injury and cerebrovascular accident or stroke.

TRAUMATIC BRAIN INJURY

Traumatic brain injury (TBI) has been defined as "an insult to the brain caused by an external force that may produce diminished or altered states of consciousness, which results in impaired cognitive abilities or physical functioning" (National Head Injury Foundation, 1989). Such injuries, which result from a blunt impact to the head, are termed closed head injuries. TBIs may also result from penetration by a sharp instrument or a missile. These injuries, termed "open head injuries," result in a more focal pattern of neurological deficit. This pattern differs from that associated with closed head injuries, where pathology tends to be more diffuse, resulting in a more complex array of cognitive, behavioral, and emotional changes. This chapter focuses on the impact and management of closed head injuries.

Epidemiology of TBI

The incidence of TBI in the United States is estimated to be 1.5 to 2 per 1,000 population (Morton & Wehman, 1995; Kraus & McArthur, 1999). Estimates from the state of Victoria, Australia, suggest an incidence of approximately 1 per 1,000 population rate in Australia (Fortune & Wen, 1999). The most common causes of TBI in more than 70% of cases are motor vehicle accidents, where the person is injured as the occupant of a car or motorcycle or as a pedestrian. Cycling accidents, falls, assaults, and sporting injuries are the next most common causes (Kraus & McArthur, 1999). Perhaps related to these causative factors is the fact that these injuries occur predominantly in young people under 30 years, most commonly in the age group 15–24 years, with a second peak in the older age groups, who tend to be injured as pedestrians or as a result of falls. Two to three males are injured for every female. A higher proportion than usual have lower socioeconomic status and a history of learning difficulties or poor academic performance, substance abuse, and other psychiatric problems and unemployment (Bond, 1984; Fortune & Wen, 1999; Haas, Cope, & Hall, 1987; Kraus & McArthur, 1999; Rimel & Jane, 1984).

Although approximately 80% of these injuries are classified as mild, with a period of unconsciousness less than an hour, survivors of a moderate or severe TBI have persistent and sometimes lifelong cognitive and behavioral impairments. TBI is thus the leading cause of acquired disability in adolescents and young adults. Even mild head injuries can result in persisting physical, psychosocial, and/or cognitive disabilities in a proportion of individuals, and therefore the significance of the incidence of these injuries should not be overlooked (Voller et al., 1999; Ponsford et al., 2000).

Pathophysiology of TBI

Blunt trauma to the head associated with acceleration or deceleration forces results in a combination of translation and rotation, causing widespread injury of both a primary and a secondary nature. Contusions occur where the brain has contact with bony skull protuberances in the basal and polar frontal and temporal regions (see Figure 9.1). Shearing strains occur between tissues of different density, where gray and white matter tracts meet, causing lesions in areas such as the midbrain reticular formation, cerebellar peduncles, basal ganglia, hypothalamus, fornices, and corpus callosum (Graham, 1999; Povlishock & Christman, 1995).

Diffuse axonal injury (DAI) may result from both biomechanical forces, causing axotomy or axonal stretching, and neurochemical causes (Gentleman,

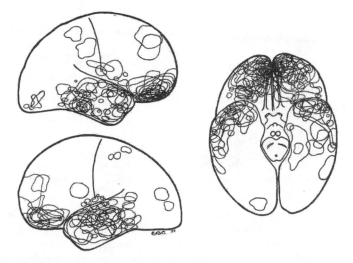

FIGURE 9.1. Most common sites of cerebral contusion following TBI. From Courville (1945). Copyright 1945 by Pacific Press Publishing Association, Inc. Reprinted by permission.

1999). Whereas focal lesions result from translational or linear trauma, diffuse axonal injury is said to be more commonly caused by rotational forces, as might occur following a motor vehicle accident and sporting injuries where a blow has rotated the head (Anderson, Northam, Hendy, & Wrennall, 2001). Common sites of diffuse axonal injury are shown in Figure 9.2. As Turner and Levine (Chapter 7, this volume) have pointed out, DAIs may be surrounded by many intact axons (15 per 1,000 axons damaged in a typical motor vehicular accident injury; Povlishock, 1993), creating some potential for neuroplastic changes. Axonal changes occur over at least 48 hours after injury. As noted by Kolb and Cioe (Chapter 1, this volume), changes in ion gradients across the plasma membrane result in release of amino acid neurotransmitters, such as glutamate and aspartate, and cause an influx of calcium, which activates enzymes that kill the neuron from within. Blood-borne and injury-produced charged particles of oxygen and iron, called free radicals, are also highly toxic to injured neurons. Further damage to neurons may occur secondary to rupture of blood vessels, a drop in blood pressure or respiratory failure, which can cause a drop in levels of oxygen and glucose—elements all cells need to survive. The hippocampus and the thalamus are differentially sensitive to hypoxia. Graham et al. (1989) reported ischemic damage to the hippocampus and the basal ganglia in around 80% of fatal head injury cases.

As described by Kolb and Cioe (Chapter 1, this volume), over the first 24 hours, edema or swelling results from both extracellular fluid accumulation, es-

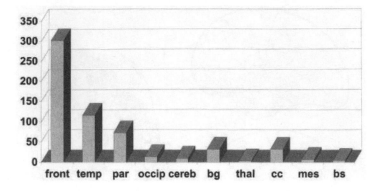

FIGURE 9.2. Frequency and site of traumatic microbleeds according to 10 brain areas. Shown is the total number of traumatic microbleeds in each brain area (front, frontal lobe; temp, temporal lobe; par, parietal lobe; occip, occipital lobe; cereb, cerebellum; bg, basal ganglia; thal, thalamus; cc, corpus callosum; mes, mesencephalon; bs, brain stem). From Scheid, Preol, Gruber, Wiggins, and Yves von Cramon (2003). Copyright 2003 by the American Society of Neuroradiology. Reprinted by permission.

pecially in the white matter, and astrocytic swelling (Nieto-Sampedro & Cotman, 1985). This swelling, together with changes in cerebral blood volume, results in elevated intracranial pressure. It acts to put pressure on the brain, causing further neuronal dysfunction and injury. There are also changes in the metabolism and/or glucose utilization, which can affect the functioning of tissue in the damaged area and otherwise intact areas and may persist for days. As a result of all these mechanisms, neurons and glial cells continue to die off in the first 24–48 hours after injury. Some neurons are killed instantly, some die later, others have long-term shock. Some more distal neurons begin to degenerate 48 hours after the trauma due to changes in blood flow, metabolism, pH, and edema—a process called secondary degeneration. This can go on for weeks or months. Some cells look normal and do not die but remain weakened and more vulnerable to stress and dysfunction throughout life. Through a process known as diaschisis, some areas related to but sometimes quite distal to the damaged area suffer a temporary loss of function due to the sudden withdrawal of excitation or inhibition. Beginning soon after injury, but continuing for months, microglia clear away debris, and adjacent astrocytes and fibroblasts isolate the surface of the injury and produce a scar that prevents axons from re-entering the injured area.

Due to these multiple mechanisms of injury, neuronal damage resulting from TBI tends to be heterogeneous. Moderate to severe injuries generally result in widespread, bilateral injury, with a preponderance of lesions in the frontal and temporal regions, as well as the basal ganglia and the hippocampus, the midbrain reticular formation, fornices, corpus callosum, hypothalamus, and cerebral peduncles.

As noted by Kolb and Cioe (Chapter 1, this volume), treatments for cerebral injury can be directed at different targets in the postinjury cascade. Neuroprotectants may be used to block calcium channels or prevent ionic imbalance. Other drugs, such as anti-inflammatories, can be used to reduce swelling or to enhance metabolic activity. However, while these interventions have been shown to be reduce brain damage in experimental models of brain injury, it is proving difficult to translate such findings into improved outcome for human patients (Teasdale, Maas, Iannotti, Ohrman, & Unterberg, 1999). This may reflect the number and complexity of injury mechanisms occurring simultaneously following TBI.

Initially TBI results in a period of loss or clouding of consciousness, followed by posttraumatic amnesia (PTA), which may last from seconds to many months. The initial depth of coma, as measured by the Glasgow Coma Scale (GCS) (Teasdale & Jennett, 1976) and the duration of PTA are said to be the best indicators of injury severity (Bishara, Partridge, Godfrey, & Knight, 1992; Jennett & Teasdale 1981; Ponsford, Olver, Curran, & Ng, 1995). Depending on the location and extent of injury to the brain, a broad range of sensorimotor disabilities may result from TBI. Motor deficits can take the form of weakness or paralysis on one or both sides of the body, incoordination of muscle movements (ataxia), loss of fine and gross motor dexterity, poor balance, and reduced physical endurance. Injury to the nerves that supply the motor apparatus responsible for the production of speech may result in dysarthria or dyspraxia. Swallowing disorders (dysphagia) may also occur. A broad range of sensory disturbances affecting smell, vision, hearing or taste, touch, or proprioception may be caused by cranial nerve lesions, or injury to subcortical or cortical sensory pathways. Tinnitus and vertigo are also common symptoms, especially following mild head injuries (Jennett & Teasdale, 1981).

Following mild TBI a range of symptoms tends to occur in the first few hours, days, or weeks. These symptoms include headache, dizziness, sensitivity to noise and/or bright lights, tinnitus, blurred or double vision, restlessness, insomnia, reduced speed of thinking, concentration and memory problems, fatigue, irritability, anxiety, and depression. In the majority of cases these symptoms resolve over a period from 1 to 4 weeks, although there are a group of approximately 20% who experience persisting symptoms, due to a variety of factors, including injury severity, presence of other injuries or stressors and preinjury psychological adjustment (Ponsford et al., 2000).

Moderate to severe TBI commonly results in a range of more lasting cognitive and behavioral changes. The nature and severity of these vary widely depending on the nature of the injury, which can affect any cognitive domain, including attention, memory, language, and visuospatial or executive functions. The most common cognitive changes reflect frontotemporal and/or DAI. Impairments of attention and speed of information processing, as outlined by Ponsford and Willmott (Chapter 3, this volume) are particularly common. Learning and memory difficulties will depend on which parts of the memory system have been damaged. Although the hippocampus is certainly very vulnerable to the effects of hypoxia, it is relatively unusual to see a complete amnesic syndrome following TBI. More commonly there is some impairment of episodic memory, perhaps more in one modality than in another. Even more commonly one sees memory impairment typically associated with frontal lobe lesions, where encoding and retrieval are inefficient and unreliable but recognition memory is relatively preserved. As noted by Glisky (Chapter 4, this volume), there may be problems with source memory or memory for temporal order, or in difficult recall tasks that require strategic processes. Working memory may also be affected by frontal lobe lesions. Any or all of a range of executive difficulties are particularly common, including impaired planning and problem solving, "goal neglect," impaired abstract thinking, and mental flexibility. The capacity for verbal regulation of behavior may be affected, with difficulty following through with one's intentions, impulsivity, or loss of initiative. Reduced frustration tolerance, irritability, aggression, sexual disinhibition, and socially inappropriate behavior are also common, as is self-centerdness. Communication problems include excessive talking or verbosity, poor turn-taking skills in conversation, and a tendency to repeat oneself or have difficulty keeping to the point. Word-finding difficulties and impaired auditory processing are also common. Mood swings may occur, or there may be a flatness of affect. There is a tendency of lack insight into or awareness of these changes.

The early recovery after TBI tends to be quite rapid as there is resolution of temporary physiological changes, such as edema, vascular disruption, intracranial pressure changes, and biochemical alterations, which have caused functional rather than structural axonal disruption. Recovery following TBI follows a negatively accelerating curve which is most rapid in the first 3 to 6 months but may continue for several years. Indeed, the time frame over which improvement occurs following severe TBI appears to be somewhat longer than is the case following stroke. This probably reflects the fact that the mechanisms of injury differ and neuronal injury is more diffuse and extensive and tends to be bilateral. Processes such as remyelination may occur over long periods. Some long-term improvement may also result from the development of compensatory processes. The vast majority of patients make a good physical recovery, with over 90% being independently mobile at 1 year postinjury (Ponsford, Olver, & Curran 1995; Ponsford, Olver, Nelms, Curran, & Ponsford, 1999). This might reflect the fact that individual lesions are smaller, though more diffuse, and it is less common for an entire area such as the motor cortex to be wiped out. Some cognitive impairments, such as dysphasia and unilateral spatial neglect, show the same tendency to resolve, again suggesting different causative mechanisms from those associated with cerebrovascular accident. It is possible that some of these early impairments result from temporary dysfunction associated with metabolic changes.

However, results of numerous outcome studies have indicated that many cognitive and behavioral changes do persist in the majority of cases, particularly impairments of attention and speed of information processing, memory, and executive function, as well as behavioral control and regulation (Ponsford, Sloan, & Snow, 1995). These cause problems with employment or study, pursuit of leisure activities, and personal and social relationships (Hoofien, Gilboa, Vakil, & Donovick, 2001; Koskinen, 1998; Oddy, Coughlan, Tyerman, & Jenkins, 1985; Ponsford, Olver, & Curran, 1995; Ponsford, Olver, Curran, & Ng, 1995; Tate, Lulham, Broe, Strettles, & Pfaff, 1989). The failure to achieve such important developmental goals as completing a course of study, holding down a job, and having a social network and close personal relationships tends to result, in the long term, in loss of self-esteem, anxiety and depression, and social isolation (Elsass & Kinsella, 1987; Fryer, 1989; Hoofien et al., 2001; Oddy, 1984; Tyerman & Humphrey, 1984). These young people often remain dependent on their families for support and assistance (Hoofien et al., 2001; Jacobs 1988; Olver, Ponsford, & Curran, 1996), creating a significant long-term burden (Brooks, Campsie, Symington, Beattie, & McKinlay, 1986; Hoofien et al., 2001). The major source of family stress appears to be changes in cognition, behavior, and personality (Brooks, Campsie, Symington, Beattie, & McKinlay, 1987; Kreutzer, Gervasio, & Camplair, 1994; McKinlay, Brooks, Bond, Martinage, & Marshall, 1981; Ponsford, Olver, Ponsford, & Nelms, 2003).

Rehabilitation Following TBI

A great deal of research has and continues to be devoted to the development of acute management strategies, pharmacological interventions, and stem cell therapies to reduce morbidity and mortality or enhance recovery following TBI. Much has been achieved through rapid transportation to specialized trauma centers and institution of methods to prevent secondary brain damage caused by elevated intracranial pressure or hypoxia. However, given the diffuse nature of these injuries, which affect so many brain regions and neurotransmitter systems through multiple injury mechanisms, progress in developing effective interventions of a pharmacological nature or stem cell therapies has been very slow and seems unlikely to have a major impact in the near future (Teasdale, 2002).

In view of this and the fact that these predominantly young people are facing a unique range of difficulties with so many important aspects of what is likely to be a normal lifespan, the importance of developing effective rehabilitative interventions for individuals with TBI cannot be overestimated. As Kolb concludes in Chapter 2, rehabilitative therapy should be delivered early in the postinjury recovery phase, in order to take maximal advantage of the brain's plastic state and to ensure that changes occurring are functionally beneficial to the injured person. Maladaptive patterns of movement or behavior can be extremely difficult to reverse as they are well entrenched. Because of the complex and interactive nature of the impairments following TBI, multidimensional programs are certainly more likely to be effective, for reasons outlined in detail later. Evidence presented in Chapters 3, 4, and 8 (in this volume) suggests that pharmacological therapies may also be of assistance in treating disorders of memory, attention, and behavior.

Factors Influencing Outcome/Response to Therapy

In Chapter 1 Kolb and Cioe identified a number of factors influencing response to injury and recovery. Some of these are pertinent to TBI. From a demographic point of view, there is one very positive influence. Those injured tend to be young and are unlikely to suffer coexisting medical conditions which might complicate recovery. Given that age is one of the more significant factors influencing outcome following TBI, with older age (> 45) being associated with poorer outcomes (Ponsford, Olver, Curran, & Ng, 1995), younger age represents a significant advantage.

In the case of children, the relationship between age and outcome is more complex. According to Kolb and Cioe (Chapter 1), recovery is very poor during the period of neural migration and relatively good during the periods of mitosis and synaptogenesis. Babies injured during the third trimester, when there is extensive migration, are likely to have more devastating injuries, whereas those injured around 8–12 months of age, the peak period of synaptogenesis, may show greatest potential for cerebral plasticity. In children, some functions (e.g., language), show greater potential for plasticity than others. Certain functions undergoing rapid development at the time of injury may be more affected than others (Anderson et al., 2001). There is also evidence to suggest that children injured in infancy or early childhood fail to develop certain functions, such as executive skills, so there may be a growing disability over time (Anderson et al., 2001; Dennis, Barnes, Donnelly, Wilkinson, & Humphreys, 1996). The findings of Anderson and Moore (1995) suggest that children injured in the preschool years show poorer outcomes than those injured later in childhood.

Negative prognostic indicators for recovery following TBI include a history of learning difficulties, low IQ, unemployment, lower socioeconomic status, substance use, or psychiatric problems. Unfortunately, these appear to occur in a greater than average proportion of individuals who sustain TBI (Bond, 1984; Fortune & Wen, 1999; Haas et al., 1987; Kraus & McArthur, 1999; Rimel & Jane, 1984).

There is clearly wide variability in the nature, location, and extent of lesions resulting from TBI. Where lesions are confined to a small area and are surrounded by intact neural tissue, as might occur in some cases of DAI, there should be greater potential for neuronal/dendritic reorganization. Thus mild to moderate cases of TBI show greatest potential for recovery, and this is borne out in the results of outcome studies (Anderson, Catroppa, Morse, Haritou, & Rosenfeld, 2000; Rapoport, McCauley, Levin, Song, & Feinstein, 2002). However, in the majority of those with severe TBI, the neuronal injury is widespread, with a great deal of scarring and loss of many neuronal connections. In these cases there may not be a great deal of intact tissue and hence little potential for dendritic growth or synaptic change.

Nevertheless, recovery does occur in many cases over very long periods after injury and there is clear evidence of response to rehabilitation (e.g., Burke, Wesolowski, & Guth, 1988; Fryer & Haffey, 1987; Mills, Nesbeda, Katz, & Alexander, 1992; Sander, Roebuck, Struchen, Sherer, & High, 2001; Seale et al., 2002). According to Robertson and Murre (1999), this improvement most probably occurs via compensation from other intact neural circuits or through use of external supports. As Glisky has pointed out (Chapter 4, this volume), the potential for rehabilitation will to some extent depend on which components of a functional system have been damaged and which other systems remain intact. Disorders of executive and social function show relatively poor recovery following TBI and have thus far proved to be relatively resistant to rehabilitative efforts. According to Kolb (1995), this may reflect the fact these are species–specific behaviors that require the integration of a complex range of functions, involving diverse brain regions, including perception, working memory, attention, intuition, self-monitoring, emotional control, and many others. It may be more difficult to reorganize such complex neural networks. This explanation is speculative, however.

From the perspective of the nature of impairments, unfortunately the most common cognitive and behavioral impairments associated with TBI can also place limitations on the effective implementation of rehabilitation. Fatigue, lowered arousal, slowed thinking, distractibility, and memory problems limit the injured person's ability to actively participate in and benefit from rehabilitative therapy. Impaired verbal regulation of behavior and initiative interfere with generalization of what is practiced in therapy sessions. Behavioral changes, such as lowered frustration tolerance, irritability, self-centeredness, and attention seeking or disinhibited behavior can make the task of the therapists and nursing staff extremely frustrating and stressful and in some instances can result in premature discharge from or denial of therapy. Probably the greatest problem is lack of self-awareness, which means that the injured person sets unrealistic goals and may not see the point of rehabilitation (thereby being an unwilling participant).

Individuals who have realistic self-awareness and are willing and motivated to cooperate in therapy are better candidates for rehabilitation. The absence of behavior change and absence of executive dysfunction, particularly impaired self-regulation, also represent positive prognostic indicators. However, given that this is the exception rather than the rule, TBI rehabilitation programs need to be adapted to maximize gains in the face of all these difficulties, in the manner suggested herein. These principles of the REAL (rehabilitation for everyday adaptive living) approach, are outlined in greater detail by Ponsford, Sloan, and Snow (1995).

Ways of Maximizing Outcomes from Rehabilitation Following TBI

1. *Teamwork.* The effects of TBI are complex and have a significant impact on one another. For example, a physiotherapist's capacity to work with a TBI person's gait and balance problems is likely to be significantly affected if that person does not remember or follow through with instructions, is distracted by the activities of a busy physiotherapy department, behaves in a demanding and attention-seeking fashion and/or makes sexually inappropriate comments. Gains from physiotherapy will be extremely limited if therapists in other settings are not able to prompt the injured person to use the correct gait pattern. As a consequence, all members of the rehabilitation team need be aware of all the problems of the individual with TBI and of appropriate management strategies so that such problems are dealt with in a consistent fashion. They need to formulate goals and priorities for treatment together with the injured person and family and adhere to these as a team. They need to share their expertise with one another and with the family. They also need to share their frustrations and uncertainties. Good interdisciplinary teamwork can thus alleviate some of the stress created by working with such complex, challenging, and frequently tragic problems. Opportunities for regular communication and participation in decision making are essential. Good team coordination is also important.

2. *Involvement of the injured individual and family.* Due to their lack of self-awareness, many individuals with TBI are unwilling or passive participants in the rehabilitation process. Their motivation for therapy may be limited. Their families, delighted that the injured relative has survived, might show little concern about the cognitive and behavioral changes that will create so much stress after the injured person has returned home. Both parties hope for a full recovery and tend to set unrealistic goals. As a consequence, it is very tempting and indeed common for therapists to set rehabilitation goals on behalf of the injured person and family. Negotiating goals and future plans which are realistic but also meaningful to those injured and their families is often laborious and stressful. It involves taking the perspective and using the language of the injured person to maximize his or her involvement, self-awareness, and cooperation. It is this individual, after all, who will be confronting the consequences of the injury for many years to come. Webb and Glueckhauf (1994) found that program participants who actively participated in setting and monitoring their attainment of goals showed superior goal attainment and maintenance of gains.

The use of methods such as Goal Attainment Scaling to set goals and monitor outcomes from therapy may facilitate this process (Kiresuk & Sherman, 1968; Malec, 1999). Close others need to be actively involved in the therapy process and trained to implement interventions. They can be invaluable cotherapists.

3. *Focusing therapy on functional goals that are relevant to the injured person's lifestyle.* The manifestations of TBI are complex and difficult to separate from the qualities of the individual who has sustained the injury. The process of goal setting will be facilitated by a comprehensive assessment of the preinjury personality, values, life roles, activities, and priorities of the injured person. To maximize the relevance and effectiveness of intervention, the processes of assessment, goal setting, and intervention should focus directly on these activities in the context in which they are usually performed. This will also maximize the likelihood that the injured person and family will participate in goal setting and see the relevance of rehabilitation activities, and it will facilitate awareness of change. There is evidence that individuals with TBI, even those with quite severe cognitive impairments, are able to learn skills or acquire knowledge with repeated practice. However, those with executive impairments have great difficulty generalizing from one situation or task to another. They may lack the capacity to implement strategies learned in the abstract into real-life situations. Therefore, whether intervention takes the form of intensive training, development of compensatory strategies or environmental supports, these are most likely to be of lasting benefit if they are applied in the real-world context. Moreover, the findings of Nudo and colleagues (Nudo, Barbay, & Kleim, 2000; Nudo, Plautz, & Frost, 2001) have indicated that repetitive practice is more beneficial if directed toward learning of a functional and meaningful skill, thus taking advantage of the relatively well-preserved semantic memory system. Goals need to be stated and outcomes measured in concrete terms which are meaningful to the individual and measurable over a set time frame. Methods such as Goal Attainment Scaling lend themselves to such an approach (Kiresuk & Sherman, 1968; Malec, 1999).

4. *Assess the precise nature of cognitive impairments.* From information presented in each of the chapters in this book it will be clear that each of the brain's cognitive functions is multifaceted. It is very important to assess precisely which aspects of cognitive function are impaired and, if possible, identify their neurological correlates using neuroimaging techniques as a basis for planning interventions most likely to be effective.

5. *Maximize recovery of function.* Every attempt should be made to maximize recovery by providing therapy which is initially directed at restitution of function as soon as possible following injury. There is clear evidence from the physical and sensory point of view that facilitation of movement and sensation in the affected limb may bring about some restitution of function in that limb. Whether this is also possible for more complex cognitive functions which are mediated by several brain regions is less clear. With the development of more

sophisticated and dynamic neuroimaging techniques it will, it is hoped, be possible to examine more closely whether and how different types of stimulation impact on cerebral organization and the functional consequences of any changes that do occur. One example was provided by Turner and Levine (Chapter 7, this volume). In a PET study, Levine et al. (2002) demonstrated increased areas of brain activation in individuals with TBI relative to controls during performance of a cued recall task. These were thought to reflect either cortical disinhibition resulting from deafferentation or functional compensation for inefficient memory processes. Clearly further work will be required to understand the mechanisms underlying such changes.

6. *Facilitate adaptation.* Given the extensive nature of damage associated with severe TBI, there will be a limit to which spontaneous recovery and restitution of function result in recovery. In the majority of cases, the injured person is left with residual disabilities which affect different aspects of his or her lifestyle. It is important to use whatever means possible to facilitate adaptation to limitations, to maximize the person's ability to perform previous life roles. This may involve learning strategies to maximize performance of tasks; learning new ways of performing tasks or interacting with others; using external aids, training others to provide prompting, supervision, or assistance; or modifying the tasks themselves or the environment. Chapters 3–8 outline in detail methods of achieving this. In evidenced-based reviews of cognitive rehabilitation studies conducted to date, many of those approaches proven effective have been of a compensatory nature, involving such interventions as training in the use of a memory notebook and the use of an external paging system known as the Neuropage (Carney, Chestnut, Maynard, Mann, & Hefland, 1999; Cicerone et al., 2000; Schmitter-Edgecombe, Fahy, Whelan, & Long, 1995; Wilson, Evans, Emslie, & Malinek, 1997).

7. *Use methods of training which maximize attention to task and learning.* Attentional difficulties are common following TBI. Animal studies have shown that active attention to a task is necessary for learning and cerebral reorganization to occur (Recanzone, Schreiner, & Merzenich, 1993). If this is also true in humans, then therapy is most likely to be effective if applied in a quiet, one-on-one fashion, and in frequent, short sessions rather than infrequent, lengthy sessions. It is also important to use what has been learned from the cognitive psychology literature to maximize learning on the part of the injured person. These methods are described by Glisky (Chapter 4, this volume). The first is the *spaced retrieval technique*, which involves repeated practice at retrieving information at gradually increasing retention intervals (Schacter, Rich, & Stampp, 1985). The second is the use of *perceptual priming methods*, such as the vanishing cues technique (Glisky, Schacter, & Tulving, 1986), which take advantage of intact implicit learning mechanisms in amnesic individuals. The third is *errorless learning*, which involves provision of maximal cueing throughout the learning process so that learning occurs without errors. This method

has been shown to be more effective in teaching memory-impaired individuals names of unfamiliar people than a learning process that allows the person to guess the correct response (Wilson, Baddeley, Evans, & Shiel, 1994). However, caution needs to be exercised here. Evans et al. (2000) found no advantage in the use of errorless learning in learning routes and programming an electronic organizer. As discussed in some detail by Nadeau and Gonzalez Rothi (Chapter 5, this volume), errorless learning may be of most use in treatment when there is only one correct response, but it may be of less value when redifferentiation of procedural or semantic representations is required. Fourth, it is well known that memory-impaired individuals frequently have intact procedural learning abilities, which means that motor skills may be learned through repeated practice. Finally, although it is difficult to teach individuals with TBI who have severe cognitive impairment to use mnemonic strategies, for those with less severe memory impairments, good awareness and motivation, the use of mnemonic strategies might assist in learning specific information. Approaches such as the PQRST technique (Glasgow, Zeiss, Barrera, & Lewinsohn, 1977) may be useful compensatory means of maximizing retention of material which has to be read, particularly for students.

   8. *Facilitate emotional adjustment in injured person and family.* There has now been extensive documentation of the psychological adjustment difficulties of individuals who sustain TBI at all levels of severity, with anxiety and/or depression occurring in up to 46% of those with moderate to severe injuries (Bowen, Neumann, Conner, Tennant, & Chamberlain, 1998; Fann, Katon, Uomoto, & Esselman, 1995; Hoofien et al., 2001; Kinsella, Moran, Ford, & Ponsford, 1988; Kreutzer, Seel, & Gourley, 2001; McCleary et al., 1998; Ponsford et al., 1999; Seel et al., 2003; Tyerman & Humphrey, 1984). The degree of emotional distress does not appear to be significantly related to the severity of injury. Although McCleary et al. (1998) found that those who were depressed had lower Glasgow Outcome Scores, Ponsford, Anson, and Curran (2003) reported only modest correlations between depression and anxiety and the extent of residual handicap. Anxiety and depression levels were more strongly associated with the coping style of the injured person (Curran, Ponsford, & Crowe, 2000). Other factors associated with post-TBI depression include a previous history of psychiatric disturbance, younger age, unemployment, lower education, and poor social functioning (Bowen et al., 1998; Fann et al., 1995; Jorge et al., 1993). Injury to the left dorsolateral frontal region or left basal ganglia has been associated with early-onset, transient depression, supporting theories that early depression reflects disruption of frontostriatal circuits that regulate mood (Jorge et al., 1993). Later-onset depression is thought to be associated with psychosocial factors. There have been few studies evaluating pharmacological treatment of post-TBI depression, but there is some evidence of positive response to tricyclic and nontricyclic antidepressants (Rosenthal, Christensen, & Ross, 1998; Wroblewski, Joseph, & Cornblatt,

1996). In light of these findings, it would appear that provision of emotional support represents an essential component of the rehabilitation process. It is important that the injured person is assisted in coming to terms with changes and rebuilding a positive self-image. This is an extremely complex and challenging process, which has been discussed in detail by George Prigatano (Prigatano et al., 1986; Prigatano, 1999) and Yehuda Ben Yishay (Ben Yishay et al., 1978). The extent to which such goals can be achieved depends on many factors, including preinjury personality, severity of cognitive impairment, and undoubtedly also the quality of therapeutic input the individual receives. Whether it is possible to facilitate more adaptive coping styles remains to be seen (Ponsford et al., 2003). Depression and anxiety also occur at higher than average rates in the relatives in those with moderate to severe TBI, particularly those in a direct caregiving role, of whom more than 30% exhibit clinically significant anxiety and/or depression (Ponsford et al., 2003). The presence of emotional and family adjustment problems appears to be most strongly associated with the presence of cognitive and behavioral changes in the injured person and is most evident in those directly responsible for the care of their injured relative (Ponsford et al., 2003). Thus, the provision of supportive counseling or family therapy, as well as practical supports such as attendant care, day activities, and assistance in coping with behavior problems, may alleviate the caregiver's burden, although the impact of specific family interventions has not been evaluated in a controlled fashion.

9. *Evaluate the effectiveness of interventions.* We know so little of the impact of the many interventions suggested in this book, yet it is relatively rare to see their effectiveness being evaluated. This is, in reality, a difficult task, due to the diffuse and variable nature of injuries and impairments, the multifocal nature of the rehabilitation process, difficulties separating the effects of therapy from those of therapist attention, spontaneous recovery or practice effects on repeated measures, and a lack of agreement over meaningful outcome measures. Increased implementation of randomized controlled trials to evaluate different approaches to rehabilitation is to be encouraged. However, given the inherent differences in lifestyles and priorities of individuals with TBI, not to speak of the heterogeneity of their injuries, it is always going to be difficult to find outcome measures which are meaningful and sensitive to change across individuals. The use of single-case designs lends itself to a rehabilitation approach that focuses on the needs and lifestyle of the individual. As Wilson (1987) has pointed out, therapy can be tailored to the individual's needs and the approach changed if it is not working. The most important aspect is to arrive at a meaningful measure of whatever is being treated, take baseline recordings, and continue these throughout the intervention and over a follow-up period. This allows one to evaluate continuously the person's responses to the intervention while controlling for the effects of practice or spontaneous recovery. It is also possible to ascertain reasons for failure to respond to treatment and thus

establish sources of variability either in procedures or in the injury-related or personal characteristics of the person being treated.

10. *Take a long-term view.* Recovery following TBI occurs over a very lengthy time frame. However, long-term outcome studies have shown that the cognitive, behavioral, and emotional changes persist over very long periods (Hoofien et al., 2001; Koskinen, 1998; Olver et al., 1996; Rappaport, Herrero-Backe, Rappaport, & Winterfield, 1989; Tate et al., 1989, Thomsen, 1984). Moreover, the problems and needs of these predominantly young people change across their lifespan. Psychological adjustment difficulties frequently do not develop until after such individuals have left rehabilitation and experienced some of the common psychosocial consequences, such as difficulty holding down a job, maintaining a social network, and forming and holding close personal relationships. Their needs change as they face different life stages. For example, the needs of a young teenager who is still living with his parents and attending school are quite different from those of the same person 5 years later, when he is wanting to live independently, hold down a job, and form a close personal relationship. Simply training a person to be independent in activities of daily living and setting up that person in work, study, or avocational activities does not guarantee successful adaptation. Services need to be available to provide relevant input as different issues arise. The extent to which a person with TBI is able to play a meaningful role in the community is also likely to be determined by the availability of practical and emotional supports. Families are often the only support available to those injured over the long term, and the families also need continuing support in this role.

Approaches to Rehabilitation

The most common problems in individuals with TBI include impairments of attention and speed of information processing, learning and memory, planning, self-regulation, and behavioral control and regulation, including social skills, as well as disorders of self-awareness. These disorders and approaches to their rehabilitation have been comprehensively discussed in previous chapters, to which the reader is referred. Clearly, a very comprehensive assessment is necessary to isolate precisely the nature of specific impairments. The approach taken to therapy should depend on the nature and extent of cognitive and behavioral impairment, particularly skills in the domains of memory, self-monitoring, and awareness of deficits in the injured person. For those functioning at very low levels in these and other respects, environmental manipulation and behavioral approaches are likely to be most effective in reducing disability and handicap. For individuals with some degree of self-awareness, capacity for self-regulation and memory function, the various self-instructional or strategy training approaches have the potential to be effective. Those with less extensive injuries and cognitive deficits are more likely to benefit from all types of intervention, particularly those involving self-generated strategies, but also including restorative training approaches, which may facilitate neuronal regrowth or reorganization. Any strategies or training approaches used are most likely to be of lasting benefit if they are relevant to and applied directly in real-world settings.

A number of studies have demonstrated that significant and lasting gains may be made by focusing directly on functional skills involved in the roles normally performed by the injured person (e.g., Burke et al., 1988; Fryer & Haffey, 1987; Mills et al., 1992; Sander et al., 2001; Seale et al., 2002). These gains have been made at any time after injury and despite the presence of ongoing cognitive impairments. The approach to intervention needs to be flexible, with a number of different techniques usually being employed to deal with different problems encountered in a given individual.

In the domain of attention, which is one of the most common cognitive impairments following TBI, interventions may take the following forms. For those with low levels of arousal, memory, self-awareness, and executive function it will be necessary to alter the environment or the tasks in order to maximize the attentional performance of the injured person. These tasks are outlined in Chapter 3, but may include removing sources of distraction, providing frequent rest breaks, providing alerting signals at regular intervals, simplifying the task, or simply slowing it down. Pharmacological interventions might also be considered to increase arousal, attentional capacity, or speed of information processing. At the next level, it may be possible to train the person to perform everyday activities which place demands on his or her attention more efficiently, by providing intensive training in components of the task. For those with some degree of self-awareness and self-monitoring capacity, self-instructional strategies may be taught, but these strategies will depend on the specific nature of the attentional problem. They might include time pressure management (Fasotti, Kovacs, Eling, & Brouwer, 2000) and strategies for dividing attention between tasks, focusing attention when reading, or increasing alertness. Chapter 3 reviews in detail evidence regarding the effectiveness of these strategies.

In the domain of memory, interventions may be applied at similar levels. For those with very severe amnesic problems, modification of the task or the environment will be necessary. A variety of external aids may be applied, ranging from those that are externally programmed, such as the NeuroPage (Wilson et al., 1997), to those that require more active involvement of the injured person, such as diaries, checklists, or electronic memory aids. Training in the use of these aids needs to be conducted in an intensive and systematic fashion and applied in the context of the person's daily lifestyle. Close others may be invaluable cotherapists in seeing that these aids are used. In Chapter 4, Glisky has discussed how memory-impaired individuals may be trained to perform important daily tasks using implicit learning procedures such as the vanishing cues technique or errorless learning. At the next level, mnemonic strategies may be useful for some individuals to assist them in learning important information or to enhance the depth of encoding of material they have to read (e.g., the PQRST technique).

In the domains of executive function and self-awareness, there are also a range of levels of intervention. For those with very little self-awareness or capacity for self-monitoring, provision of external prompting and structure will be required. The environment and tasks can be simplified to reduce the demands on planning and initiative. At the next level, provision of checklists to be followed when performing daily home- or work-related tasks until a routine is learned may be of considerable benefit. For those with some capacity for self-regulation "goal management training" or training in problem-solving strategies to be followed in a range of situations has the potential to be successful (Cicerone & Wood, 1987; Levine et al., 2000; von Cramon, Matthes von Cramon, & Mai, 1991). Similarly, programs to enhance self-awareness need to be tailored to the individual's cognitive abilities, as suggested by Sohlberg (2000). Chapter 7 reviews evidence regarding the effectiveness of these approaches.

Social and behavior problems present the greatest challenge to rehabilitation professionals working with individuals with TBI and, in the long-term, families. They represent possibly the greatest barrier to social reintegration. In Chapter 8, Alderman has outlined approaches to the management of behavior problems. Any intervention should be based on a comprehensive assessment, taking into account all factors that may be contributing to the behavioral change, including personality factors, developmental or emotional factors, and environmental factors as well as the brain injury itself. As suggested by Alderman, the philosophy of management should be to maximize the desirable behavior using the least intrusive means. Behavior problems occurring as a result of agitation in the acute recovery stage are generally best managed by environmental manipulation (Ponsford, 1995). At later stages of recovery, pharmacological intervention may be appropriate. Behavior modification techniques, including stimulus-control methods, chaining and shaping, and response–consequence learning technologies (Wood, 1990) have been shown to be very effective both in reducing inappropriate behavior and in skill building to maximize independence in carrying out daily activities. As Alderman points out, these techniques need to be delivered within a highly structured environment to produce good outcomes, and in severe cases, they are probably most effectively administered within specialized units. However, the implementation of fundamental behavioral principles to reinforce appropriate behavior and skills and to withdraw attention from inappropriate or undesirable behavior can and should be incorporated into all rehabilitation programs.

For those individuals with TBI who have anger management problems but are aware of and motivated to overcome them, cognitive-behavioral techniques can be successful and family members may be invaluable as cotherapists. However, as with other forms of intervention, lack of self-awareness and problems with self-monitoring represent major barriers to the success of such interventions. Manchester and Wood (2001) have described the use of a more intensive and structured form of cognitive therapy to enhance self-awareness of socially inappropriate behavior and implement the use of so-called concrete cognitive restructuring strategies (CCRS) in which alternatives to dysfunctional automatic beliefs are identified by the therapist and taught through mass practice. Such techniques are highly specialized and would need to be applied in an intensive fashion to be successful. However, there is no doubt that the development of more appropriate social skills, in terms of verbal and nonverbal communication and behavior, represents one of the greatest challenges for those involved in rehabilitation of individuals with TBI, as it is a major cause of their long-term social isolation and failure to establish successful personal relationships.

CEREBROVASCULAR ACCIDENT

The term "cerebrovascular accident" (CVA), or "stroke," is used to refer to neurological disorders in which brain injury is caused by a vascular mechanism. This is one of the leading causes of death and chronic disability resulting from neuronal injury (Kandel, Schwartz, & Jessell, 2000).

Epidemiology of CVA

The incidence of stroke has been estimated at two first-ever-strokes-per-1,000-population overall (Bamford et al., 1988; Caroloei et al., 1997; Ellekjaer, Holmen, Indredavik, & Terent, 1997; Hankey, 2002), the rate rising significantly with age, so that for the age group 45–85 the incidence is four-per-1,000-population annually (Hewer & Tennant, 2003). Three-quarters of stroke cases occur in individuals over 65 (Hankey, 2002). It is thus the highest cause of disability in those over 45 years. Men and women are affected in roughly equal numbers (Hankey, 2002). The rate of recurrence of stroke is 5% per annum. In a study by Geddes et al. (1996), the proportion reporting ongoing disability and dependency varied significantly across age groups, with 24.7% of those ages 55–64 reporting ongoing disability, as opposed to 75.3% of those age 85 years or over.

There are two categories of CVA: *ischemic* and *hemorrhagic*. *Ischemic stroke* occurs when insufficient blood flow deprives neural tissue of oxygen and glucose, causing an area of cerebral infarction. This may result from occlusion caused by a thrombosis or an embolus or as a result of a systemic reduction in blood flow. A thrombosis is a blood clot which can form over areas where atherosclerotic plaque has been deposited. This may occur anywhere in the vascular system, causing stenosis or blockage of large extracranial arteries such as the internal carotid or the vertebral arteries, or may affect small deep penetrating arteries. They are most common where arteries branch or bifurcate—at the origin of the internal carotid artery, the upper end of the vertebral arteries, the lower portion of the basilar artery, the stem of the middle cerebral artery, or the posterior artery. Emboli may detach and travel from thrombi further down the arterial tree or from the heart to block smaller vessels, such as the retinal arterioles, causing amaurosis fugax or loss of vision in one eye. A systemic reduction in blood flow caused by cardiac arrest or shock can also lead to ischemia, especially in the border zones between major cerebral vessels, such as the middle and posterior cerebral arteries (Adams, Victor, & Ropper, 1997; Netter, 1986; Walsh & Darby, 1999). More than 80% of CVAs occur as a result of ischemia (Hankey, 2002).

In *hemorrhagic* stroke, bleeding into the brain tissue or subarachnoid space causes injury by exerting pressure on or displacing cerebral tissue. This bleeding may result from many causes, including TBI. However, the three most common causes are hypertensive intracerebral hemorrhage, ruptured aneurysm, and ruptured arteriovenous malformation. *Hypertensive intracerebral hemorrhages* arise mainly from the penetrating branches of the middle cerebral, posterior cerebral, and basilar arteries, causing damage in the basal ganglia, thalamus, cerebellar hemispheres, pons, and subcortical areas. Due to the sparing of cortex, symptoms tend to be of a neurological or physical rather than a behavioral or cognitive nature. *Aneurysms* are most common on the Circle of Willis, and the most common sites of rupture are the anterior communicating artery and the middle cerebral bifurcation. *Arteriovenous malformations* are developmental malformations, the rupture of which may cause intracerebral or subarachnoid bleeding (Adams et al., 1997; Walsh & Darby, 1999).

The brain regions affected by ischemic stroke, while tending to follow the distribution of the arteries affected, may vary from very large areas, such as when a stenosis occurs at the bifurcation of the middle cerebral artery, to very small areas when an embolus occludes a single distal branch. The size and locus of infarction resulting from stenosis or occlusion are also determined by the distribution of collaterals and anastomoses in and around the affected region and the speed with which occlusion occurs, which determines the time allowed for collateral channels to open (Adams et al., 1997). The pathophysiological mechanisms set in train when a CVA occurs are in some ways similar to those occurring as a result of TBI, although the same mechanical forces are not operating to cause diffuse axonal injury, axotomy, or contusion. As outlined by Kolb and Cioe (Chapter 1, this volume) the primary mechanism of neuronal injury caused by stroke, which also operates following TBI, is ischemia. Ischemia causes changes in the cell membrane, release of glutamate, and an influx of toxic amounts of calcium into the cells. Edema or swelling, along with changes in the metabolism and/or utilization of glucose, cause more widespread dysfunction and sometimes secondary degeneration of neurons. "Diaschisis" may also result in temporary loss of function in areas adjacent to or quite distant from the area in which the ischemia occurred. As shown by Aimola Davies (Chapter 6, this volume), these factors may be most significant in determining the initial pattern of impairment following stroke, a pattern that may bear only limited resemblance to that once they have dissipated.

A number of treatments have and continue to be trialed with a view to blocking some of these processes. Antagonists to glutamate receptors have been shown to be beneficial in blocking excitotoxicity in experimental paradigms of focal brain ischemia in rats. Unfortunately, these paradigms have not yet been successfully translated into the clinical situation in humans (Larner & Sofroniew, 2003). Nimodipine is a calcium channel ion blocker which has been shown to prevent ischemic neurological deficits following aneurysmal subarachnoid hemorrhage. Unfortunately trials of nimodipine in ischemic stroke have failed to show improved patient outcomes, but it may nevertheless be helpful in some cases (Larner & Sofroniew, 2003). Trials of the 21-aminosteroid tirilazad mesylate in acute neural injury (ischemia, subarachnoid hemorrhage, and central nervous system trauma) have also failed to improve patient outcomes (Bath, Iddenden, Bath, & Orgogozo, 2001). As for TBI, the failure of these treatments, used individually, to demonstrate a clinically significant impact on recovery is perhaps not surprising, given that numerous mechanisms are operating simultaneously to cause neuronal damage.

Major Stroke Syndromes and Their Consequences

The manifestations of CVA may vary considerably due to a number of factors, most notably variations in the efficiency of collateral circulation and as a result of individual differences in vasculature. As already mentioned, there are also generally distal effects of a temporary nature, due to metabolic changes or "diaschisis." Finally there are frequently other cognitive disorders present, perhaps as a result of a previous vascular episode or as a result of some other degenerative process that may also be taking place or as a result of aging. The syndromes discussed next are described in greater detail by Adams et al. (1997), Bogousslavsky and Caplan (1995), and Bradshaw and Mattingley (1995).

Middle Cerebral Artery Syndromes

The middle cerebral arteries supply the premotor, motor, and somatosensory cortex; the language areas in the dominant hemisphere; dorsolateral prefrontal areas; the temporal lobes and parietal lobes; the globus pallidus; caudate nucleus; and internal capsule (see Figure 9.3). A stroke in the distribution of the middle cerebral artery may therefore result in any or all of the following impairments: contralateral hemiparesis (worse in the face and arm than the leg)

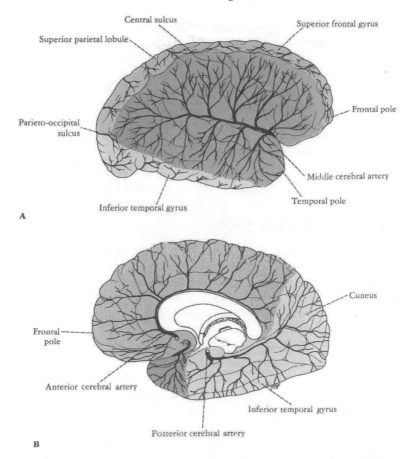

FIGURE 9.3. Areas supplied by the cerebral arteries. (A) the lateral surface of the right cerebral hemisphere. (B) The medial surface of the right cerebral hemisphere. From Snell (1997). Copyright 1997 by Lippincott Williams & Wilkins. Reprinted by permission.

and hemisensory loss, horizontal gaze palsy and contralateral homonymous hemianopia, and, if the anterior trunk is affected, any of the impairments associated with lesions in the dorsolateral prefrontal areas, including perseveration, poor planning and conceptual ability, working-memory difficulties, and impaired self-awareness (Anderson & Damasio, 1995). In addition to these problems occurring following middle cerebral artery (MCA) stroke in either hemisphere, in the dominant hemisphere there may be expressive and/or receptive dysphasia—with motor speech disorders associated with damage to Broca's area and receptive difficulties including word deafness, as well as jargon speech and anomia associated with lesions in the central and parieto-occipital cortex—as well as dysgraphia, verbal memory difficulties, dyscalculia, left–right disorientation, finger agnosia, and/or right-sided neglect and/or visuospatial difficulty, which tends to be less severe than that seen following nondominant hemisphere stroke. Following nondominant MCA stroke, there may be awareness deficits, termed anosognosia, unilateral spatial neglect, constructional and dressing dyspraxia, visuospatial disorientation, nonverbal/visuospatial memory difficulties, and problems with nonverbal aspects of communication, such as prosody, facial expression, and gesture (Adams et al., 1997; Bradshaw & Mattingley, 1995). Lacunar infarcts resulting from occlusion of perforating arteries supplying the interior of the hemisphere cause primarily motor or sensory deficits involving the face, arm, and leg.

Anterior Cerebral Artery Stroke

The anterior cerebral arteries (ACA) supply the anterior third of the medial aspect of the hemisphere, including the medial frontal and parietal lobes, the diencephalic nuclei, anterior commissure, corpus callosum, internal capsule, and basal ganglia (see Figure 9.3). This is also the territory affected by ruptured aneurysms of the anterior cerebral and anterior communicating arteries (ACoA). The vast majority (85–95%) of aneurysms develop at the anterior portion of the cerebral arterial supply (DeLuca & Diamond, 1995) and tend to cause bilateral medial frontal damage. CVA in the ACA territory may cause contralateral paralysis of the foot and leg, contralateral grasp reflex, gait disorders, urinary incontinence, adynamia/ abulia, and executive dysfunction, including cognitive inflexibility, perseveration, difficulty with self-monitoring, planning, decision making and concept formation, and distractibility, as well as reduced self-awareness (Adams et al., 1997; Bottger, Prosiegel, Steiger, & Yassouridis, 1998; DeLuca & Diamond, 1995; see also Turner & Levine, Chapter 7, this volume). Difficulties with initiation of speech (akinetic mutism) may also occur. Dominant hemisphere damage may result in language disturbance characterized by a paucity of spontaneous speech but relatively preserved repetition and comprehension (transcortical motor or dynamic aphasia) and ideomotor apraxia. ACA infarctions involving the mesial and orbital frontal regions may result in personality change, disinhibition, and apathy. Infarction of hypothalamic and septal regions following rupture and repair of ACoA aneurysms may produce an impairment similar to Korsakoff psychosis, including amnesia and confabulation (Bradshaw & Mattingley, 1995).

Posterior Cerebral Artery Stroke

The posterior cerebral arteries (PCA) branch from the basilar artery, part of the vertebrobasilar system. They supply the medial and inferior aspect of the temporal lobes, the occipital lobes, part of the hippocampus and the subthalamus,

thalamus and hypothalamus, and splenium of the corpus callosum (see Figure 9.3). CVA in this territory may result in a contralateral homonymous hemianopia, cortical blindness, visual agnosias, distorted visual images, and/or memory loss. If it occurs in the dominant hemisphere, there may be alexia without agraphia, and color anomia or agnosia, simultanagnosia, and, where lesions involve the occipitotemporal region, transcortical sensory aphasia, in which speech is fluent and paraphasic, comprehension is poor, but repetition is intact. If the infarction occurs in the nondominant hemisphere, one may see agnosia for faces, as well as unilateral spatial neglect and constructional dyspraxia where the lesions encroach on the parietal area, as well as hemisensory loss (thalamic syndrome), paralysis of vertical gaze, and extrapyramidal movement disorders (Adams et al., 1997; Bradshaw & Mattingley, 1995).

Watershed Infarctions

Watershed infarctions occur due to vascular insufficiency in two or more arterial systems. They may affect the occipitoparietal region at the junction of the ACA, MCA, and PCA territories, between the MCA and either the ACA or the PCA alone or between the superficial and deep branches of the MCA in the region of the putamen, the caudate nucleus, and the internal capsule.

Clearly, many physical disabilities form long-term barriers to independence following stroke. Of the cognitive impairments, disorders of language and visuospatial function are the most handicapping consequences of MCA infarcts, executive and self-regulatory problems following ACA stroke or ACoA, and visual impairments following PCA stroke.

Recovery Following CVA

The recovery course following CVA varies widely across individuals, because of differences in lesion location, the extent of more widespread disruption of metabolic function, and each person's preexisting condition. There may also be individual differences in vasculature and in cerebral organization of function, particularly in left-handers. Unlike TBI, age represents a negative prognostic factor following CVA, as the majority of cases are over 65 years of age and many are much older than this. A significant proportion may have impairments due to previous vascular episodes or due to coexisting conditions, such as Alzheimer's disease or Parkinson's disease.

On the positive side, some elderly people are potentially better equipped psychosocially to deal with an acquired disability than young people who sustain TBI, because they have already attained many important life goals, may already have retired from the work force, and have a supportive spouse and/or adult children. This, of course, is not always the case, and a significant proportion of elderly stroke victims do experience depression and social isolation. Although behavioral and executive problems certainly occur, especially in association with CVA in the ACA, or more commonly ACoA aneurysms, these problems are relatively less common following stroke than TBI, whereas problems with communication or visuospatial orientation are far more common. Finally, the community arguably recognizes and accepts the nature of poststroke disability to a greater extent than is the case for TBI, and more comprehensive community services exist to cater to the needs of people with poststroke disability.

In most cases, spontaneous recovery takes place in the early days, weeks, and months following the CVA, with most recovery occurring within 3–6 months. Motor function improves at a progressively slower pace over the first year (Kelly-Hayes et al., 1989). The time frame for recovery following stroke is generally shorter than that following TBI, possibly because damage is less diffuse and possibly because of differing mechanisms of injury, which might result in qualitatively different morphological adaptations. As with TBI, much of the early recovery is likely to reflect the resolution of edema or reperfusion of the ischemic penumbra. However, some evidence also suggests that other areas take over the functions of the damaged area. As Cohen and Hallett (2003) point out, the existence of corticomotoneuronal connections from various cortical motor areas provides a basis for such a recovery mechanism in the motor system. Sprouting from surviving fibers to establish new synaptic contacts may contribute to recovery at later stages. As for TBI, this will depend on the extent of the lesion, with very extensive lesions showing a much poorer likelihood of improvement. The severity of initial neurological impairment is a useful predictor of outcome (Heinemann, Roth, Cichowski, & Bets, 1987).

As outlined by Kolb (Chapter 2, this volume), functional imaging studies after stroke have demonstrated the recruitment of cortical areas along the edge of the injured zone, and larger than usual areas of motor cortex tend to be activated. There is also evidence of activation of more extensive areas of the cortex, including premotor and parietal areas and the cerebellum, and activation may be bilateral. Cases showing good motor recovery tend to show robust activation in the sensorimotor cortex of the affected hemisphere, when the affected hand moves (Cohen & Hallett, 2003). Indeed, the presence of intact primary sensorimotor cortex represents a good prognostic factor for functional improvement, even if there is initially a hemiparesis. The vast majority of studies demonstrating neural plasticity have focused on motor and sensory functions. However, there is some evidence of activation of relevant areas in the opposite hemisphere in patients with language disturbance. The presence of intact regions, such as Wernicke's area, represents a good prognostic sign. The larger the area of infarction and the older the person, the poorer the capacity for reorganization.

It would appear from the work of Taub and colleagues (Taub et al., 1993; Taub & Morris, 2001), Nudo and colleagues (Nudo, Wise, SiFuentes, &

Milliken, 1996; Nudo, Plautz, & Millikan, 1997), and others that, at least as far as sensorimotor function is concerned, therapy for or forced use of the impaired limb increases the likelihood that adjacent areas will take over the functions of that limb and minimizes loss of function arising from disuse. Therapy thus appears to be necessary to maximize return of function, although in light of the findings of Schallert and colleagues (Kozlowski, James, & Schallert, 1996), discussed by Kolb and Cioe (Chapter 1, this volume), it is unclear how early or how intense this therapy should be. Kozlowski et al.'s (1996) findings suggested that intense therapy in the first few days poststroke may be unwise, although in practice patients are rarely ready to participate in therapy at this stage. It is also unclear whether such stimulation will enhance the return of *cognitive* functions following stroke or TBI. In Chapter 2, Kolb has presented some evidence to suggest that therapy or stimulation may potentiate the production of neurotrophic factors, which, in turn, enhances synaptic changes and functional improvement (Witt-Lajeunesse & Kolb, 2003). It is important to note that simple repetitive exercise was not sufficient to produce such changes in animals. The stimulation needed to involve the learning of a motor or a mental task. As Kolb notes in Chapter 2, "Studies of laboratory animals have consistently shown that the single most successful treatment strategy for optimizing functional recovery is placing animals in complex, stimulating environments" (e.g., Johansson & Belichenko, 2002).

Rehabilitation Following CVA

All this evidence provides support for the importance of providing intensive skilled rehabilitative therapy designed to address the multiple areas of impairment associated with stroke. Wade (2003) provides comprehensive evidence, based on review of seven randomized controlled trials, one meta-analysis, and one systematic review, published between 1994 and 1998, which shows overwhelmingly that treatment by a specialized stroke service, where staff have expertise in managing stroke, work together as a coordinated team, and undergo regular education and training, results in reduced mortality, lower incidence of stroke recurrence, and faster recovery, shorter hospital stay, fewer nursing home discharges, and lower levels of emotional distress in patient and carer than unspecialized, uncoordinated services. The use of standardized protocols and a structured process of discharge planning have been shown to result in shorter length of stay and/or less morbidity and readmission. Outpatient therapy should also be delivered by a specialized team.

Wade (2003) also reviews studies demonstrating that, as in the case of TBI, short- and long-term goal setting and review, involving the patient and family, represents an important part of the rehabilitation process. This should form the basis from which therapy is planned. A broad range of motor and sensory changes may be present, the most common including hemiparesis, hemisensory loss, dysarthria, and dysphagia. Studies of therapeutic approaches have so far had mixed findings, although there is some support for early muscle and gait retraining (Wade, 2003) and for training on functional tasks (Nelson et al., 1996; Dean & Shepherd, 1997). Parry, Lincoln, and Vass (1999) demonstrated a positive impact of an additional 2 hours of weekly physiotherapy for the arm over 5 weeks on outcome in patients with less severe impairments, but benefits were not evident in more severely impaired patients. This supports the view that severity of impairment affects response to therapy.

Any cognitive function may be impaired as a result of CVA. However, given the frequency with which the territory of the MCA is affected, the most common and disabling problems are disorders of language and visuospatial function. Subarachnoid hemorrhage resulting from ruptured aneurysms of the ACoA results in problems associated with frontal lobe dysfunction and may be managed similarly to those resulting from TBI, as outlined earlier in this chapter.

Rehabilitation of Speech and Language Disorders

The prevalence of persisting speech and language disorders following stroke has been estimated at 50% (Douglas, Brown, & Barry, 2002). The evidence regarding effectiveness of aphasia therapy has been very mixed. A number of studies published in the 1980s indicated no significant differences in outcome according to the nature of therapy offered (group vs. individual, operant vs. "normal" therapy), and one particularly influential study by Lincoln et al. (1984), a randomized controlled trial (RCT) in 327 patients, showed no differences in outcome between those receiving "normal speech therapy" over 0–48 hours and those receiving no therapy. This study had quite an influence on attitudes to speech therapy. However, as Howard (1986) and Byng and Jones (2003) have pointed out, these studies did not fully describe either the nature of the aphasic disorders or the therapy delivered, and outcome was measured on global measures of language and communication. Greener, Enderby, and Whurr's (1999) Cochrane review, which included only RCTs, concluded that none of the trials conducted contained sufficient detail to allow complete description or analysis, so that no conclusion could be drawn as to the effectiveness or ineffectiveness of aphasia therapy. However, one more recent RCT by Elman and Bernstein-Ellis (1999) did demonstrate a significant impact of group communication treatment in adults with chronic aphasia. Other recent reviews including a broader range of evidence have reached more positive conclusions. Rohey (1994, 1998) demonstrated clear treatment advantages in both acute and chronic recovery stages and concluded that treatment time exceeding 2 hours per week was associated with greater gains than shorter treatment. On the basis of their review of 41 studies, Cicerone et al. (2000) recommended language therapy following left-hemisphere stroke as a practice standard in both acute and postacute rehabilitation.

Byng, Pound, and Parr (2000) conducted a study of the concerns of people with aphasia, showing that these are less about the specific nature of their language difficulties but more about the impact of it on their lifestyle, their self-esteem, and their ability to communicate effectively with others in the roles that are important to them. Thus, as with other cognitive impairments, aphasic impairments must be seen within a psychosocial framework, and interventions need to focus on enhancing participation in life roles and psychosocial adjustment, rather than simply treating an impairment, although this might represent an important component of the intervention. Intervention might also include the development of strategies to find a way around impairments, and working with conversational partners and close others to enhance the aphasic individual's communicative interactions.

Traditional classification systems of aphasic syndromes, such as Broca's aphasia, transcortical motor aphasia, and global aphasia (the so-called nonfluent aphasias), Wernicke's, transcortical sensory and conduction aphasia (the so-called fluent aphasias), and anomic aphasia, are based largely on symptomatology and the anatomical location of the lesion. They assume that the underlying cause of the symptoms is the same. However, more recently, cognitive neuropsychologists have argued that this is not the case (Nickels & Best, 1996), and therefore application of the same therapeutic interventions might not be expected to result in success in all cases. Cognitive neuropsychologists have developed an approach that involves examining precisely which components of the language processing system are affected and directing therapy very specifically at these components. This is still impairment-oriented therapy. However, a number of single-case studies have demonstrated significant gains from such therapy, as described by Byng and Jones (2003). It is difficult to conduct group studies of this type of intervention, as the focus of the intervention and hence also the outcome measures will vary from one case to the next. However the publication of replication studies is adding support for the approach.

In Chapter 5 (this volume), Nadeau and Gonzalez Rothi have proposed a parallel distributed processing model of language and made numerous suggestions regarding therapy targeted at specific impairments, based on this model. Most of these involve massed practice, aimed at strengthening or reestablishing connections or knowledge. These have considerable plausibility, although they have yet to be tested. Nadeau and Gonzalez Rothi suggest, for example, that naming therapy, the most common approach to therapy for anomia, might be most appropriate for patients with no phonological function, who do not respond to phonemic cues. On the other hand, in those with some ability to respond to phonemic cueing, and hence partial integrity of the acoustic–articulatory motor pathway, it is suggested that phonological therapy might improve naming. Where there is semantic impairment, the suggested goal of therapy is to strengthen representations of features that distinguish concepts from each other and/or provide direct training in the semantic features of objects, methods employed with some success by Raymer and Rothi (2000). Whether working-memory capacity can be increased by pharmacological means or by retraining, as they suggest, remains to be seen, but this is suggested as a means of alleviating grammatic impairment. Massed practice has been shown to improve concept manipulation skills, with generalization across exemplars of particular manipulations but not a generic improvement in the ability to manipulate concepts (Thompson, 2001).

Another form of therapy also discussed by Nadeau and Gonzalez Rothi is constraint-induced language therapy (CILT). This more pragmatic form of therapy seeks to engage patients in intensive language production in long sessions, thereby providing massed practice in a pragmatic setting (Pulvermuller et al., 2001; Maher et al., 2003) to address their naming, phonological sequencing, or grammatic impairments. This therapy also has yet to be fully evaluated, but preliminary findings are encouraging (Maher et al., 2003). The challenge would appear to be how to achieve the most useful practice content for patients with differing impairments who are being treated together.

Clearly the important principles in applying language therapy are those relevant to all cognitive impairments—careful analysis of the impairment, its impact on the ability of the person to communicate when performing roles important to them, and design of an intervention which may target the specific impairment as intensively as possible but might, particularly in the later stages, also involve the development of compensatory strategies, modifying the interactions of others or the environment. Future RCTs need to be conducted with more homogeneous groups, where the therapy is carefully described and can be replicated, using outcome measures which relate to the goal of therapy but also to the functional communication of the dysphasic individual.

Rehabilitation of Disorders of Spatial Attention

As already outlined, a broad range of visuoperceptual and visuospatial disorders may be associated with stroke in the middle cerebral or posterior arteries. MCA stroke can cause contralateral homonymous hemianopia or quadrantanopia. Compensation for visual field defects usually develops reasonably well over time, although those with lesions extending into the posterior thalamus and parieto-occiptal region may have difficulty. The question as to whether visual fields can be enlarged by stimulation of the blind areas with light stimuli, and visual scanning improved by training, as claimed by Zihl and von Cramon (1979) and Zihl (1995), has remained open for some time. However results of more recent well controlled studies suggest that computer-mediated visual restitution training may result in enlarged visual fields, particularly in those with optic nerve lesions, but also in those with post-chiasmic brain injury (Kasten, Wust, Behrens-Baumann, & Sabel, 1998). Kasten, Muller-Ohring and Sabel (2001) showed that the gains were maintained up to 2 years later, although not all patients had been able to use the gains to improve their function in everyday life.

As with attentional training, there have been numerous attempts at perceptual retraining, as discussed in chapter six. The same issues and criticisms apply to evaluations of this form of training as have been discussed at length in relation to the training of attention (i.e., that patients trained on perceptual tasks tend to get better at these tasks, or similar tasks, but there is little evidence of generalization to everyday activities). The training needs to extend to the performance of tasks that have to be performed day-to-day, such as dressing, feeding, meal preparation, reading, crossing roads, shopping, and generally getting around in the community.

Unilateral spatial neglect represents one of the greatest impediments to functional independence following stroke. As discussed in Chapter 6, there is some evidence to suggest that scanning training using behavioral cueing may be effective in severe cases of neglect, if administered systematically over a long period. Again, the effect is likely to be manifested on tasks similar to those trained, so it seems most sensible to train on functionally meaningful tasks. As Aimola Davies points out in Chapter 6, it is also important to consider not just whether the individual with unilateral neglect can redirect his or her attention contralesionally, but also whether attention can be maintained at the new location. A number of other techniques show some promise. Robertson and colleagues (Robertson & North, 1992; Robertson, North, & Geggie, 1992) have suggested that activation of the left hand in the left side of space (in the absence of movement of the contralateral hand) produces a more powerful activation of the brain's representation for that side of space. This has been shown to result in improvement in neglect on a range of everyday tasks. Kalra, Perez, Gupta, and Wittink (1997) found that it resulted in earlier discharge from hospital, and Robertson, McMillan, McLeod, Edgeworth, and Brock (2002) found that it resulted in improvements in contralesional limb movements that were maintained at 18–24 month follow-up. As discussed in Chapter 6, this finding is consistent with other studies indicating benefits from unilateral activation of the hemiplegic side (e.g. Taub et al., 1993), suggesting that the damaged hemisphere might be inhibited by activation of the undamaged hemisphere. The finding that active simultaneous limb movements abolish the effectiveness of single contralesional limb movements is important and needs emphasis, given that some approaches to therapy emphasize bilateral symmetry of movement. If the limb is to be activated by the individual with unilateral neglect, however, the presence of some degree of motor control on the hemiplegic side is necessary.

Another approach also discussed in Chapter 6 is based on the theory that the right hemisphere mediates arousal or sustained attention and that this contributes to neglect. Robertson, Tegner, Tham, Lo, and Nimmo-Smith (1995) used cognitive-behavioral techniques to train patients with neglect in a self-alerting procedure, which apparently had an impact not only on sustained attention but also on their neglect. The extent to which patients could be trained to follow through with this procedure in their daily lives has not yet been evaluated, however. As with other cognitive strategies, it could only be applied in situations in which there was some degree of self-awareness of the problem and some capability for behavioral self-monitoring. Alternatively, some external means of alerting might be maintained. As Aimola Davies points out in Chapter 6, the presence of anosognosia may well play a role in neglect and, along with impairment of alertness or sustained attention, may in turn interfere with attempts at intervention.

Two other important recent developments are discussed by Aimola Davies in Chapter 6. The first of these is the use of leftward deviating wedge prism lenses to produce a right-sided bias and hence reduce left-sided neglect (Frassinetti, Angeli, Meneghello, Avanzi & Ladavas, 2003; Mattingley, 2002; McIntosh, Rossetti, & Milner, 2002; Michel et al., 2003; Rossetti et al., 1998). This is a relatively simple measure, involving little time and expensive equipment and minimal cognitive effort on the part of the patient. It appears to have a significant impact on scanning behavior, and gains have been maintained for up to 5 weeks after treatment (Frassinetti et al., 2003). Another approach is the application of a standard electromechanical vibrator to the left neck muscles of patients while they engage in visual search exercises (Schindler, Kerheff, Karnath, Keller, & Goldenberg, 2002). Three weeks of daily treatment have been shown to result in lasting benefits. Much further research has yet to be conducted to examine the practical applicability of these approaches, but they appear to be promising methods of redirecting attention in unilateral spatial neglect.

One final issue concerns the timing of instituting interventions for neglect. On the one hand, there is evidence suggesting that early, intensive rehabilitation is desirable. On the other hand, there is significant potential for spontaneous resolution of unilateral spatial neglect in a proportion of cases. Arguably, it could be better to wait and see whether resolution is going to occur before instituting costly and time-consuming rehabilitation programs. This argument might also apply to the resolution of language deficits following stroke. As Aimola Davies argues in Chapter 6, the decision as to when to begin therapy should ultimately depend on an assessment of the person's level of awareness of the problem and his or her capacity to sustain attention to therapy.

Disorders of Nonspatial Attention and Memory

Disorders of nonspatial attention, particularly slowed information processing and problems with alertness, may also be associated with any form of stroke. As outlined in Chapter 3, attentional problems appear to be particularly common following anterior CVA, which tends to result in problems with focusing, dividing, and switching of attention. Thalamic stroke has also been shown to cause some difficulties with focusing of attention. Robertson, Ridgeway, Greenfield, and Parr (1997) have shown that impairment of sustained attention was associated with poorer recovery of function after right-hemisphere stroke.

Interventions for these problems have been discussed in the earlier section of this chapter on TBI. Lincoln, Majid, and Weyman (2000) conducted a Cochrane review of cognitive rehabilitation for attention deficits after stroke and concluded that there was some evidence that training improves alertness and sustained attention. However, none of the studies demonstrated generalization to functional activities. These studies are reviewed in detail in Chapter 3, along with a range of other intervention strategies. It does seem important to take into account attentional difficulties in the delivery of therapy. Gains will be maximized if therapy is delivered when patients are at their highest level of arousal, in a quiet and distraction-free environment. In those who have difficulty sustaining attention, therapy should be given in frequent short bursts rather than lengthy sessions.

Memory problems will depend on the site of the CVA, with verbal memory difficulties more evident following dominant MCA stroke and nonverbal or visual memory problems more evident when the stroke is on the nondominant hemisphere. Once again, anterior CVA tends to result in inefficient memorization and recall, with confabulation being very commonly associated with ruptured aneurysms of the anterior communicating artery (ACoA). ACoA aneurysms also result in a range of other executive and behavioral changes. All these problems should be dealt with as discussed in relation to TBI. As Majid, Lincoln, and Weyman (2000) concluded in a Cochrane review, there is currently insufficient evidence to support or refute the effectiveness of cognitive rehabilitation for memory problems after stroke.

Depression Following Stroke

Midbrain lesions may result in periods of easily provoked tearfulness, which should not be confused with depression. However, emotional changes, most particularly depression, are also common following stroke. A review of 14 studies by Whyte and Mulsant (2002) showed that prevalence rates of major depression vary with the time poststroke and are highest in the first 6 months, ranging from 9–37% at 1–2 months poststroke to 9–34% at 6 months poststroke, decreasing by 50% to 5–16% at 1 year and 19–21% at 2 years poststroke. Those who develop depression within days following a stroke are more likely to show spontaneous remission, whereas those developing it 7 weeks poststroke or later are less likely to recover spontaneously (Andersen, Vestergaard, & Lauritzen, 1994).

There has been a continuing debate over the causes of poststroke depression. Some have proposed a primary biological mechanism, in which ischemia disrupts frontostriatal circuits which regulate mood. Robinson and colleagues (Robinson, Kubos, Starr, Rao, & Tr, 1984; Robinson, Lipsey, Rao, & Price, 1986; Starkstein, Robinson, & Price, 1988) have suggested that left anterior and left basal ganglia lesions close to the frontal pole are associated with poststroke depression. This association has been disputed by other researchers, and a meta-analysis by Carson et al. (2000) revealed no association between poststroke depression and left anterior or left-hemispheric lesions. Any apparent association appears to be stronger in the first 6 months and psychosocial factors, such as social isolation, play an increasing role in later-onset depression (Hermann & Wallesch, 1993). Others propose that depression occurs as a consequence of the social and psychological stress of adjusting to an acquired disability Overall it appears that the causes of poststroke depression are multifactorial. Level of disability and occurrence of major life events are the strongest predictors of poststroke depression, with family psychiatric history also being a predictor.

There is evidence that poststroke depression can respond to pharmacological intervention with either tricyclic antidepressants or serotonin reuptake inhibitors. According to a review by Whyte and Mulsant (2002), antidepressants appear to be well-tolerated in stroke patients and over 60% respond to medication, with no particular class of antidepressant showing a clear advantage. No randomized trials have been conducted in the use of psychostimulants with stroke patients. However the results of two retrospective chart reviews and one open-label study suggest that methylphenidate is generally safe and well-tolerated and has a positive effect (Whyte & Mulsant, 2002). ECT has also been shown to be successful (Currier, Murray, & Welsh, 1992). Evidence regarding the effectiveness of psychological therapies, such as cognitive-behavioral therapy (CBT), is less clear. Whereas a pilot study by Lincoln, Flannaghan, Sutcliffe, and Rother (1997) found CBT to be effective, a follow-up RCT found no significant differences between patients receiving CBT and an attention placebo control group (Lincoln & Flannaghan, 2003). The provision of early screening and pharmacological treatment of depression, as well as long-term psychosocial support, would appear to be important in order to minimize poststroke depression. Stroke survivors in active rehabilitation have been shown to have lower rates of depression (Kotila, Numminen, & Waltimo, 1998).

As with TBI, stroke places a significant burden on caregivers. In a study of 222 co-resident spouses of stroke patients by Blake and Lincoln (2000), 37% showed significant levels of strain, which was associated with negative affectivity, carer mood on the General Health Questionnaire—12, and caregivers' perceptions of the patient's independence in activities of daily living. Stroke support services offering information, emotional support, and liaison with other services to stroke patients and their caregivers have been established in many countries. Results of an RCT evaluating such a service in the United Kingdom, indicated that it increased knowledge of stroke and support services and satisfaction with services provided, but it did not have a significant impact on mood, independence in activities of daily living, or caregiver strain (Lincoln, Francis, Lilley, Sharma, & Summerfield, 2003). Given the many factors contributing to these variables this is not surprising.

CONCLUSIONS

An understanding of the unique pathophysiological and recovery mechanisms of TBI and stroke is essential to fully understand how different rehabilitative interventions should be applied. Each has unique demographic factors which have a significant impact on the effects of injury, recovery, and long-term adjustment. In the case of TBI, the youth of those sustaining the injuries might maximize potential for recovery, but it also interferes with attainment of important life goals, causing long-term loss of self-esteem in many cases. The high incidence of premorbid learning difficulties or poor academic performance, substance abuse, and other psychiatric problems and unemployment also limits potential to benefit from rehabilitation. More significant following TBI, however, are the cognitive, behavioral, and emotional changes that occur, often in the absence of residual physical disability. These problems with attention, memory, executive function, and behavioral control interfere in seemingly subtle but dramatic ways with the rehabilitation process, return to work, and school and leisure activities and affect social and personal relationships, having a very significant long-term negative impact on psychosocial adjustment. Highly specialized and individualized approaches to rehabilitation are necessary to make gains. There is a need to assess the individual's preinjury abilities, interests, and goals and to ensure that rehabilitation goals are relevant to and shared by the injured person and family. It is also important to take a very long-term view of the rehabilitation process and to educate the family and others as to optimal management of any problems. Finally, in many cases lifelong support will be necessary.

In the case of stroke, one is dealing with issues pertaining to the elderly—the presence of concurrent medical conditions which may interfere with recovery, greater physical handicap, for which intensive physical therapy is recommended, communication problems in those with dysphasia, and practical problems in activities of daily living in those with unilateral spatial neglect and/or physical disabilities. For some elderly people, social isolation and depression also become significant problems. Approaches to therapy are more directly focused on physical impairments and regaining independence in activities of daily living.

In the case of both TBI and CVA, there is a need for early intensive intervention by a specialized team of therapists experienced with that condition. It is important to focus on the individual's goals to maximize motivation and to ensure that any training conducted is functionally relevant. It is also essential to conduct a detailed assessment in order to establish precisely which elements of a function have been impaired and which remain intact, as a basis for formulating therapy. If the goal of therapy is to rebuild new functional circuits, it will need to be carried out as intensively as possible, but also in a manner that maximizes attention to tasks. Such therapy is recommended particularly in cases in which lesions are less extensive. Provision of assessment and therapy for psychological problems occurring during the course of recovery is also important, as is ongoing psychosocial support for the brain-injured person and his or her close others. There is clear evidence that rehabilitative interventions are effective, but we still know relatively little about which specific interventions are appropriate in which conditions. Pharmacological interventions also show promise, but, again, the research evidence in support of these interventions is limited. Therefore, the highest priority must be given to conducting RCTs and single-case studies, evaluating the effectiveness of specific interventions of both a behavioral and a pharmacological nature.

REFERENCES

Adams, R. D., Victor, M., & Ropper, A. H. (1997). Cerebrovascular diseases. In *Principles of neurology* (6th ed., pp. 777–873). New York: McGraw-Hill.

Andersen, K., Vestergaard, K., & Lauritzen, L. (1994). Effective treatment of poststroke depression with the selective serotonin reuptake inhibitor citalopram. *Stroke, 25,* 1099–1104.

Anderson, S. W., & Damasio, A. R. (1995). Frontal-lobe syndromes. In J. Bogousslavsky & L. Caplan (Eds.), *Stroke syndromes* (pp. 140–144). New York: Cambridge University Press.

Anderson, V., Catroppa, C., Morse, S., Haritou, F., & Rosenfeld, J. (2000). Recovery of intellectual ability following TBI in childhood: Impact of injury severity and age at injury. *Paediatric Neurosurgery, 32,* 282–290.

Anderson, V., & Moore, C. (1995). Age at injury as a predictor of outcome following paediatric head injury. *Child Neuropsychology, 1,* 187–202.

Anderson, V., Northam, E., Hendy, J., & Wrennall, J. (2001). *Developmental neuropsychology. A clinical approach.* Hove, East Sussex, UK: Psychology Press.

Bamford, J., Sandercock, P., Dennis, M., Warlow, C., Jones, L., McPherson, K., et al. (1988). A prospective study of acute cerebrovascular disease in the community: The Oxfordshire Community Stroke Project. 1981–1986. 1. Methodology, demography and incident cases of first ever stroke. *Journal of Neurology, Neurosurgery and Psychiatry, 51,* 1373–1380.

Bath, P. M., Iddenden, R., Bath, F. J., & Orgogozo, J. M. (2001). Tirilazad for acute ischemic stroke. *Cochrane Database of Systematic Reviews, 4,* CD002087.

Ben-Yishay, Y., Ben-Nachum, Z., Cohen, A., Gross, Y., Hofien, A., Rattok, Y., et al. (1978). Digest of a two-year comprehensive clinical rehabilitation research program for out-patient head injured Israeli veterans (Oct. 1975–Oct. 1977). In *Working approaches to remediation of cognitive deficits in brain damaged persons* (Rehabilitation Monograph No. 59, pp. 1–61). New York: Institute of Rehabilitation Medicine, New York University Medical Center.

Bishara, S. N., Partridge, F. M., Godfrey, H., & Knight, R. G. (1992). Post-traumatic amnesia and Glasgow Coma Scale related to outcome in survivors in a consecutive series of patients with severe closed-head injury. *Brain Injury, 6,* 373–380.

Blake, H., & Lincoln, N. B. (2000). Factors associated with strain in co-resident spouses of patients following stroke. *Clinical Rehabilitation, 14*(3), 307–314.

Bogousslavsky, J., & Caplan, L. (Eds.). (1995). *Stroke syndromes.* New York: Cambridge University Press.

Bond, M. (1984). The psychiatry of closed head injury. In N. Brooks (Ed.), *Closed head injury: Psychological, social and family consequences* (pp. 148–178). London: Oxford University Press.

Bottger, S., Prosiegel, M., Steiger, H. -J., & Yassouridis, A. (1998, July). Neurobehavioral disturbances, rehabilitation outcome, and lesion site in patients after rupture and repair of anterior communicating artery aneurysm. *Journal of Neurology, Neurosurgery and Psychiatry, 65*(1), 93–102.

Bowen, A., Neumann, V., Conner, M., Tennant, A., & Chamberlain, M. A. (1998). Mood disorders following traumatic brain injury: Identifying the extent of the problem and the people at risk. *Brain Injury, 12*(3), 177–190.

Bradshaw, J. L., & Mattingley, J. B. (1995). *Clinical neuropsychology: Behavioral and brain science.* San Diego: Academic Press.

Brooks, D. N., Campsie, L., Symington, C., Beattie, A., & McKinlay, W. (1986). The five-year outcome of severe blunt head injury: A relative's view. *Journal of Neurology, Neurosurgery, and Psychiatry, 49,* 764–770.

Brooks, N., Campsie, L., Symington, C., Beattie, A., & McKinlay, W. (1987). The effects of severe head injury on patient and relative within seven years of injury. *Journal of Head Trauma Rehabilitation, 2*(3), 1–13.

Burke, W. H., Wesolowski, M. D., & Guth, M. L. (1988). Comprehensive head injury rehabilitation: An outcome evaluation. *Brain Injury, 2,* 313–322.

Byng, S., & Jones, E. (2003). Therapy for language impairment in aphasia. In R. J. Greenwood, M. P. Barnes, T. M. McMillan, & C. D. Ward (Eds.), *Handbook of neurological rehabilitation* (2nd ed., pp. 365–376). Hove, East Sussex, UK: Psychology Press.

Byng, S, Pound, C., & Parr, S. (2000). Living with aphasia: A framework for therapy interventions. In I. Papathanasiou (Ed.), *Acquired neurological communication disorders: A clinical perspective* (pp. 49–75). London: Whurr.

Carney, N., Chestnut, R. M., Maynard, H., Mann, N. C., Hefland, M. (1999). Effect of cognitive rehabilitation on outcomes for persons with traumatic brain injury: A systematic review. *Journal of Head Trauma Rehabilitation, 14,* 277–307.

Caroloei, A., Marini, C., DiNapoli, M., DiGianfilippo, G., Santalucia, P., Baldassarre, M., et al. (1997). High stroke incidence in the prospective community-based L'Aquila registry (1994–1998): First year's results. *Stroke, 28,* 2500–2506.

Carson, A., MacHale, S., Allen, K., Lawrie, S., Dennis, M., House, A., et al. (2000). Depression after stroke and lesion location: A systematic review. *Lancet, 356,* 122–126.

Cicerone, K. D., Dahlberg, C., Kalmar, K., Langenbahn, D. M., Malec, J. F., Bergquist, T., et al. (2000). Evidence-based cognitive rehabilitation: Recommendations for clinical practice. *Archives of Physical Medicine and Rehabilitation, 81,* 1596–1615.

Cicerone, K., & Wood, J. (1987). Planning disorder after closed head injury: A case study. *Archives of Physical Medicine and Rehabilitation, 68,* 111–115.

Cohen, L. G., & Hallett, M. (2003). Neural plasticity and recovery of function. In R. J. Greenwood, M. P. Barnes, T. M. McMillan & C. D. Ward (Eds.), *Handbook of neu-*

rological rehabilitation (2nd ed., pp. 99–111). Hove, East Sussex, UK: Psychology Press.

Courville, C. B. (1945). *Pathology of the central nervous system.* Nampa, ID: Pacific Press.

Curran, C. A., Ponsford, J. L., & Crowe, S. (2000). Coping strategies and emotional outcome following traumatic brain injury: A comparison with orthopaedic patients. *Journal of Head Trauma Rehabilitation, 15*(6), 1256–1274.

Currier, M., Murray, G., & Welsh, C. (1992). Electroconvulsive therapy for poststroke depressed geriatric patients. *Journal of Neuropsychiatry and Clinical Neuroscience, 4,* 140–144.

Dean, C. M., & Shepherd, R. B. (1997). Task-related training improves performance of seating reaching tasks after stroke. A randomized controlled trial. *Stroke, 28,* 722–728.

DeLuca, J., & Diamond, B. J. (1995). Aneurysm of the anterior communicating artery: A review of the neuroanatomical and neuropsychological sequelae. *Journal of Clinical and Experimental Neuropsychology, 17,* 100–121.

Dennis, M., Barnes, M. A., Donnelly, R. E., Wilkinson, M., & Humphreys, R. P. (1996). Appraising and managing knowledge: Metacognitive skills after childhood head injury. *Developmental Neuropsychology, 12,* 77–103.

Douglas, J., Brown, L., & Barry, S. (2002). Is aphasia therapy effective? Exploring the evidence in systematic reviews. *Brain Impairment, 3*(1), 17–27.

Ellekjaer, H., Holmen, J., Indredavik, B., & Terent, A. (1997). Epidemiology of stroke in Innherred, Norway, 1994–1996: Incidence and 30–day case fatality rate. *Stroke, 28,* 2180–2184.

Elman, R., & Bernstein-Ellis, E. (1999). The efficacy of group communication treatment in adults with chronic aphasia. *Journal of Speech, Language and Hearing Research, 42,* 411–419.

Elsass, L., & Kinsella, G. (1987). Social interaction after severe closed head injury. *Psychological Medicine, 17,* 67–78.

Evans, J. J., Wilson, B. A., Schuri, U., Andrade, J., Baddeley, A., Bruna, O., et al. (2000). A comparison of "errorless" and "trial-and-error" learning methods for teaching individuals with acquired memory deficits. *Neuropsychological Rehabilitation, 10*(1), 67–101.

Fann, J. R., Katon, W. J., Uomoto, J. M., & Esselman, P. C. (1995). Psychiatric disorders and functional disability in outpatients with traumatic brain injuries. *American Journal of Psychiatry, 152*(10), 1493–1499.

Fasotti, L., Kovacs, F. Eling, P. A. T. M., & Brouwer, W. H. (2000). Time Pressure Management as a compensatory strategy after closed head injury. *Neuropsychological Rehabilitation, 10*(1), 47–65.

Fortune, N., & Wen, X. (1999). *The definition, incidence and prevalence of acquired brain injury in Australia.* Canberra: Australian Institute of Health and Welfare.

Frassinetti, F., Angeli, V., Meneghello, F., Avanzi, S., & Ladavas, E. (2003). Long-lasting amelioration of visuospatial neglect by prism adaptation. *Brain, 125*(Pt. 3), 608–623.

Fryer, J. (1989). Adolescent community integration. In P. Bach-y-Rita (Ed.), *Traumatic brain injury* (pp. 255–286). New York: Demos.

Fryer, L. J., & Haffey, W. J. (1987). Cognitive rehabilitation and community readaptation: Outcomes from two program models. *Journal of Head Trauma Rehabilitation, 2*(3), 51–63.

Geddes, J. M., Fear, J., Pickering, A., Tennant, A., Hillman, M., & Chamberlain, M. A. (1996). Prevalence of self-reported stroke in a population in Northern England. *Journal of Epidemiological and Community Health, 50,* 140–143.

Gentleman, D. (1999). Improving outcome after traumatic brain injury—Progress and challenges. *British Medical Bulletin, 55*(4), 910–926.

Glasgow, R. E., Zeiss, R. A., Barrera, M., & Lewinsohn, P. M. (1977). Case studies on remediating memory deficits in brain damaged individuals. *Journal of Clinical Psychology, 33,* 1049–1054.

Glisky, E. L., Schacter, D. L., & Tulving, E. (1986). Learning and retention of computer related vocabulary in memory-impaired patients: Method of vanishing cues. *Journal of Clinical and Experimental Neuropsychology, 8,* 292–312.

Graham, D. I. (1999). Pathophysiological aspects of injury and mechanisms of recovery. In M. Rosenthal, J. Kreutzer, E. R. Griffith, & B. Pentland (Eds.), *Rehabilitation of the adult and child with traumatic brain injury* (3rd ed., pp. 19–41). Philadelphia: Davis.

Graham, D. I., Ford, I., Adams, J. H., Doyle, D., Teasdale, G. M., Lawrence, A. E., et al. (1989). Ischemic brain damage is still common in fatal non-missile head injury. *Journal of Neurology, Neurosurgery, and Psychiatry, 52,* 346–350.

Greener, J., Enderby, P., & Whurr, R. (1999, December). Speech and language therapy for aphasia following stroke (Cochrane Review). In *The Cochrane Library, Issue 4.* Oxford, UK: BMJ Books/Update Software.

Haas, J. F., Cope, D. N., & Hall, K. (1987). Premorbid prevalence of poor academic performance in severe head injury. *Journal of Neurology, Neurosurgery, and Psychiatry, 50,* 52–56.

Hankey, G. J. (2002). *Stroke* (Vol 1). Edinburgh, Scotland: Churchill Livingstone.

Heinemann, A. W., Roth, E. J., Cichowski, K., & Bets, H. B. (1987). Multivariate analysis of improvement and outcome following stroke rehabilitation. *Archives of Neurology, 44,* 1167–1172.

Hermann, M., & Wallesch, C. (1993). Depressive changes in stroke patients. *Disability Rehabilitation, 15*(2), 55–66.

Hewer, R. L., & Tennant, A. (2003). The epidemiology of disabling neurological disorders. In R. J. Greenwood, M. P. Barnes, T. M. McMillan & C. D. Ward (Eds.), *Handbook of neurological rehabilitation* (2nd ed., pp. 5–14). Hove, East Sussex, UK: Psychology Press.

Hoofien, D., Gilboa, A., Vakil, E., & Donovick, P. J. (2001). Traumatic brain injury 10–20 years later: A comprehensive outcome study of psychiatric symptomatology, cognitive abilities and psychosocial functioning. *Brain Injury, 15*(3), 189–209.

Howard, D. (1986). Beyond randomized controlled trials: the case for effective case studies of the effects of treatment in aphasia. *British Journal of Disorders of Communication, 21,* 89–102.

Jacobs, H. E. (1988). The Los Angeles Head Injury Survey: Procedures and preliminary findings. *Archives of Physical Medicine and Rehabilitation, 69,* 425–431.

Jennett, B., & Teasdale, G. (1981). *Management of head injuries.* Philadelphia: Davis.

Johansson, B. B., & Belichenko, P. V. (2002). Neuronal plasticity and dendritic spines: Effect of environmental enrichment on intact and postischemic rat brain. *Journal of Cerebral Blood Flow and Metabolism, 22,* 89–96.

Jorge, R. E., Robinson, R. G., Arndt, S. V., Starkstein, S. E., Forrester, A. W., & Geisler, F. (1993). Depression following traumatic brain injury: A 1-year longitudinal follow-up. *Journal of Affective Disorders, 27*(4), 233–243.

Kalra, L., Perez, I., Gupta, S., & Wittink, M. (1997). The influence of visual neglect on stroke rehabilitation. *Stroke, 28*(7), 1386–1391.

Kandel, E. R., Schwartz, J. H., & Jessell, T. M. (2000). *Principles of neural science* (4th ed.). New York: McGraw Hill.

Kasten, E., Muller-Oehring, E., & Sabel, B. A. (2001). Stability of visual field enlargements following computer-based restitution training—Results of a follow-up. *Journal of Clinical and Experimental Neuropsychology, 23*(3), 297–305.

Kasten, E., Wust, S., Behrens-Baumann, W., & Sabel, B. A. (1998) Computer-based training for the treatment of partial blindness. *Nature Medicine, 4*(9), 1083–1087.

Kelly-Hayes, M., Wold, P. A., Kase, C. S., Gresham, G. E., Kannel, W. B., & D'Agostino, R. B. (1989). Time-course of functional recovery after stroke: The Framingham study. *Journal of Neurological Rehabilitation, 3,* 65–70.

Kinsella, G., Moran, C., Ford, B., & Ponsford, J. (1988). Emotional disorder and its assessment within the severe head injured population. *Psychological Medicine, 18,* 57–63.

Kiresuk, T. J., & Sherman, R. E. (1968). Goal attainment scaling. A general method for evaluating comprehensive mental health programs. *Community Mental Health Journal, 4,* 443–453.

Kolb, B. (1995). *Brain plasticity and behavior.* Hillsdale, NJ: Erlbaum.

Koskinen, S. (1998). Quality of life 10 years after a very severe traumatic brain injury: The perspective of the injured and the closest relative. *Brain Injury, 12*(8), 611–618.

Kotila, M., Numminen, H., & Waltimo, O. (1998). Depression after stroke: Results of the FINNSTROKE study. *Stroke, 29*(2), 368–372.

Kozlowski, D. A., James, D. C., & Schallert, T. (1996). Use-dependent exaggeration of neuronal injury after unilateral sensorimotor cortex lesions. *Journal of Neuroscience, 16*(15), 4776–4786.

Kraus, J. F., & McArthur, D. L. (1999). Incidence and prevalence of and costs associated with traumatic brain injury. In M. Rosenthal, E. R. Griffith, J. S. Kreutzer & B. Pentland (Eds.), *Rehabilitation of the adult and child with traumatic brain injury* (pp. 3– 17). Philadelphia: Davis.

Kreutzer, J. S., Gervasio, A. H., & Camplair, P. S. (1994). Patient correlates of caregivers' distress and family functioning after traumatic brain injury. *Brain Injury, 8,* 211–230.

Kreutzer, J. S., Seel, R. T., & Gourley, E. (2001). The prevalence and symptom rates of depression after traumatic brain injury: A comprehensive examination. *Brain Injury, 15*(7), 563–576.

Larner, A. J., & Sofroniew, M. V. (2003). Mechanisms of cellular damage and recovery. In R. J. Greenwood, M. P. Barnes, T. M. McMillan, & C. D. Ward (Eds.), *Handbook of neurological rehabilitation* (2nd ed., pp. 71–98). Hove, East Sussex, UK: Psychology Press.

Levine, B., Cabeza, R., McIntosh, A. R., Black, S. E., Grady, C. L., & Stuss, D. T. (2002). Functional reorganisation of memory after traumatic brain injury: A study with H(2)(15)0 positron emission tomography. *Journal of Neurology, Neurosurgery and Psychiatry, 73*(2), 173–81.

Levine, B., Robertson, I. H., Clare, L., Carter, G., Hong, J., Wilson, B. A., et al. (2000). Rehabilitation of executive functioning: An experimental-clinical validation of goal management training. *Journal of International Neuropsychological Society, 6*(3), 299–312.

Lincoln, N. B., & Flannaghan, T. (2003). Cognitive behavioral psychotherapy for depression following stroke: A randomized controlled trial. *Stroke, 34*(1), 111–115.

Lincoln, N. B., Flannaghan, T., Sutcliffe, L., & Rother, L. (1997). Evaluation of cognitive behavioral treatment for depression after stroke: A pilot study. *Clinical Rehabilitation, 11*, 114–122.

Lincoln, N. B., Francis, V. M., Lilley, S. A., Sharma, J. C., & Summerfield, M. (2003). Evaluation of a Stroke Family Support Organiser: A randomized controlled trial. *Stroke, 34*(1), 116–121.

Lincoln, N. B., Majid, M. J., & Weyman, N. (2000). Cognitive rehabilitation for attention deficits following stroke. *Cochrane Database of Systematic Reviews, 4*, CD002852.

Lincoln, N. B., McGuirk, E., Mulley, G. P., Lendrem, W., Jones, A. C., & Mitchell, J. R. (1984). Effectiveness of speech therapy for aphasic stroke patients. A randomized controlled trial. *Lancet, 1*(8388), 1197–1200.

Maher, L. M., Kendall, D., Swearengin, J. A., Pingel, K., Holland, A., & Roth, L. J. G. (2003). Constraint induced language therapy for chronic aphasia: Preliminary findings. *Journal of the International Neuropsychological Society, 9*, 192.

Majid, M. J., Lincoln, N. B., & Weyman, N. (2000). Cognitive rehabilitation for memory deficits following stroke. *Cochrane Database of Systematic Reviews 3*, CD002293.

Malec, J. F. (1999). Goal Attainment Scaling in rehabilitation. *Neuropsychological Rehabilitation, 9*(3/4), 253–275.

Manchester, D., & Wood, R. L. (2001). Applying cognitive therapy in neuropsychological rehabilitation. In R. L. Wood & T. M. McMillan (Eds.), *Neurobehavioral disability and social handicap following traumatic brain injury* (pp. 157–174). Hove, East Sussex, UK: Psychology Press.

Mattingley, J. B. (2002). Visuomotor adaptation to optical prisms: A new cure for spatial neglect? *Cortex, 38*(3), 277–283.

McCleary, C., Satz, P., Forney, D., Light, R., Zaucha, K., Asarnow, R., et al. (1998). Depression after traumatic brain injury as a function of Glasgow Outcome Score. *Journal of Clinical and Experimental Neuropsychology, 20*(2), 270–279.

McIntosh, R. D., Rossetti, Y., & Milner, A. D. (2002). Prism adaptation improves chronic visual and haptic neglect: A single case study. *Cortex, 38*(3), 309–320.

McKinlay, W. W., Brooks, D. N., Bond, M. R., Martinage, D. P., & Marshall, M. M. (1981). The short-term outcome of severe blunt head injury as reported by relatives of the injured persons. *Journal of Neurology, Neurosurgery, and Psychiatry, 44*, 527–533.

Michel, C., Pisella, L., Halligan, P., Luaute, J., Rode, G., Boisson, D., et al. (2003). Simulating unilateral neglect in normals using prism adaptation: Implications for theory. *Neuropsychologia, 41*(1), 25–39.

Mills, V. M., Nesbeda, T., Katz, D. I., & Alexander, M. P. (1992). Outcomes for traumatically brain-injured patients following post-acute rehabilitation programs. *Brain Injury, 6*, 219–228.

Morton, M. V., & Wehman, P. (1995). Psychosocial and emotional sequelae of individuals with traumatic brain injury: Literature review and recommendation. *Brain Injury,* *9,* 285–299.

National Head Injury Foundation Task Force on Special Education. (1989). An educator's manual: What educators need to know about students with traumatic brain injury. Southborough, MA: Author.

Nelson, D. L., Konosky, K., Fleharty, K., Webb, R., Newer, K., Hazbourn, V. P., et al. (1996). The effects of an occupationally embedded exercise on bilaterally assisted supination in persons with hemiplegia. *American Journal of Occupational Therapy,* *50,* 639–646.

Netter, F. H. (1986). Cerebrovascular disease. In *The CIBA collection of medical illustrations* (Vol. 1, Pt. II, pp. 49–87). West Caldwell, NJ: CIBA.

Nickels, L., & Best, W. (1996). Therapy for naming disorders (part 1): Principles, puzzles and progress. *Aphasiology,* *10,* 21–47.

Nieto-Sampedro, M., & Cotman, C. W. (1985). Growth factor induction and temporal order in central nervous system repair. In C. W. Cotman (Ed.), *Synaptic plasticity* (pp. 407–456). New York: Guilford Press.

Nudo, R. J., Barbay, S., & Kleim, J. A. (2000). Role of neuroplasticity in functional recovery after stroke. In H. S. Levin & J. Grafman (Ed.), *Cerebral reorganization of function after brain damage* (pp. 168–197). Oxford, UK: Oxford University Press.

Nudo, R. J., Plautz, E. J., & Frost, S. B. (2001). Role of adaptive plasticity in recovery of function after damage to motor cortex. *Muscle and Nerve,* *24,* 1000–1019.

Nudo, R. J., Plautz, E. J., & Millikan, G. W. (1997). Adaptive plasticity in primate motor cortex as a consequence of behavioral experience and neuronal injury. *Seminars in Neuroscience,* *9,* 13–23.

Nudo, R. J., Wise, B. M., SiFuentes, F., & Milliken, G. W. (1996). Neural substrates for the effects of rehabilitative training on motor recovery after ischemic infarct. *Science,* *272,* 1793.

Oddy, M. (1984). Head injury and social adjustment. In N. Brooks (Ed.), *Closed head injury: Psychological, social and family consequences* (pp. 108–122). London: Oxford University Press.

Oddy, M., Coughlan, T., Tyerman, A., & Jenkins, D. (1985). Social adjustment after closed head injury: A further follow-up seven years after injury. *Journal of Neurology, Neurosurgery, and Psychiatry,* *48,* 564–568.

Olver, J. H., Ponsford, J. L., & Curran, C. A. (1996). Outcome following traumatic brain injury: A comparison between 2 and 5 years after injury. *Brain Injury,* *10*(11), 841–848.

Parry, R. H., Lincoln, N. B., & Vass, C. D. (1999). Effect of severity of arm impairment on response to additional physiotherapy early after stroke. *Clinical Rehabilitation,* *13*(3), 187–198.

Ponsford, J. L. (1995). Assessment and management of behavior problems. In J. Ponsford, S. Sloan, & P. Snow, *Traumatic brain injury: Rehabilitation for everyday adaptive living* (pp. 165–194). London: Erlbaum.

Ponsford, J., Anson, K., & Curran, C. (2003). Facilitating adaptive coping following traumatic brain injury. *Journal of the International Neuropsychological Society,* *9*(2), 291.

Ponsford, J. L., Olver, J. H., & Curran, C. (1995). A profile of outcome two years following traumatic brain injury. *Brain Injury,* *9,* 1–10.

Ponsford, J. L., Olver, J. H., Curran, C., & Ng, K. (1995). Prediction of employment status two years after traumatic brain injury. *Brain Injury, 9,* 11–20.

Ponsford, J., Olver, J., Nelms, R., Curran, C., & Ponsford, M. (1999). Outcome measurement in an inpatient and outpatient traumatic brain injury rehabilitation program. *Neuropsychological Rehabilitation., 9*(3/4), 517–534.

Ponsford, J., Olver, J., Ponsford, M., & Nelms, R. (2003). Long-term adjustment of families following traumatic brain injury where comprehensive rehabilitation has been provided. *Brain Injury, 17*(6), 453–468.

Ponsford, J. L., Sloan S., & Snow P. (1995). *Traumatic brain injury: Rehabilitation for everyday adaptive living.* London: Erlbaum.

Ponsford, J., Willmott, C., Rothwell, A., Cameron, P., Kelly, A. M., Nelms, R., et al. (2000). Factors influencing outcome following mild traumatic brain injury in adults. *Journal of the International Neuropsychological Society, 6*(5), 568–579.

Povlishock, J. T. (1993). Pathobiology of traumatically induced axonal injury in animals and man. *Annals of Emergency Medicine, 22*(6), 980–986.

Povlishock, J. T., & Christman, C. W (1995). The pathobiology of traumatically induced axonal injury in animals and humans: A review of current thoughts. *Journal of Neurotrauma, 12,* 555–564.

Prigatano, G. P. (1999). *Principles of neuropsychological rehabilitation.* New York: Oxford University Press.

Prigatano, G. P., Fordyce, D. J., Zeiner, H. K., Roueche, J. R., Pepping, M., & Wood, B. C. (1986). *Neuropsychological rehabilitation after brain injury.* Baltimore: Johns Hopkins University Press.

Pulvermüller, F., Neininger, B., Elbert, T., Mohr, B., Rockstroh, B., Koebbel, P., et al. (2001). Constraint-induced therapy of chronic aphasia after stroke. *Stroke, 32,* 1621–1626.

Rappaport, M., Herrero-Backe, C., Rappaport, M. -L., & Winterfield, K. M. (1989). Head injury up to 10 years later. *Archives of Physical Medicine and Rehabilitation, 70,* 885–892.

Rapoport, M., McCauley, S., Levin, H., Song, J., & Feinstein, A. (2002). The role of injury severity in neurobehavioral outcome 3 months after traumatic brain injury. *Neuropsychiatry, Neuropsychology and Behavioral Neurology, 15*(2), 123–132.

Raymer, A. M., & Rothi, L. J. G. (2000). The semantic system. In S. E. Nadeau, L. J. Gonzalez Rothi, & B. Crosson (Eds.), *Aphasia and language: Theory to practice* (pp. 108–132). New York: Guilford Press.

Recanzone, C. H., Schreiner, C. E., & Merzenich, M. M. (1993). Plasticity in the frequency representation of primary auditory cortex following discrimination training in adult monkeys. *Journal of Neuroscience, 13*(1), 87–103.

Rimel, R. W., & Jane, J. A. (1984). Patient characteristics. In M. Rosenthal, E. R. Griffith, M. R. Bond, & J. D. Miller (Eds.), *Rehabilitation of the head injured adult* (pp. 9–20). Philadelphia: Davis.

Robertson, I. H., McMillan, T. M., MacLeod, E., Edgeworth, J., & Brock, D. (2002). Rehabilitation by limb activation training reduces left-sided motor impairment in unilateral neglect patients: A single-blind randomized control trial. *Neuropsychological Rehabilitation, 12,* 439–454.

Robertson, I. H., & Murre, J. M. J. (1999). Rehabilitation of brain damage: Brain plasticity and principles of guided recovery. *Psychological Bulletin, 125,* 544–575.

Robertson, I. H., & North, N. (1992). Spatio-motor cueing in unilateral neglect. The role of hemispace, hand and motor activation. *Neuropsychologia, 30,* 553–563.

Robertson, I. H., North, N., & Geggie, C. (1992). Spatio-motor cueing in unilateral neglect. Three single case studies of its therapeutic effectiveness. *Journal of Neurology, Neurosurgery and Psychiatry, 55,* 799–805.

Robertson, I. H., Ridgeway, V., Greenfield, E., & Parr, A. (1997). Motor recovery after stroke depends on intact sustained attention. A 2–year follow-up study. *Neuropsychology, 11*(2), 290–295.

Robertson, I. H., Tegner, R., Tham, K., Lo, A., & Nimmo-Smith, I. (1995). Sustained attention training for unilateral neglect: Theoretical and rehabilitation implications. *Journal of Clinical and Experimental Neuropsychology, 17,* 416–430.

Robinson, R., Kubos, K., Starr, L., Rao, K., & T, T. P. (1984). Mood disorders in stroke patients: Importance of location of lesion. *Brain, 107,* 81–93.

Robinson, R., Lipsey, J., Rao, K., & Price, T. (1986). Two-year longitudinal study of poststroke mood disorders: Comparison of acute-onset with delayed-onset depression. *American Journal of Psychiatry, 143*(10), 1238–1244.

Rohey, R. (1994). The efficacy of treatment for aphasic persons: A meta-analysis. *Brain and Language, 47,* 582–608.

Rohey, R. (1998). A meta-analysis of clinical outcomes in the treatment of aphasia. *Journal of Speech, Language and Hearing Research, 41,* 172–187

Rosenthal, M., Christensen, B. K., & Ross, T. P. (1998). Depression following traumatic brain injury. *Archives of Physical Medicine and Rehabilitation, 79*(1), 90–103.

Rossetti, Y., Rode, G., Pisella, L., Farne, A., Li, L., Boisson, D., et al. (1998). Prism adaptation to a rightward optical deviation rehabilitates left hemispatial neglect. *Nature, 395* (6698), 166–169.

Sander, A. M., Roebuck, T. M., Struchen, M. A., Sherer, M., & High, W. M., Jr. (2001). Long-term maintenance of gains obtained in postacute rehabilitation by persons with traumatic brain injury. *Journal of Head Trauma Rehabilitation, 16*(4), 356–373.

Schacter, D. L., Rich, S. A., & Stampp, M. S. (1985). Remediation of memory disorders: Experimental evaluation of the spaced retrieval technique. *Journal of Experimental and Clinical Neuropsychology, 7,* 79–96.

Scheid, R., Preol, C., Gruber, O., Wiggins, C., & von Cramon, D. Y. (2003). Diffuse axonal injury associated with chronic brain injury: Evidence from T_2*-weighted gradient-echo imaging at 3T. American *Journal of Neuroradiology, 24,* 1049–1056.

Schindler, I., Kerheff, G., Karnath, H-O, Keller, I., & Goldenberg, G. (2002). Neck muscle vibration causes lasting recovery in spatial neglect. *Journal of Neurology, Neurosurgery, and Psychiatry, 73,* 412–419.

Schmitter-Edgecombe, M., Fahy, J., Whelan, J., & Long, C. (1995). Memory remediation after severe closed head injury: Notebook training versus supportive therapy. *Journal of Consulting and Clinical Psychology, 63,* 484–489.

Seale, G. S., Caroselli, J. S., High, W. M. Jr., Becker, C. L., Neese, L. E., & Scheibel, R. (2002). Use of community integration questionnaire (CIQ) to characterize changes in functioning for individuals with traumatic brain injury who participated in a post-acute rehabilitation program. *Brain Injury, 16*(11), 955–967.

Seel, R. T., Kreutzer, J. S., Rosenthal, M., Hammond, F. M., Corrigan, J. D., & Black, K. (2003). Depression after traumatic brain injury: A National Institute on Disability and Rehabilitation Research Model Systems multicenter investigation. *Archives of Physical Medicine and Rehabilitation, 84*(2), 177–184.

Snell, R. S. (1997). *Clinical neuranatomy for medical students* (4th ed.). Philadelphia: Lippincott-Raven.

Sohlberg, M. M. (2000). Assessing and managing unawareness of self. *Seminars in Speech and Language, 21*(2), 135–150.

Starkstein, S., Robinson, R., & Price, T. (1988). Comparison of patients with and without poststroke major depression matched for size and location of lesion. *Archives of General Psychiatry, 45,* 247–252.

Tate, R. L., Lulham, J. M., Broe, G. A., Strettles, B., & Pfaff, A. (1989). Psychosocial outcome for the survivors of severe blunt head injury: The results from a consecutive series of 100 patients. *Journal of Neurology, Neurosurgery, and Psychiatry, 52,* 117–126.

Taub, E., Miller, N. E., Novack, T. A., Cook, E. W., Fleming, W. C., Nepomuceno, C. S., et al. (1993). Technique to improve chronic motor deficit after stroke. *Archives of Physical Medicine and Rehabilitation, 74,* 347–354.

Taub, E., & Morris, D. M. (2001). Constraint-induced movement therapy to enhance recovery after stroke. *Current Atherosclerosis Reports, 3,* 279–86.

Teasdale, G. (2002, October). *TBI: History and challenges for the future.* Paper presented at First Joint Symposium of the National and International Neurotrauma Societies, Tampa, FL.

Teasdale, G., & Jennett, B. (1976). Assessment and prognosis of coma after head injury. *Acta Neurochirurgica, 34,* 45–55.

Teasdale, G. M., Maas, A., Iannotti, F., Ohman, J., & Unterberg, A. (1999). Challenges in translating the efficacy of neuroprotective agents in experimental models into knowledge of clinical benefits in head injured patients. *Acta Neurochirurgica—Supplementum, 73,* 111–116.

Thompson, C. K. (2001). Treatment of underlying forms: A linguistic specific approach to sentence production deficits in agrammatic aphasia. In R. Chapey (Ed.), *Language intervention strategies in aphasia and related neurogenic communication disorders* (4th ed., pp. 605–625). Philadelphia: Lippincott Williams & Wilkins.

Thomsen, I. V. (1984). Late outcome of very severe blunt head injury: A ten to fifteen year second follow-up. *Journal of Neurology, Neurosurgery, and Psychiatry, 47,* 260–268.

Tyerman, A., & Humphrey, M. (1984). Changes in self concept following severe head injury. *International Journal of Rehabilitation Research, 7,* 11–23.

Voller, B., Benke, T., Benedetto, K., Schnider, P., Auff, E., & Aichner, F., (1999). Neuropsychological, MRI and EEG findings after very mild traumatic brain injury. *Brain Injury, 613,* 821–827.

von Cramon, D. Y., Matthes von Cramon, G., & Mai, N. (1991). Problem-solving deficits in brain-injured patients: A therapeutic approach. *Neuropsychological Rehabilitation, 1*(1), 45–64.

Wade, D. T. (2003). Stroke rehabilitation: The evidence. In R. J. Greenwood, M. P. Barnes, T. M. McMillan & C. D. Ward (Eds.), *Handbook of neurological rehabilitation* (2nd ed., pp. 487–504). Hove, East Sussex, UK: Psychology Press.

Walsh, K., & Darby, D. (1999). *Neuropsychology. A clinical approach* (4th ed.). Edinburgh, Scotland: Churchill Livingstone

Webb, P. M., & Glueckhauf, R. L. (1994). The effects of direct involvement in goal set-ting on rehabilitation outcome for persons with traumatic brain injuries. *Rehabili-tation Psychology, 39,* 179–188.

Whyte, E. M., & Mulsant, B. H. (2002). Post stroke depression: Epidemiology, patho-physiology, and biological treatment. *Biological Psychiatry, 52*(3), 253–264.

Wilson, B. A. (1987). Single-case experimental designs in neuropsychological rehabilita-tion. *Journal of Clinical and Experimental Neuropsychology, 9,* 527–544.

Wilson, B. A., Baddeley, A. D., Evans, J., & Shiel, A. (1994). Errorless learning in the re-habilitation of memory impaired people. *Neuropsychological Rehabilitation, 4,* 307–326.

Wilson, B. A., Evans, J. J., Emslie, H., & Malinek, V. (1997). Evaluation of NeuroPage: A new memory aid. *Journal of Neurology, Neurosurgery and Psychiatry, 63,* 113–115.

Witt-Lajeunesse, A., & Kolb, B. (2003). *Therapy and bFGF interact to stimulate recov-ery after cortical injury.* Manuscript in preparation.

Wood, R. L. (1990). Conditioning procedures in brain injury rehabilitation. In R. L. Wood (Ed.), *Neurobehavioral sequelae of traumatic brain injury* (pp. 153–174). London: Taylor & Francis.

Wroblewski, B. A., Joseph, A. B., & Cornblatt, R. R. (1996). Antidepressant pharmaco-therapy and the treatment of depression in patients with severe traumatic brain in-jury: A controlled prospective study. *Journal of Clinical Psychiatry, 57*(12), 582–587.

Zihl, J. (1995). Visual scanning behavior in patients with homonymous hemianopia. *Neuropsychologia, 33,* 287–303.

Zihl, J., & von Cramon, D. (1979). Restitution of visual function in patients with cerebral blindness. *Journal of Neurology, Neurosurgery and Psychiatry, 42,* 312–322.

Concluding Comments

Jennie Ponsford

So how far have we come since the speculation, outlined in the introduction to this text, of John Hughlings-Jackson in 1888 and Karl Lashley in 1938 regarding mechanisms of recovery? It could be argued that we have not come very far, as similar issues are still the focus of discussion and research. However, whereas their comments were speculative, based largely on clinical observation of patients recovering from neurological injury, we now have a vast amount of scientific evidence that answers many of the questions they raised, summarized in Chapters 1 and 2. Kolb and Cioe have elucidated the manner in which neurons communicate and form functional systems. There is now a large body of knowledge regarding physiological processes associated with brain injury and reparative responses, including regeneration, sprouting, denervation supersensitivity, reactive synaptogenesis, and neural and glial genesis. As Kolb and Cioe point out in Chapter 1, although none of these reparative processes will completely replace the lost tissue, there is often an associated behavioral improvement. It is extremely important that clinicians understand these processes and use therapeutic interventions that can enhance them, in order to maximize functional improvement after injury. Factors that influence processes of injury and repair include the age of the person sustaining the injury, the mechanism of injury, hormone levels, genetic factors, and the extent to which functions are localized. Again, an understanding of these factors has the potential to enhance clinical practice.

For many years it was thought that the central nervous system had little capacity for repair after injury. In Chapter 2, Kolb has shown that environmental and other events, including behavioral therapies, can alter the organization of the normal and the injured brain. He argues that rehabilitation programs should be designed to facilitate such plastic changes. From the research of Taub and Morris (2001) regarding the impact of forced use versus lack of use of a hemiparetic limb, and the finding of Robertson and North (1994) that active simultaneous hand movements abolish the positive effects of contralesional limb movements, it seems possible that some rehabilitation approaches could actually interfere with plasticity. Hence the importance of therapists being cognizant of these findings. It is also important to understand the constraints which localization of function place on recovery of function. Kolb is quite clear in stating his belief that the principal mechanism of functional improvement after injury, at this point in time, is compensation rather than recovery resulting from neuronal regeneration. Achievement of the latter awaits further basic research on mechanisms stimulating neural generation.

Kolb reviews results of functional imaging studies which show that stroke patients tend to activate larger areas of cortex when making movements, and there may be bilateral cortical activation. However, the capacity for reorganization declines with increasing area of infarction and increasing age, with considerable interindividual variability. In animal studies, administration of neurotrophic factors stimulates functional improvement and synaptic reorganization following ischemic lesions in the motor cortex. The impact of some neurotrophins on synaptic reorganization may be stimulated by therapy, a fact that clearly supports the impact of rehabilitation. The work of Nudo and Kleim and their colleagues suggests that therapy is necessary to maintain the functions of the undamaged cortex and the movements it represents and can also enable compensation for the affected body parts (Nudo, Barbay, & Kleim, 2000). Whether such findings with sensory and motor functions can be extended to cognitive functions remains to be seen, but the prospect is exciting.

Factors that influence recovery following cerebral injury and response to therapy include age, time since injury, intelligence, handedness, sex, and personality. The final factor is that of experience. As Kolb acknowledges in Chapter 2, although there is clear evidence that provision of rehabilitation enhances recovery, there is little scientific evidence to provide guidance as to the optimal timing or duration of therapy and the specific nature of interventions for different types of problems. He concludes, however, that provision of fairly intensive stimulation in dedicated units is desirable. He also advocates the use of psychomotor stimulants to facilitate plastic changes in the brain.

Each of the ensuing five chapters focuses on an aspect of cognition—nonspatial attention, memory, language, visuospatial attention, and executive function and self-awareness, followed by a chapter on behavior. Evidence presented shows that each of the cognitive functions is multidimensional, with different aspects represented in widely separated cortical regions, forming highly complex and dynamic networks. The parallel distributed processing model of language put forward by Nadeau and Gonzalez Rothi particularly exemplifies this aspect. Careful assessment of each aspect of these functional networks, as well as the integrity of other cognitive abilities and neuronal systems, is necessary as a basis for planning rehabilitative intervention. Further development of more sensitive and consistently used assessment tools in each of these domains, particularly attention and executive function, clearly represents an important part of this process. As Glisky has pointed out in Chapter 4, the potential for rehabilitation will depend on which aspects of the system are damaged, how extensively, and which are preserved. In the case of attention and memory, some aspects of the functional system may remain intact—automatic processing in the case of attention and procedural memory or implicit learning in the case of memory. These intact abilities can be used as a means of overcoming weaknesses and methods of achieving this have been discussed in Chapters 3 and 4. In the case of language difficulties, the most common of which is anomia, identification of which specific pathways are affected will determine whether therapy takes a semantic focus, a phonological focus, or a more traditional naming therapy focus. Glisky and colleagues have demonstrated that techniques may need to be applied differently, depending on the individual's strengths and weaknesses. For those with frontal lesions, error reduction appears to be more important, whereas for those with medial temporal damage there is a need to provide explicit links between information being learned and related information in the knowledge system as part of the training process. It is also important to establish what tasks need to be performed by the injured person and to focus interventions directly on these tasks or their components, as generalization from meaningless tasks or drills may be very limited.

Much of the cognitive rehabilitation work conducted to date has been reviewed in these chapters. Some interventions have been applied on an ad hoc basis, under the constraints imposed by the demands of the clinical setting and without a great deal of analysis of the specific nature and extent of disruption to functional systems. However, in each of the cognitive domains a number of theoretically based approaches have been formulated that show considerable promise based on available evidence. It is to be hoped that the theoretical models presented in this book, together with more sophisticated assessment instruments and neuroimaging techniques, will enable more individualized and effective interventions to be designed. Above all, these interventions need to be more widely applied in rehabilitation settings than they have been to date. The gulf between the exciting experimental work being conducted and day-to-day clinical practice is still very large.

If the approach to intervention selected is retraining, from the evidence presented by Kolb, it would appear that the training will need to be conducted early in the recovery period, in an intensive and systematic fashion which maximizes attention to task and ideally is functionally relevant. While the aim of such training might be restitution of function, this is only a realistic goal if damage to the brain system is incomplete and there are some intact neurons which can reconnect. If the lesion is large, compensation from other intact neural circuits is more likely to be successful. Indeed, in such cases the provision of intensive training may result in the development of such compensatory processes. On the other hand, Nadeau and Gonzalez Rothi have argued that even a damaged network still contains a great deal of information, so that the task of therapy is to refine network knowledge rather than to reestablish it.

Compensatory processes may also be facilitated more explicitly as in the use of cognitive-behavioral alerting strategies to maximize alertness and attention to tasks, mnemonic strategies to increase the depth of efficiency of encoding of information, redirection strategies such as use of prism lenses for unilateral spatial neglect, or the use of goal management strategies. Once again, the choice of intervention should be based on a detailed assessment, to ensure that strategies being taught are tapping into relatively intact abilities, and that the injured person has the cognitive abilities (particularly attention, memory, self-awareness, and self-monitoring capabilities) to support the learning and application of such strategies. Turner and Levine emphasize this in their review of interventions for executive dysfunction in Chapter 7. Motivation is also a crucial factor, so that selection of meaningful goals and tasks is very important. Where these are deficient and awareness of deficits is lacking, it is arguably more appropriate to rely on externally guided compensatory systems. In Chapter 4, Glisky has noted the importance of using training methods which maximize retention.

For those individuals with very extensive injuries who show limited response to rehabilitative therapy, the focus needs to shift toward manipulation of the environment, tasks and interactions of others in order to maximize independence and participation in daily life roles. This applies as much in the domains of language, spatial attention, executive function, and behavior as it does in attention and memory, and examples of such interventions have been given throughout this volume. It might involve reducing environmental distractions, using an externally programmed memory aid, training close others to be more effective conversational partners for a dysphasic individual, behavioral cueing or alerting for the person with unilateral spatial neglect, external prompting to move from one task or aspect of a task to another in the person with executive difficulties, and modifying the environment or other people's responses to minimize agitation in a behaviorally disturbed individual. There is a large body of research evidence supporting the efficacy of these approaches. It is, however, just as important to base the design of such interventions on a careful analysis of the nature of the impairment and residual strengths so that these may be harnessed most effectively.

As far as pharmacological interventions are concerned, there is some evidence that dopaminergic agents may enhance aspects of attention and initiation. However, the impact of these and other medications on the person's day-to-day functioning and the extent to which the effects can be maintained in the long term has not been determined. The potential impact of psychostimulants combined with behavioral therapy in the more acute stages of recovery is an area that warrants further controlled investigation. Drug treatments to increase acetylcholine in the brain have been used with modest effects in patients with early Alzheimer's disease. Many other potential pharmacological interventions are still in the experimental stages and have not yet been tested in humans. With the increased implementation of randomized controlled trials, the body of knowledge in this domain is likely to expand significantly in coming years. However, given the number of different mechanisms often operating simultaneously to cause pathology in conditions such as stroke and traumatic brain injury, and the large number of neurotransmitter systems involved, it may not be realistic to expect a single drug to have a significant impact on recovery and outcome.

In Chapter 8, Alderman has demonstrated that influences on behavior are as numerous as are the brain regions involved in regulating cognitive functions. A broad range of organic lesions may be associated with behavior disorders. However, there are many other potential influences on behavior that are less commonly recognized by clinicians— such as premorbid personality factors, reactive factors, denial or lack of awareness, postinjury learning, environmental factors, and cognitive impairments themselves. Many of these factors may be operating simultaneously. Thus the assessment of behavior change is no less complex a task than is the assessment of cognition. It is essential to accurately establish all factors contributing to a behavior problem and to use this as a basis for designing intervention. A limited amount of evidence supports the use of pharmacological agents in managing behavior problems. However, as with their application to cognitive dysfunction, there is a need for much further evaluative research. Other treatment approaches for behavioral problems need to be determined by the nature of the causative factors and the severity of other cognitive impairments, with psychotherapeutic approaches being suitable only for those with some degree of self-awareness, memory, and executive control, and behavior modification being more appropriate in the absence of these skills.

Different etiologies of brain impairment have unique pathophysiological and recovery mechanisms. Demographic factors, such as age, gender, and socioecomic background, as well as the presence of preexisting psychiatric or other medical conditions, also interact significantly with response to injury, recovery, and rehabilitation. An understanding and evaluation of the potential influence of each of these factors is crucial. Most important, we must understand that we are dealing with human beings, whose individual personalities, life goals, coping styles, and emotional responses have a very significant impact on motivation for rehabilitation and outcome. These must be evaluated and addressed as part of the intervention process. The effectiveness of different approaches to maximizing motivation and dealing with emotional responses remains as unclear as that of all other interventions. There is still limited evidence supporting the efficacy of psychotherapeutic and cognitive-behavioral interventions, partly due to the lack of well-designed studies. The method of intervention for psychological problems will depend on the person's psychiatric history and on his or her cognitive strengths and weaknesses, as well as his or her coping styles. Factors such as social support and availability of other practical assistance also appear to minimize long-term emotional distress in the injured person and his or her relatives.

One of the most important challenges that remains is to establish, in a meaningful but objective manner, the impact of all these rehabilitative interventions. Which aspects are effective? What impact do they have on plasticity? What is the optimal timing, focus, and duration of therapy? What is the impact on the person's lifestyle, and how should this be assessed? How is the person feeling emotionally? In many instances the therapy approaches suggested in these chapters, while having a logical theoretical basis, have not been tested empirically. For example, we do not know yet whether it is possible to retrain working memory, either by pharmacological or behavioral means, as suggested by Nadeau and Gonzalez Rothi as a means of overcoming grammatic impairment, although there have been some promising findings which suggest this might be possible. Similarly, constraint-induced language therapy, while conceptually analogous to constraint induced limb activation, remains to be fully explored and evaluated. We also do not know whether goal management training can be reliably implemented by brain-injured individuals in daily life over long periods of time. It seems unlikely that these interventions will prove successful in all cases, and due to heterogeneity of response, results of randomized controlled trials evaluating these interventions may not be positive. It is therefore even more important to establish who responds to a particular intervention and why, and the reasons for failure in other cases.

Although early delivery of therapy is generally advocated, numerous factors will influence the optimal timing and mode of therapeutic intervention, including the mechanism of injury, rate of spontaneous recovery, level of alertness and sustained attention in the injured person, and his or her level of self-awareness and motivation.

There is still considerable variability in the manner whereby rehabilitative interventions are evaluated. Findings presented in Chapters 3 and 7 show that although it is relatively easy to demonstrate gains on the task which is the focus of training and on similar neuropsychological measures, it is generally much more difficult to demonstrate an impact on the daily lifestyle of the injured person. Whereas this is arguably the most meaningful level at which to measure outcome, everyday living tasks are inherently complex and their performance is determined by many factors other than just one cognitive function which might be the focus of therapy. Relying solely on global outcome measures may well doom many controlled trials to failure. It is important to use a range of outcome measures. A great deal of work is needed in the development of measures that reflect meaningful cognitive and behavioral change.

This attempt to bridge the gap between neurobiology and clinical practice has undoubtedly raised as many questions as it has answered. Do animal models of injury and cognitive impairment apply to humans? How can we more effectively simulate the complexities of traumatic injuries? Will it be possible to stimulate reorganization of cognitive functions in the same manner as sensorimotor functions? How and when should this be done? Clearly, numerous challenges face cognitive neuroscientists and rehabilitation practitioners. There have been many exciting developments in recent years which have not yet made their way into clinical settings. It is only by working together that we will find solutions and achieve our ultimate goal of enhancing quality of life for individuals with brain injury.

REFERENCES

Nudo, R. J., Barbay, S., & Kleim, J. A. (2000). Role of neuroplasticity in functional recovery after stroke. In H. S. Levin & J. Grafman (Eds.), *Cerebral reorganization of function after brain damage* (pp. 168–197). Oxford, UK: Oxford University Press.

Robertson, I. H., & North, N. T. (1994). One hand is better than two: Motor extinction of left hand advantage in unilateral neglect. *Neuropsychologia, 32,* 1–11.

Taub, E., & Morris, D. M. (2001) Constraint-induced movement therapy to enhance recovery after stroke. *Current Arteriosclerosis Reports, 3,* 270–286.

Index